RCGPLearning
Essential CPD for primary care

Mapping Uncertainty in Medicine

What do you do when you don't know what to do?

Avril Danczak, Alison Lea and Geraldine Murphy

Illustrations by
Andy Howarth

RCGP Royal College of General Practitioners

Reprinted in 2026 with permission from the original pubishers by Consultation Skills Ltd

ISBN: 978-1-0369-5243-3

The Royal College of General Practitioners was founded in 1952 with this object:

'To encourage, foster and maintain the highest possible standards in general practice and for that purpose to take or join with others in taking steps consistent with the charitable nature of that object which may assist towards the same.'

Among its responsibilities under its Royal Charter the College is entitled to:

'Diffuse information on all matters affecting general practice and issue such publications as may assist the object of the College.'

British Library Cataloguing-in-Publication Data
A catalogue record for this book is available from the British Library

Published by the Royal College of General Practitioners, 2016
30 Euston Square, London NW1 2FB

Designed and typeset by Prepress Projects Ltd, Perth, UK

Indexed by Jim Henderson

In the varied topography of professional practice, there is a high, hard ground, overlooking a swamp. On the high ground, manageable problems lend themselves to solution through the application of research-based theory and technique. In the swampy lowland, messy, confusing problems defy technical solution. The irony of this situation is that the problems of the high ground tend to be relatively unimportant to individuals or society at large, however great their technical interest may be, while in the swamp lie the problems of greatest human concern. The practitioner must chose. Shall he remain on the high ground where he can solve relatively unimportant problems according to prevailing standards of rigor, or shall he descend to the swamp of important problems and non-rigorous inquiry?

Donald A. Schön[i]

i Schön DA. *Educating the Reflective Practitioner: toward a new design for teaching and learning in the professions*. San Francisco, CA: Jossey-Bass, 1987.

Contents

Foreword *ix*
Preface *xi*
About the authors *xv*
Acknowledgements *xvii*

Part I Uncertainty in medicine 1

1 Thinking about uncertainty in medical practice 5

2 How to use this book 11

Part II Mapping uncertainty in medicine 21

The Analysing Quadrant 25

3 Introduction to uncertainty in the Analysing Quadrant 27

4 Functional ways through uncertainty in the Analysing Quadrant 41

5 The clinical setting, assessment and teaching methods for uncertainty in the Analysing Quadrant 63

The Networking Quadrant 69

6 Introduction to uncertainty in the Networking Quadrant 71

7 Functional ways through uncertainty in the Networking Quadrant 77

8 The clinical setting, assessment and teaching methods for uncertainty in the Networking Quadrant 95

The Negotiating Quadrant 99

9 Introduction to uncertainty in the Negotiating Quadrant 101

10 Functional ways through uncertainty in the Negotiating Quadrant 105

11 The clinical setting, assessment and teaching methods for uncertainty in the Negotiating Quadrant 131

THE TEAM-WORKING QUADRANT 135

12 Introduction to uncertainty in the Team-working Quadrant 137

13 Functional ways through uncertainty in the Team-working Quadrant 143

14 The clinical setting, assessment and teaching methods for uncertainty in the Team-working Quadrant 165

Part III Mapping the psychology of uncertainty 171

15 The psychological themes that underpin clinicians' responses to uncertainty 175

16 Mapping the psychology of uncertainty against the Analysing, Networking, Negotiating and Team-working Quadrants 187

Part IV Mapping uncertainty in medical training 207

17 Training clinicians to deal with uncertainty 211

18 Assessment using the Map of Uncertainty in Medicine 219

19 Educational methods for training for uncertainty 227

20 Educational skills for uncertainty in training 237

21 Learning about uncertainty 249

Part V Exploring uncertainty from the patient's perspective 261

22 The impact of uncertainty on patients 265

23 Mapping uncertainty from the patient's perspective 277

24 Conclusion 299

Index *307*

Foreword

Every medical student starts his training in a blur of uncertainty – but he assumes that the years of training ahead will resolve that blur, as his knowledge and skills become honed in the furnace of medical school and clinical practice. Every Foundation Doctor on her first day braces herself for the unpredictable shift ahead – when she is certain to be busy, but assumes she will not know what to do with most of the demands made on her. And every GP starting morning surgery is only certain that by midday he will have been mystified several times (at least!) – both by what is wrong with his patients, and by how people cope with the challenges that life throws at them.

Certainty in medicine is an illusion, just as it is in everyday life. A brilliant and experienced surgeon hits a wildly aberrant artery during an operation. A fit young man is rushed into resus from the football field with no cardiac rhythm restored. A baby of normal intrauterine growth pops out from a normal delivery sporting the unforgiving signs of Pierre Robin syndrome. And a woman who you have known as a patient for years bursts into tears and confesses her husband is bullying her, with occasional acts of direct violence. But once we have acknowledged that life is uncertain, and we just have to get on with it, there is still the professional challenge to answer – what we can actually do with that uncertainty in clinical practice?

The authors of this book, all practising GPs and educators, have braved this challenge and offer us tools to help us through the labyrinth. They describe a modern paradigm. They take us beyond discussions of sensitivity and specificity or predictive value into the means that we can use to resolve dilemmas – discussing with others, using the team, acknowledging the uncertainties with patients, and being disciplined in our own analyses and actions. They encourage conscious acknowledgement and classification of the roots of our uncertainties. They discourage using ways out to resolve our own uncertainty that do not benefit the patient – for example, excessive blood tests or referrals. They also encourage physician wellbeing – by making uncertainty an issue of conscious competence rather than unconscious stress and anxiety.

Why should you read it? Because it reminds us all that as professionals our job is to reduce uncertainty – by systematic history and exam, by diagnostic reasoning, and by conscious labelling of where our uncertainties remain. It is also a very human book – reassuring in its acceptance of limits to our knowledge and skills, while challenging us to apply logic to Schön's swampy lowland and climb out wherever we can.

If you are uncertain at the end of a consultation, make a note; there will be more you can do to resolve the situation. At the same time, accept it. And keep this book by you – it will make sense of your uncertainties.

Prof. Amanda Howe MD MEd FRCGP FAcadMed DCH DRCOG
President-Elect, World Organisation of Family Doctors (WONCA)
Former Vice Chair (Professional Development)
Royal College of General Practitioners

Preface

'What do you do when you don't know what to do?'

While writing this book we have asked this question of many clinicians, from the most junior to the most senior, from academics to jobbing GPs. We always get an immediate response, a wry smile, a grin of relief that told us that every clinician faces this challenge. Those who are most honest will reveal that they face this pretty much every day: sometimes with patients, colleagues, trainees or non-clinical staff, often with families, patients with complex needs or when working on call or out of hours.

Our book is about this, the moment when you don't know what to do, and we refer to this as 'uncertainty in medicine'. As clinicians, all our training, education, continuous professional development, guidelines, protocols and multidisciplinary team meetings are supposed to 'design out' uncertainty and tell us what to do. Strangely, uncertainty doesn't go away with all this effort. Although we know more about medicine than ever, our uncertainty about the way forwards can often seem greater too. In primary care, uncertainty is the norm, as we negotiate the 'swampy lowlands' of daily practice where information is by turns limited, confusing, contradictory, lost, inaccurate and ambiguous. Sometimes we are dealing with complex comorbidities that interact in unknown ways. Sometimes there can seem to be too much information to make sense of. Surrounded by ever increasing scientific knowledge and with limited time, it is hard to decide the best option for the individual patient we are caring for. We hope that this book will help clinicians cope with uncertainty a little more easily.

If you want get straight to work, turn to **Chapter 2** 'How to use this book' (see p. 11), which explains a practical Map of Uncertainty in Medicine (MUM), and an algorithm that will highlight which chapter in Part II is likely to help you most.

Part II 'Mapping uncertainty in medicine' demonstrates how to use the MUM to understand and manage uncertainty.

Part III 'Mapping the psychology of uncertainty' explores the psychological aspects of uncertainty, including the reasons why clinicians find it so unpleasant to be uncertain.

Part IV 'Mapping uncertainty in medical training' covers the teaching and learning of strategies for managing uncertainty and the issues that arise when the uncertainty is about training matters, when it is the educator who 'does not know what to do'.

Part V 'Exploring uncertainty from the patient's perspective' considers the impact of uncertainty from the patient's point of view, as they face the challenges of illness and even death. Understanding uncertainty from the patient's point of view will, we hope, help clinicians react more sensitively.

In our **Conclusion** we argue for a greater acceptance that uncertainty is normal in medical practice as it is in life, and that uncertainty is something we can sensitively share with our patients. More collaborative relationships can result from such an approach, to the benefit of clinicians and patients alike.

WHO is this book for?

We hope that any clinician who is interested in the 'What do you do when you don't know what to do?' question (hereinafter referred to as WDYDWYDKWTD) will find this book useful. It will be especially helpful if you teach, train or supervise other clinicians, because they too will often come to you with WDYDWYDKWTD questions. Associates-in-Training in general practice will probably find this book especially useful, because uncertainty is the specialty of general practice! Advanced Nurse Practitioners face many of the same issues and may find this book helpful too. Reflective junior doctors who wish to be less fazed by the variability and complexity of medical practice, especially in any generalist setting (core medical or surgical training, psychiatry or Accident and Emergency), can apply the principles to their work and to their training.

WHAT is this book for?

The purpose of this book is to help clinicians think about WDYDWYDK WTD in a proactive and structured way. We hope that this will reduce the sense of shame and helplessness we all feel when we get stuck, help us to work more effectively with colleagues and patients, and lead to a more confident application of our skills and knowledge, to the rich and glorious variability of the humans beings in our care. Challenges will come in every setting, from an apparently routine family planning clinic (when a patient unexpectedly asks for a guarantee that her tablets are vegan), to the delicate management required to treat a frail patient who has complex comorbidities.

WHEN is the best time to use this book?

This book is an aid to reflection and learning, and how to manage things over time. It is not a manual you can use in the consultation like checking a drug dose in the BNF (sorry!). Rather, it will be useful when reflecting on a difficult situation afterwards and starting to think how to manage similar situations better next time or when you next see the patient. However, if you use the principles of this book regularly, you will find them starting to embed themselves in your brain and you will develop an important clinical skill, which is called metacognition. This rather off-putting word simply means that you are able to think about thinking, or, in even simpler terms, that you can choose what kind of thinking process will help you. For example, in a patient with a swollen leg, choosing to use the appropriate decision rules (the Wells score) will be the most helpful if you want to get an accurate diagnosis. However, you will need to choose negotiating or explaining skills to get a reluctant patient with needle phobia and a DVT to accept blood tests or heparin injections.

WHERE might you use this book?

Have this book on your desk, of course. Make sure it is handy when you are reflecting on your work, studying alone, in groups or with a tutor, or when you are having case discussions. The principles will be useful for secondary and primary care clinicians alike.

HOW can you use this book?

Start with Chapter 2 'How to use this book' (see p. 11). Uncertainty is classified into different types there, using an algorithm. This will help you to identify which type of uncertainty you are dealing with. Then use the relevant chapter of the book to identify the knowledge, skills and attitudes that will help unlock uncertain situations. For experienced clinicians, identifying the skills will be enough to help kick-start the process. For less experienced clinicians, identifying the skill needed may then come with the painful realisation that you don't have that skill … worry not, if you know what you want to learn, your teachers will help. A 'known unknown' is easier to remedy than an 'unknown unknown'!

Each part of the MUM contains distilled wisdom and skills, which very experienced clinicians use unconsciously. For the rest of us, using the MUM is a short cut to their expertise. It is always good to have your MUM with you in tricky situations.

Avril Danczak, Alison Lea and Geraldine Murphy

About the authors

Dr Avril Danczak BSc MBBS FRCP FRCGP FAoME PGCE is a GP in Central Manchester and has also worked in Zimbabwe. She has extensive experience as a postgraduate and undergraduate educator, teaching general practice to medical students, Foundation Doctors and general practice trainees (Associates-in-Training). She has also been a GP tutor organising training for experienced GPs, is involved in the North West Deanery and University Hospital of South Manchester 'Train the Trainers' courses and has been a general practice appraiser, and trainer of appraisers. She has a special interest in teaching consultation skills and in developing educational methods, and is currently involved in patient safety research.

Dr Alison Lea BSc (Hons) MBChB MSc (Primary Health Care) MRCGP works in Tameside, Greater Manchester, as a GP, Training Programme Director and GP member of Tameside and Glossop Clinical Commissioning Group. Alison has a strong educational background, having been a clinical lecturer at the Academic Unit of Primary Care, University of Leeds, prior to moving into postgraduate medical education. A theme throughout her career has been learning and teaching clinical reasoning and decision making, to clinicians at all levels.

Dr Geraldine Murphy MBChB MSc (Healthcare Ethics and Law) PGCert (Medical Education) is an Academic Clinical Fellow, currently in general practice training in Manchester. She is active in medical education, participating in undergraduate teaching at the University of Manchester and peer teaching of postgraduates. Her academic interests are focused around clinical reasoning and the use of new technology in teaching and learning.

Acknowledgements

This book could not have been thought of, started, written or finished without the help and support of many people.

A short conversation with Prof. Amanda Howe, when the concept of WDYDWYDKWTD was shyly mentioned, brought a smile of recognition to her face. She arranged a conversation there and then with Prof. Nigel Mathers, who facilitated contact with the right people at the RCGP … and so one thing led to another until we had a book. Education is not about filling a bucket, it is about lighting a fire. Thanks, Amanda, for lighting the blue touch paper!

Our colleagues on the Central and South Manchester Specialty Training Programme for General Practice, Julian Tomkinson, Anne Turner and Rebecca Baron, have been endlessly encouraging, reading early drafts with good humour and making many helpful suggestions.

Colleagues in our practices, especially Anthony Larkin, Tim Greenaway and Susie Power, have tolerated absences to write and edit, and have encouraged us to continue. Colleagues James Rangel, Aisha Awan and Erica Newbury read early versions of chapters and shared helpful reflections.

Our wonderful Associates-in-Training over several years on the Central and South Manchester and subsequently Tameside and Glossop Study Release courses have inspired us, tried out our methods, given us feedback and been true examples to us in their energy and commitment to learning how to be better GPs.

Thanks also to Barbara Meredith, Stephen Rigby, Judith Emmanuel and Steve Potter who gave helpful advice and feedback on early versions of our work.

Thanks to many people for practical things too: Gillian Nineham, our excellent and unflappable editor for the RCGP, Sherwin Dariani who kept the computers working, Matthew Creighton for IT wrangling to make the diagrams and Andy Howarth for his beautifully concise and cheerful illustrations.

Finally, yet crucially, thanks to Francis, Helen and Matthew, whose belief that the book would really be finished one day kept Avril going and to Catherine, Jack and Charlie whose pride in Alison is a very strong motivator in dark, desperate times.

We could not have done this without you all; our errors and infelicities remain our own.

PART I

Uncertainty in medicine

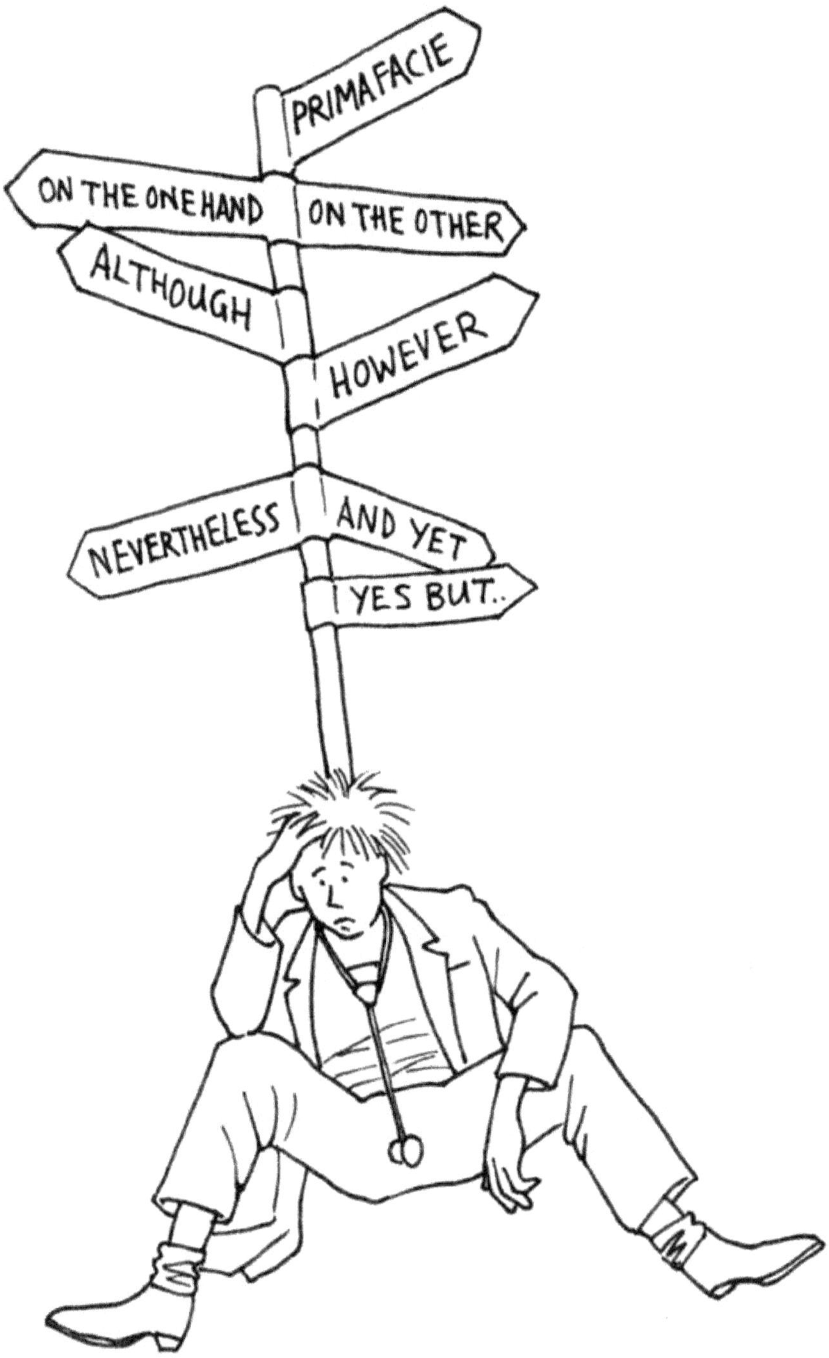
PRIMA FACIE
ON THE ONE HAND
ON THE OTHER
ALTHOUGH
HOWEVER
NEVERTHELESS
AND YET
YES BUT..

This part of the book is an introduction to uncertainty in medicine, and the moment when a clinician realises that she does not know what to do next. It is divided into two chapters.

- **Chapter 1 'Thinking about uncertainty in clinical practice'** is a general introduction to the concepts of uncertainty explored more fully in later chapters.
- **Chapter 2 'How to use this book'** explains how this book can be used as a manual, when a clinician is faced with a tricky 'what do you do when you don't know what to do' moment in his work.

Chapter 1

Thinking about uncertainty in medical practice

> Uncertainty creeps into medical practice through every pore. Whether a physician is defining a disease, making a diagnosis, selecting a procedure, observing outcomes, assessing probabilities, assigning preferences, or putting it all together, he is walking on very slippery terrain. It is difficult for non-physicians, and for many physicians, to appreciate how complex these tasks are, how poorly we understand them, and how easy it is for honest people to come to different conclusions.
>
> David Eddy[1]

Recognising the myriad uncertainties in medicine can be paralysing, no matter what your specialty is. Consider this train of issues that CANNOT BE AVOIDED in medicine.

First, as much as 90% of diagnoses are suggested by the history that the patient gives, which may be incomplete, untypical, may focus on aspects of the patient's experience that are important to her but not the most salient symptoms of disease, or may even be frankly inaccurate because the patient is embarrassed, in denial or forgetful.

Second, the symptoms the patient has may, or just as often may not, point to a particular diagnosis, syndrome or differential diagnosis.

Third, even if the story allows a reasonable differential diagnosis, the physical signs may be absent or untypical. Clinicians may even disagree about whether a particular physical sign is present or not.

Fourth, all tests and investigations have false-positive and false-negative rates, which may mean that true cases are missed, or that a positive test later turns out to be unconfirmed. Different people assessing an X-ray or interpreting a blood result may come to different conclusions, as the distinctions between 'normal' and 'abnormal' are not always clear cut.

Fifth, the treatment options for the condition may be numerous, and, even if clear cut, this patient may be the one for whom things go wrong, whose condition does not respond, or who does not cooperate with treatment, is intolerant of the treatment or cannot afford the treatment.

Sixth, many conditions require input from other team members, for example the care of a dying person at home or complex oncology treatments. Such teams may have limited capacity, certain members may turn out to be unavailable or of variable competency, and patients may not like their teams or find them hard to access.

Finally, the clinician himself may not have all the knowledge or skills needed to make the right diagnosis or assessment, and may not be able to arrange all the different elements of the treatment plan effectively.

In the face of such variables, how do clinicians ever actually *know* what to do? The uncertainty is pervasive and, to a large extent, irreducible. Enough, then, to turn most sentient humans to despair.

However, most of the time, most doctors and most of their patients can live with this uncertainty, which is after all a mere reflection of the uncertainties of life itself. What doctors are experiencing 'when they don't know what to do' is different. This type of uncertainty is experienced by doctors when they think they *ought* to know what to do, and when they have the feeling that someone else (cleverer, more senior, harder working) *would* know what to do. The 'not knowing' may be perceived as a personal failure that can feel threatening, shaming and uncomfortable. In this book we try to understand some of these situations and to help doctors find ways to cope with them better.

'What do you do when you don't know what to do?' is a question faced in other settings than health care because uncertainty is pervasive in many other fields. For example, making money remains an uncertain business; if it was more certain we could all be wealthy. The *Harvard Business Review* devoted a whole issue to managing uncertainty in September 2012 and referred to 'Leadership in a (Permanent) Crisis', a scenario that many doctors could identify with![2] In business, risk is considered to be calculable, but uncertainty is not calculable (for example, roulette is risky, but not uncertain in those terms). Dealing with uncertainty requires us to be comfortable with what cannot be calculated and with ambiguity. Scientists and doctors are not that keen on uncertainty, whereas artists celebrate it.

Doctors experience the urge to reduce what is unknowable to quantifiable probabilities and risks. This has been called 'pseudo certainty'. There is a lot of this in medicine, as we create risk stratifications for cardiovascular disease, or for the rates of response to chemotherapy, as if this will help. Faced with a patient who says, 'Will it actually help *me*?' we must recognise our uncertainty more deeply. Although we can calculate risks for populations, for any given individual the outcome remains uncertain.

Are doctors selected for their ability to tolerate ambiguity or uncertainty? Medical students who are less comfortable with ambiguity express preferences for those specialties with highly structured training and high use of technological solutions, and are uncomfortable with psychological issues. They are not keen to work with patients who are older, hypochondriacal or suffering chronic pain.[3] Moreover, students with a low tolerance for ambiguity are less likely to feel that the diagnosis and treatment of alcohol problems are not their responsibility, alcohol misuse being seen as an 'ambiguous' condition.[4] However, alcoholic patients, for whom certainty-preferring surgeons have less sympathy, will still need surgery sometimes, and all of our patients are getting older every year. So, understanding ambiguity and uncertainty are crucial issues for all doctors. Generalists in particular need to have good strategies for managing uncertainty (for example GPs, Accident and Emergency doctors, psychiatrists). They all have to deal with a great diversity of patients, often with highly complicated or uncertain conditions.

Much uncertainty in medicine might seem to be managed more effectively if we replace our ambitions to be certain about *outcomes* ('Will this patient be OK if I treat him at home rather than sending him to hospital?') with the more modest aim of having increased certainty of *process*. Developing confidence in knowing 'how to work it out' and perhaps 'I don't know right now but I will know when …' will help doctors manage uncertain situations more confidently, as long as they develop the art of being comfortable with ambiguity or uncertainty for a while.

Trusting the process of managing uncertainty works only if the process we are using is robust. The doctor must remain in touch with the outcome so that plans can be changed in response to feedback, altering clinical management as circumstances change. Our Map of Uncertainty in Medicine (MUM) can be used to ensure that the right skills are being used for the right circumstances. This means increasing certainty of *process*, which may help us to tolerate uncertainty more easily. We can try to build 'robustness into choices',[2] and understand the extent to which probability and risk create 'manageable certainty' or merely a 'pseudo certainty'. For example, assessing a patient as having a 12% cardiovascular risk may reduce uncertainties about whether or not our local health economy will approve a treatment with statins. However, treatment thresholds are decided with reference to attitudes and values, not to scientific certainties, and will not tell us whether or not the patient in front of us will actually get any benefit herself. Telling the individual that she has a 12% 'risk' is a way of expressing a pseudo certainty, because we cannot predict what will actually happen to that person. Our patient with low cardiovascular risk is not at 'no risk', and could have a heart attack tomorrow. Bad things can still happen to low-risk patients. Similarly, a high-risk patient may survive perfectly well and have no cardiovascular events at all. So should our patient at 12% 'risk' take a statin or not? The answer will depend on the patient's own attitudes to her health, as well as to what can be funded or justified by guidelines.

Doubts about how to proceed in that example mean we have to face something messier than statistics and come to terms with the implicit values that are coming into play. What is important and valued for our particular individual patient, and the decisions guided by those values, will not be found in statistics. Rather, we need to look to the skills of explanation, negotiation and shared decision making to elucidate what really matters.

In different situations of 'not knowing what to do', different skills will be needed. The skills of making sense of an unusual history from the patient are not the same as the skills needed to coordinate care for a patient who wishes to die at home, but whose spouse calls 999 three times a week because he does not agree with that plan.

Looking after patients is not like using a recipe book or a maintenance manual, or even like playing a complex computer game. We use interventions of variable effect, on a patient whose diversity (physical, psychological, social) we can only guess at, in circumstances we have little control over (social, time-scales and settings). Thus, being a doctor is not like being a mechanic but more like being at the helm of a small boat in waters of uncertain depth, current and salinity, in unpredictable weather and with a fuel tank that has no fuel gauge. Next time you ask yourself, 'What do I do when I don't know what to do?' remember that all clinicians are alongside you in spirit. Using the process described in this book will help you to 'know what to do when you don't know what to do', which is where wisdom lies.

Conclusion

Will this book remove all uncertainties or doubts about how to proceed? Probably not, although it may reduce the times when uncertainty overwhelms practitioners. The tools will help you analyse the problem, avoid some pitfalls, identify the skills you need and help you to move forwards. The rich tapestry of medicine means that, however experienced you are, you will still experience times when 'you don't know what to do'. Recognising, and even enjoying, that uncertainty is one of the charms of clinical medicine, which is often as much an art as a science.

Good luck. Let us know how you get on.

References

1. Eddy DM. Variations in physician practice: the role of uncertainty. *Health Affairs* (Millwood) 1984; **3(2)**: 74–89.
2. Nohria N, Stewart TA. Risk, uncertainty, and doubt. *Harvard Business Review*, September 2012: 8–9.
3. Geller G, Faden RR, Levine DM. Tolerance for ambiguity among medical students: implications for their selection, training and practice. *Social Science and Medicine* 1990; **31(5)**: 619–24.
4. Merrill JM, Camacho Z, Laux LF, *et al.* Uncertainties and ambiguities: measuring how medical students cope. *Medical Education* 1994; **28(4)**: 316–22.

Further reading

Schön DA. *Educating the Reflective Practitioner: toward a new design for teaching and learning in the professions.* San Francisco, CA: Jossey-Bass, 1987.

Chapter 2

How to use this book

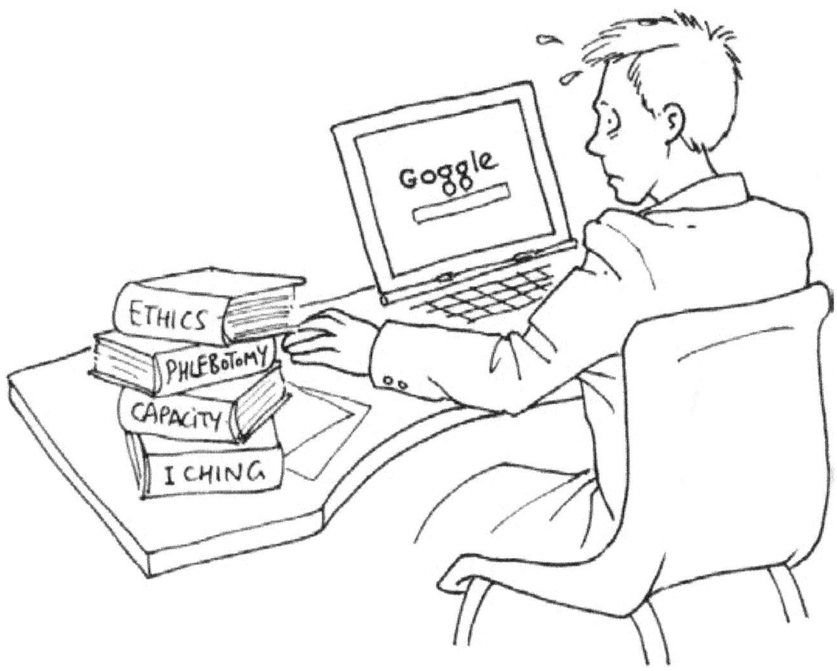

All clinicians experience moments when they 'don't know what to do'. This chapter covers:

- the stages of working out how to tackle an uncertain situation
- step one – recognising uncertainty and 'functional' and 'dysfunctional' responses
- step two – classifying uncertainty
- step three – identifying the skills needed in uncertain situations
- the MUM, and how to use it
- how the MUM approach was developed.

Map of Uncertainty in Medicine (MUM)

	INDIVIDUAL clinician/patient	GROUP working with patient
DIAGNOSTIC uncertainty	**ANALYSING** Diagnosis uncertain; one doctor, one patient. Ways forward: appropriate thinking skills and self awareness. **Skills required** • Hypothetico-deductive reasoning • Ruling in or ruling out/Diagnostic safety netting • Trust and verify • Sharing the clinical reasoning process • Using algorithms, decision rules • Exploring the emotional content of consultations • Situational awareness skills • Widening the view/functional symptoms **Examples of 'dysfunctional ways out'** • Unfocused investigations • Cognitive biases and errors **Setting should** • Enable access to decision and knowledge support • Promote CME for improving consultation and thinking skills	**NETWORKING** Diagnosis uncertain; patient and diagnostic services involved. Ways forward: targeted use of investigations, referrals and senior colleagues. **Skills required** • Holding skills • Managing expectations of investigation or referral • Understanding the referral network • Breaking good news • Dealing with exceptional circumstances • Continuing care after referral **Examples of 'dysfunctional ways out'** • Excess investigations/Over-medicalisation • Passing anxiety/responsibility on to others **Setting should** • Facilitate discussion and mutual support before referral or investigation • Ensure good information about appropriate referral options
MANAGEMENT uncertainty	**NEGOTIATING** Best management uncertain or impossible; one doctor–patient dyad. Ways forward: skills to develop dialogue with patient while maintaining ethical perspective. **Skills required** • Explaining • Negotiating • Talking about risk • Shared decision making • Why don't you? Yes, but • Motivational interviewing/behaviour change • Engaging with complex problems • Managing 'non-medical' problems • Psychosocial issues in the doctor–patient relationship **Examples of 'dysfunctional ways out'** • Blaming patient/blaming the system • Conflict/complaints **Setting should** • Enable consultation skills development • Facilitate discussion and feedback • Model/facilitate shared decision making	**TEAM-WORKING** Optimum management uncertain; patient and group (team, family, other agencies) unwilling, unable or blocking preferred management. Ways forward: best management of multidisciplinary team. **Skills required** • Creating a good team • Making meetings work/chairing skills • Managing boundaries • Being 'good enough' • Managing difficult situations • Handover skills **Examples of 'dysfunctional ways out'** • Passing the buck/blaming other teams • Withdrawal of services • Conflict **Setting should** • Value effective teamwork (including specific training in teamwork skills) • Help to manage psychological boundaries

The stages of working out how to tackle an uncertain situation

When learning how to cope with uncertain situations more effectively there are several stages to the process. Unpicking uncertainty begins with identifying uncertain situations, then classifying them (we have a useful algorithm for that on p. 15), and then, finally, selecting the right skills to manage the situation effectively, using the MUM, illustrated on p. 12. Uncertainty can be classified into *analysing*, *negotiating*, *networking* and *team-working* issues, and knowing what you are dealing with makes uncertainty a lot less daunting. Each one of these types of uncertainty is considered in detail in Part II. Initially, most people will find that this approach works best as a method to reflect on a difficult situation after the event; it is not realistic to use this manual during a consultation with a patient. However, with practice you will find that recognising uncertain situations becomes easier and you will be able to work out what kind of issue it is more quickly. Choosing the right skill becomes easier then too.

Step one – recognising uncertainty and 'functional' and 'dysfunctional' responses

Often, recognising uncertainty is straightforward for clinicians. An uncertain situation is easily recognised when you find yourself thinking something like:

> *Something is wrong, this information does not make any sense.*
>
> *I cannot get all this information to cohere together.*
>
> *I feel really uncomfortable* or *This plan isn't working, but I can't work out why.*
>
> *This feels wrong/odd* or *Why is this a problem when it has never been a problem before?*
>
> *I don't have enough time for this. What can I do safely now… .*
>
> *This approach usually works, but … .*
>
> *I am stuck, all alternatives are hopeless* or *I cannot think of anything suitable to do next!*
>
> *This is a difficult patient; she is getting cross/not cooperating/going off at a tangent.*

This point of awareness, that things are not going well, should precipitate a state of 'metacognition', a thought process that rings some kind of alarm bell internally, alerting us to unresolved uncertainty. These thoughts, and many similar ones, should highlight that uncertainty is a feature of the situation, and that *attention should be paid to that uncertainty*. This is sometimes so uncomfortable for doctors that they may not tolerate remaining in an uncertain, ambiguous position with no obvious choice of action. This can lead to the rapid choice of a 'dysfunctional way out' of the situation, which temporarily resolves the uncertainty, while not having beneficial effects in the longer term. This may happen so quickly that doctors are barely able to articulate their uncertainty.

The nature and effects of different 'dysfunctional ways out' of uncertainty are described for each type of uncertainty in Part II. 'Functional ways through' uncertainty that will generally lead to more satisfactory results are also described, with the skills needed identified. How do we know whether a plan is a 'dysfunctional way out' or a 'functional way through'?

If a decision is purposeful and deliberate, with the consequences anticipated and thought to be helpful, it is likely to be a 'functional way through'. If the decision has been made to 'get the patient out of the room', or to 'avoid making a decision', or to 'pass the buck' to another clinician or team, or if it seems to 'blame the patient' for being too difficult, then that action has the potential to be a 'dysfunctional way out'. Examples of these responses to uncertainty are discussed for each type of uncertainty in Part II.

Step two – classifying uncertainty

Having recognised that there has been a WDYDWYDKWTD moment of uncertainty, the next step is to *classify* the uncertainty. This is where the algorithm that classifies uncertainty comes in.

Answering two straightforward questions leads to a useful classification of uncertainty in clinical practice:

1 Does this uncertainty relate to an uncertain *diagnosis* or to uncertainty about *management* of the patient's care?
2 Is one *doctor–patient dyad* involved (as in a typical consultation) or is a larger *group, team or network* involved?

With the answers to these questions, use the MUM algorithm (opposite page) to identify which Quadrant of the MUM is relevant.

The MUM classifies uncertainty into four basic kinds, which form the four Quadrants of the Map:

- the *Analysing Quadrant* refers to uncertain diagnosis, when there is only one doctor–patient dyad involved
- the *Networking Quadrant* refers to uncertain diagnosis, when a larger team or network is involved
- the *Negotiating Quadrant* refers to uncertain management, when only one doctor–patient dyad is involved
- the *Team-working Quadrant* refers to uncertainties in care where a group, team or family are involved.

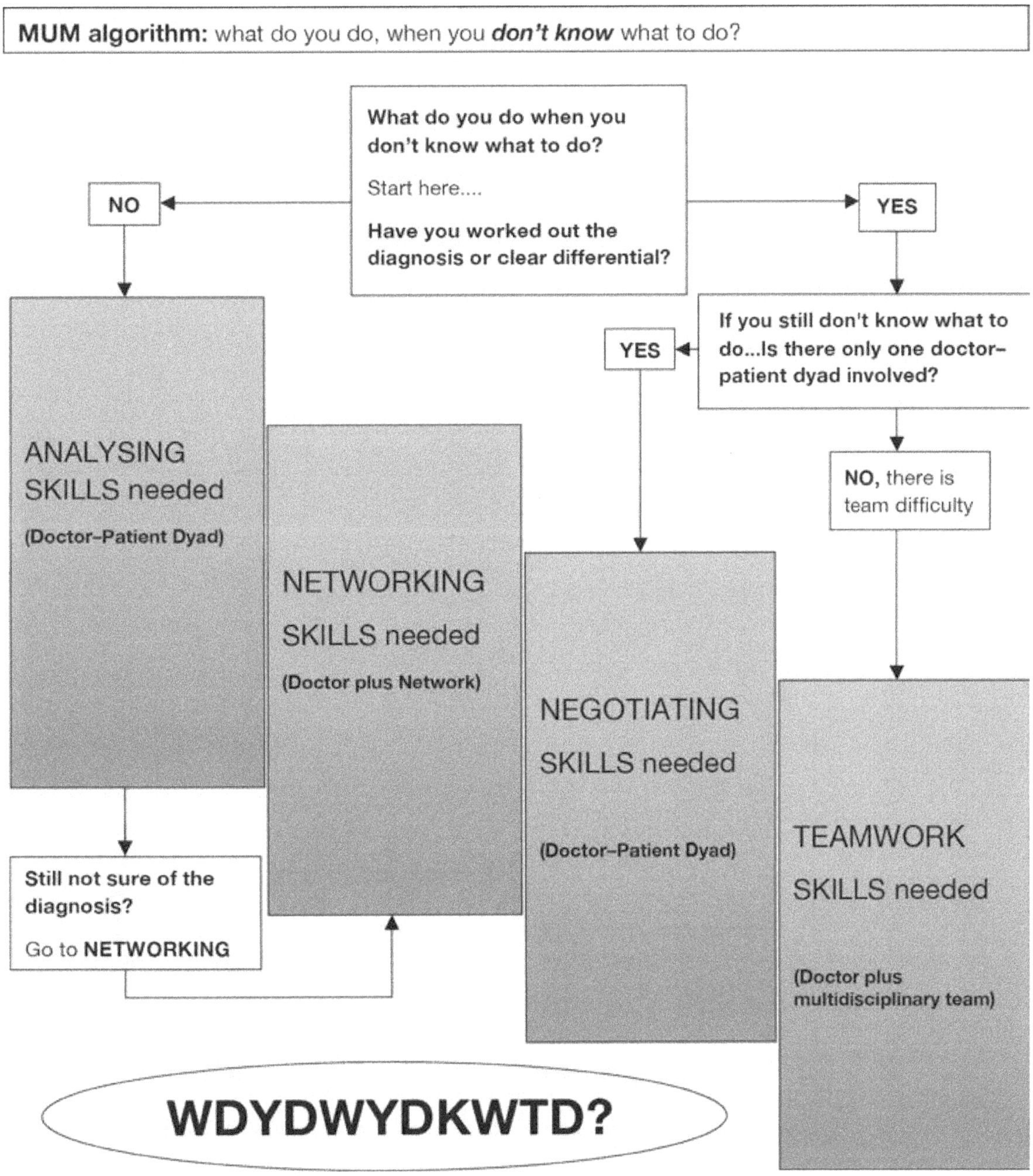

Sometimes, life being complicated, more than one Quadrant will be involved.

When you have worked out which Quadrant is relevant for the particular uncertainty in question, take an initial look at the MUM at the beginning of this chapter (p. 12). This will summarise the main issues that arise in that Quadrant.

Then go to the chapter referring to that Quadrant, which will be found in Part II. Then use the chapter in the way that works best for you. You may want to read the whole chapter, or simply select the situation and skill that seems most relevant.

Step three – identifying the skills needed in uncertain situations

In Part II, each Quadrant of the MUM is covered in detail. Tricky situations are described, with some of the 'dysfunctional ways out' that commonly occur. The skills needed to create a 'functional way through' uncertainty in each Quadrant are explained, and given clinical illustrations. For some clinicians, the skills needed will already be familiar; what is needed is to ensure the right skill is deployed at the right time. For others, the skill may be novel or rusty. It will then be necessary to learn about the nature and scope of that skill and to practise it until it becomes familiar. Most people develop skills best if they get some feedback and we encourage clinicians to seek this out. This can be by getting a colleague to observe you, by videoing consultations and watching them over again, and of course by asking patients how things went from their point of view. Training for uncertainty is covered in more detail in Part V.

The Map of Uncertainty in Medicine and how to use it

The MUM is, in effect, a summary of the whole of Part II of this book. It sets out the nature of the uncertainty in each Quadrant. Each Quadrant is set out with the same structure:

- an introduction to the nature of the uncertainty in that Quadrant
- 'dysfunctional ways out'
- examples of common situations
- 'functional ways through' common problems, identifying the right skills needed for the right situation
- how the setting can help to deal with this type of uncertainty
- suggested assessment and teaching methods
- resources for immediate use.

To illustrate WDYDWYDKWTD situations we have provided clinical scenarios that will be familiar to most doctors, and we have used a few patient narratives that thread their way through the different Quadrants, to illustrate how one individual may present different challenges in different situations. For clarity, all the clinicians are named after trees or plants and all the patients are named for minerals.

Accompanying each Quadrant in Part II are some brief observations about how best to teach and learn the particular skills needed. The settings we work in can help or sometimes hinder our learning and usage of new skills; there are also comments on how we can improve the settings we work in to help us manage uncertainty more effectively. At the end of each Quadrant section there are some resources that will be of immediate use to anyone wanting to learn more. A more wide-ranging bibliography can be found at the end of the book, for true scholars.

This book is designed to be used as a manual by all clinicians. Doctors in training, together with their supervisors and trainers, may find it particularly helpful. When teaching and learning about uncertainty, this book highlights how to recognise uncertainty, how to classify it and how to be aware of the different routes out of uncertainty that clinicians use. Decision making in uncertain situations, especially when the doctor feels that he 'doesn't know what to do', is stressful and uses a lot of mental energy. This makes for psychologically draining work. No manual can take all of the stress and uncertainty out of medical practice; as we discussed in the first chapter, uncertainty is inevitable. However, having a deeper understanding of how uncertainty impinges on practice, and having some strategies for managing uncertainty, can reduce the burden that clinical practice can place on many clinicians.

How do we know this and how did we come to write this manual?

We are all professional general practice medical educators. We teach GPs who are still in their training years in one-to-one teaching and in specialty training groups. We have also had considerable experience in the training and appraisal of more experienced clinicians. In numerous discussions with doctors of all levels of experience, uncertainty is often prominent, whether for junior doctors asking for a senior opinion or for senior doctors facing complex or difficult circumstances. We began to deliver teaching sessions about uncertainty based on asking the question, 'What do you do when you don't know what to do?' The feedback from learners and trainers was positive;

all clinicians are keen to face these matters and discuss how to manage such situations.

We explored in more detail what it is exactly that doctors face when they are in WDYDWYDKWTD situations. We recorded focus groups of GPs in their final year of training and thematically analysed their conversations, which revealed many instances of uncertainty, some of which are painfully difficult to cope with. We also observed how doctors in training recognised uncertainty, how their uncertainty related to the context in which they worked, how they responded to uncertainty and how they sometimes failed to use skills that could have helped them manage uncertainty with less stress and difficulty.[1] We came to understand the many and various 'dysfunctional ways out' of uncertainty used by clinicians.

This work brought us to several conclusions:

- not all WDYDWYDKWTD situations are the same
- uncertainty can be classified into different types – there are *analysing*, *networking*, *negotiating* and *team-working* uncertainties
- the skills needed are different for different kinds of uncertainty
- not all uncertainty is about a lack of knowledge
- uncertainty is very uncomfortable for clinicians and patients alike
- doctors sometimes impulsively jump to 'dysfunctional ways out' of uncertainty that are less effective in the longer term
- there are more 'functional ways though' uncertainty, based on applying relevant skills.

We used these insights to develop the **MUM** and the algorithm for working out which type of uncertainty the doctor is dealing with. Understanding what type of uncertainty is being faced means that doctors can start to recognise that different skills may be required at different times. Having the ability to use 'metacognition', that is, to 'think about the thinking' involved in different situations, empowers clinicians to choose from a larger repertoire of skills, matching the skill needed to the situation in a more nuanced way.

We have tested the MUM in a number of training settings, with overwhelmingly positive feedback for learners of all grades and experience, and most specialties. The Map has been used:

- in one-to-one sessions with learners
- with larger groups of specialty trainees in general practice specialty training programmes

- with groups of postgraduate general practice medical educators in the North West and nationally
- with groups of educators from a variety of hospital specialties.

We were initially rather startled to discover the degree of immediate recognition of the validity of our classification from clinicians. It felt as if there had been something there, intuitively understood, but not previously clearly articulated. The 'dysfunctional ways out' that we will describe in detail in each chapter were greeted with rueful smiles, and the 'functional ways though' accepted as the more skilful approaches.

The aim of this book is to highlight the range of skills that are needed in uncertain situations, and to help clinicians to feel that, when they have become 'stuck', they can reflect on the situation afterwards and see how they may have done something differently. In the uphill struggle of trying to cope with awkward, uncertain, difficult situations we hope that this will help clinicians to feel a little more resourceful, give them a clearer view of what is happening and make life a bit less stressful. Having a clearer focus gives more options and different routes to achieve what is needed. This increased flexibility of mind makes for more effective work.

Reference

1. Danczak A, Lea A. What do you do when you don't know what to do? GP associates in training (AiT) and their experiences of uncertainty. *Education for Primary Care* 2014; **25(6)**: 321–6.

PART II

Mapping uncertainty in medicine

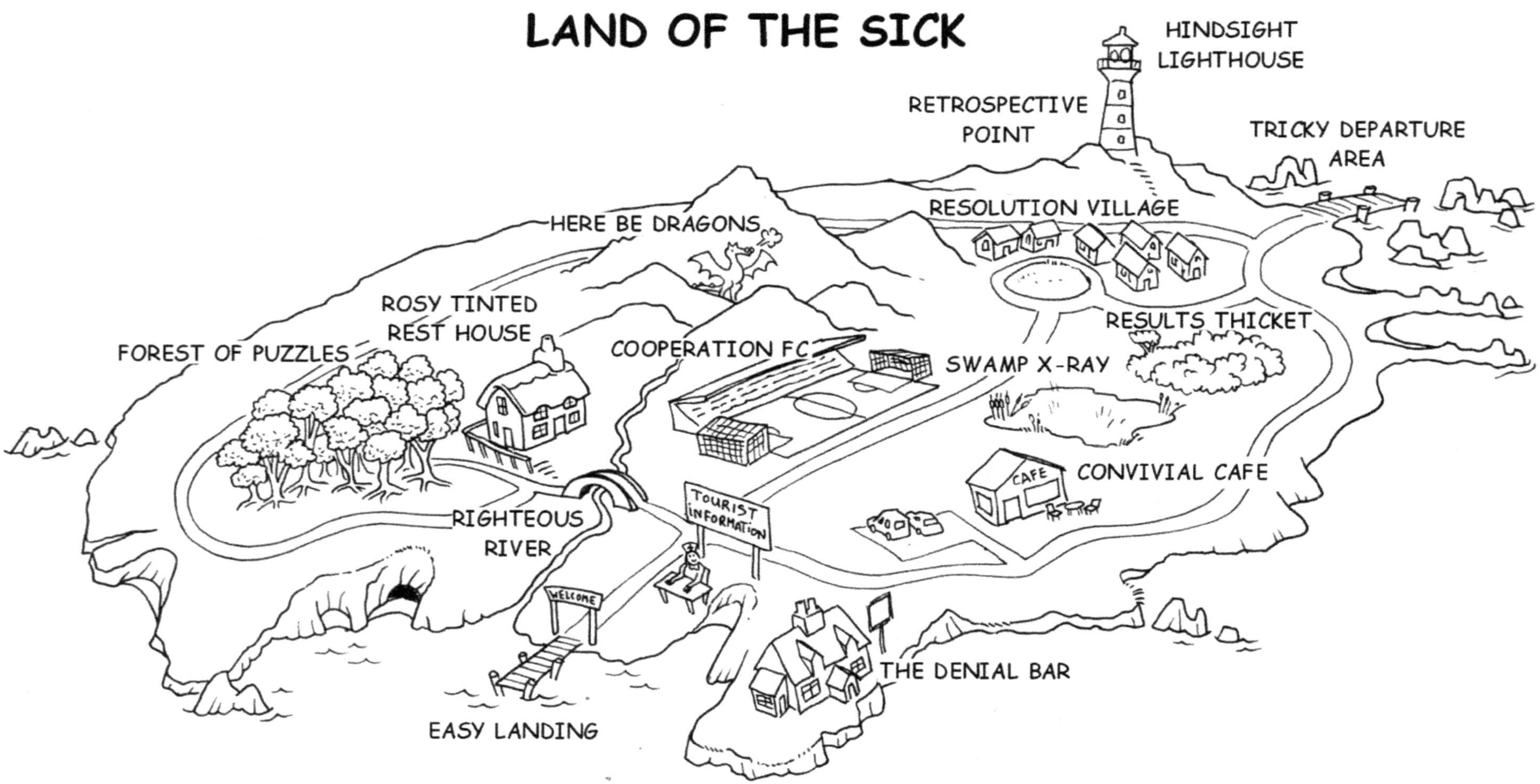
LAND OF THE SICK
HINDSIGHT LIGHTHOUSE
RETROSPECTIVE POINT
TRICKY DEPARTURE AREA
RESOLUTION VILLAGE
HERE BE DRAGONS
ROSY TINTED REST HOUSE
FOREST OF PUZZLES
COOPERATION FC
RESULTS THICKET
SWAMP X-RAY
CAFE
CONVIVIAL CAFE
TOURIST INFORMATION
RIGHTEOUS RIVER
WELCOME
THE DENIAL BAR
EASY LANDING

This part is divided into four sections that deal in turn with the:

- **Analysing Quadrant**
- **Networking Quadrant**
- **Negotiating Quadrant**
- **Team-Working Quadrant.**

The Analysing Quadrant

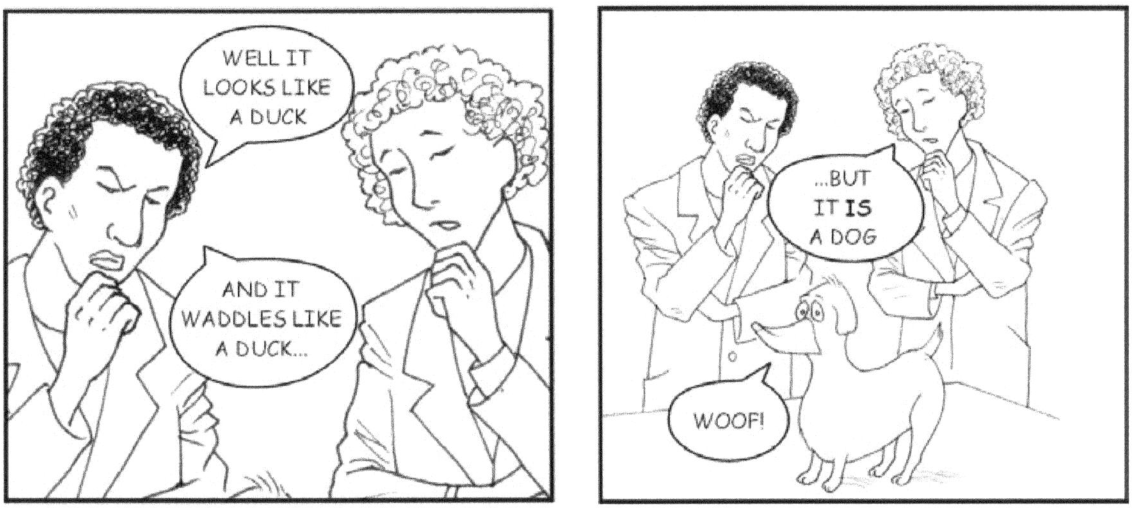
WELL IT LOOKS LIKE A DUCK
AND IT WADDLES LIKE A DUCK...
...BUT IT IS A DOG
WOOF!

The Analysing Quadrant is primarily concerned with the processes that clinicians use to make a diagnosis, which is a fundamental first step in arranging appropriate care for a patient.

Chapter 3 is an introduction to uncertainty in the Analysing Quadrant and also discusses 'dysfunctional ways out'. **Chapter 4** works through examples of common WDYDWYDKWTD situations in the Analysing Quadrant, identifying 'functional ways through' common problems, and the right skills needed for the right situation. **Chapter 5** explores how the clinical setting can help to deal with uncertainty in the Analysing Quadrant, and suggests assessment and teaching methods.

The key skills are:

- hypothetico-deductive reasoning using 'restricted rule out'
- ruling in or ruling out/diagnostic safety netting
- trust and verify
- sharing the clinical reasoning process with the patient
- using clinical guidelines, algorithms and clinical decision tools
- exploring the emotional content of the consultation
- situational awareness skills
- widening the view/explaining functional symptoms.

Chapter 3

Introduction to uncertainty in the Analysing Quadrant

> The essential unit of medical practice is the occasion when, in the intimacy of the consulting room or sick room, a person who is ill, or believes himself to be ill, seeks the advice of a doctor whom he trusts. This is a consultation, and all else in the practice of medicine derives from it.
>
> Sir James Spence (1892–1954)

This well-known quotation sums up the way that the practice of medicine starts with a consultation, the seeking of advice. Ideally, when one doctor and one patient sit down in the 'intimacy of the consulting room' to explore a medical problem, the doctor's well-honed history-taking and physical examination skills will lead to a reasonable diagnosis, which will enable a suitable management plan to be discussed. If no single diagnosis can be fixed upon, then, often, a 'working diagnosis' or differential diagnosis may, nonetheless, be enough for the doctor and patient to move forwards. For example, a patient with rectal bleeding and weight loss may have cancer, inflammatory bowel disease, radiation proctitis or none of these. However, to settle the issue and move on, the action will be clear: arrange some kind of endoscopy or imaging to resolve the issue. This is *not* a WDYDWYDKWTD situation.

Yet we do end up in WDYDWYDKWTD situations when trying to make a diagnosis. So how does this happen and what can we do about it?

The Analysing Quadrant explores the issues when the diagnosis is not known and there is mainly one doctor and one patient involved. This may be a newly presenting problem, or a follow-up of a patient whose symptoms have changed, not resolved as expected, or remain unclear in their origin. This can result in uncertainty about how to proceed, especially if the doctor is fearful of 'missing something' or when the patient has not got the answers they were looking for. In areas where they are consciously aware of incompetence, doctors readily ask for help, for example via referral. Where symptoms are non-specific, clinicians may use dysfunctional strategies (such as premature reassurance, 'There is a lot of this about') to ensure that they stay in their intellectual comfort zone, avoiding the threatening feeling of inadequacy if no diagnosis is reached. However, unconscious incompetence, which the doctor may be unaware of, while obviously leading to mistakes or errors, can also mean that doctors come up against diagnostic difficulties without being fully aware of how this situation has arisen.

This chapter covers:

- an introduction to the issues arising from uncertainty in the Analysing Quadrant
- 'dysfunctional ways out' of uncertainty in the Analysing Quadrant; common pitfalls

There are three main factors that can lead to a failure or sense of paralysis in the Analysing Quadrant:

- factors internal to the clinician
- factors external to the clinician
- patient factors.

Internal factors relate to the clinician: how they are thinking, their level of conscious and unconscious competence, their awareness of their areas of incompetence and their ability and willingness to hear, register and evaluate effectively all the information they have about the patient. This may be markedly affected by the overall physical and mental health of the clinician, her experiences of and responses to stressful situations or pressure of work. A clinician distracted by her own pain may not make accurate diagnoses. A clinician's familiarity with the setting she works in, the language she is working in and her sensitivity to local nuances of the history can also affect diagnosis. (For example, in Zimbabwe it is common to hear patients complain of 'total body pain', not a common complaint in the UK.) Furthermore, the clinician's overall level of confidence can affect her ability to remain engaged in working things out in the consultation; a clinician with low confidence in her ability may 'give up' too soon, or get fixated on only one aspect of the problem. An over-confident, senior or bored clinician may have developed reflex dysfunctional ways out, which can be more comfortable than engaging with difficult problems.

Issues external to a clinician can affect his ability to make a diagnosis. Time pressure is frequently cited,[1] remaining a major and unresolved issue. If patients have many problems for the clinician to deal with in a short time, if there are too many patients to see in the time available, if the clinician is conflicted by needing to see a patient at home, while also being expected to be in a multidisciplinary team meeting, time pressures can easily affect thinking. Having many interruptions, or too high a workload, can affect accuracy, especially in over- or under-confident clinicians. A happy mean between over- and under-confidence is not easy to achieve even after a lifetime's practice … some would say especially after a lifetime's practice! Increasingly, clinicians work in a highly regulated system, with defined pathways for certain symptom clusters or complexes. What will the clinician do if the patient's complaints don't really fit a defined pattern, or do not 'reach the threshold' defined for referral or investigation? Sometimes the best option is not available (for example following up someone personally, within a short time-scale, because a shift is ending) and sometimes the results of investigations can be misleading or presented in ways that make interpretation more difficult.

Patient factors can affect the ability of a clinician to make an accurate diagnosis. Perhaps the patient's history is unclear, complex or confusing. Patients may have more than one condition whose symptoms may overlap. Sometimes the patient's emotional or psychological issues can impede diagnosis, if, for example, she is too distressed to tell her story clearly, or if she avoids sensitive subjects (some patients with cancer will deliberately choose not to disclose worrying symptoms at first). Other, more practical, issues such as language barriers, deafness, unfamiliarity with the clinician or even dementia can all contribute to clinicians finding themselves in a WDYDWYDKWTD situation.

Recent psychological research has explored in some depth how humans think and make decisions. It is well established that people think in different ways according to the task they are trying to perform, and also the context in which they are doing the task. Historically, two main approaches have been recognised, often referred to as 'intuitive' and 'analytical'. This has been developed in recent cognitive psychology into the dual process theory, which is helpful in considering how clinicians make decisions about diagnosis.[2] This theory develops from observations that humans make decisions in one of two ways, hence 'dual process'.

The first approach is called 'Type 1 thinking'. This is the brain's preferred or default method. It is a fast, automatic, unconscious, low-effort process. For example, how do we think if we approach a house where there is a loud noise of barking, a voice says, 'Quiet Rover!' and the door shakes as if something is trying to escape? Using Type 1 thinking, we will usually make the assumption that there is a dog inside, even if we can't see through the door. This type of thinking can also be referred to as intuitive, unconscious or heuristic reasoning, and is strongly contextualised, using 'rules of thumb.' This type of thinking is based on perception, pattern recognition and orientation to the type of problem being examined.

The second method of thinking, called 'Type 2 thinking', is, by contrast, a slow, deliberate, consciously analytical process that takes a lot of effort. For example, if entering the house discussed under Type 1, no dog is to be seen, it may take a while to work out whether it was the TV on too loud, a burglar alarm recording of a dog designed to put people off, a hallucination or some other phenomenon. This more deliberate type of thinking has also been called analytical, rational or conscious reasoning. Solving a cryptic crossword clue, or Sudoku, are also examples of Type 2 thinking in practice; a deliberate problem-solving approach will yield better results than a quick guess.

Each of these methods of thinking is useful in different circumstances and has its pros and cons. Awareness of the nature of the thinking processes they are using can help clinicians to choose an effective 'thinking strategy' when faced with a tricky situation. The ability to use 'metacognition' or 'thinking about thinking' is a key skill for those clinicians who are accurately assessing their own level of competence and who are 'self-assessing' as they think about problems. Such clinicians use what Donald Schön refers to as 'reflection-in-action' to decide what type of thinking method will help them most.[3] More experienced and sophisticated diagnosticians use Type 1 thinking to recognise that patterns are atypical, or that information available cannot be explained by the intuitive diagnosis. They then use Type 2 thinking, analytic, formal, rule-based methods, to make comparisons, weigh options and generate more possibilities.

Although more junior personnel often perceive 'expert' thinkers as being 'intuitive', most experts will exhibit 'analytical' reasoning when discussing a particular situation and can freely use a mixture of intuition and analysis, moving in both directions along a continuum from intuitive to analytical thinking. Expert thinkers will vary their strategy according to the complexity of the task, how well ordered the task is, the time available and whether the task is presented visually, favouring intuition, or in an objective, quantitative form, favouring analysis.[4]

How can we apply our understanding of these two types of thinking when we are trying to make a diagnosis in a WDYDWYDKWTD situation?

Type 1 thinking includes our gut reactions, and is quick, intuitive and low effort. This is what clinicians are using when they use pattern recognition, responding quickly to familiar situations or to hazards or threats. The development of rules of thumb and other short cuts to analysis are examples of Type 1 responses. These can enable experienced practitioners to recognise syndromes or situations far more quickly than their juniors and is also a feature of those clinicians with good situational awareness.[5]

Typically, generalists (who work in settings such as Accident and Emergency, general practice or psychiatry) use the rapidly perceived, most salient features of the clinical picture to generate early hypotheses.[6] These are derived from a mixture of theoretical knowledge and previous experiences, which prompt 'intuitive' Type 1 thinking. Such hypotheses are then directly and deliberately tested using a more analytical approach, collecting specific further information until a decision threshold is reached. The Type 1 thinking is also part of the way clinicians recognise the most important features in a patient's story or identify unusual or inconsistent findings. This inner 'alarm bell' is another way that 'intuitive' Type 1 thinking works in practice.

However, Type 1 thinking has a downside: it is prone to bias, which can result in errors. Type 1 thinking is less reliable and is affected by the thinker's emotional state and the emotional responses of those around her. Additional factors include the context, perceived difficulty and the risks associated with the decision itself.[6] If an intuitive assessment does not yield an effective decision or diagnosis, this can rapidly result in a WDYDWYDKWTD situation arising if the clinician is not able to change her mode of thinking appropriately. Type 1 thinking is very specific to the situation. A radiologist may be able to spot an abnormality on a chest X-ray rapidly, using pattern recognition honed by years of experience. This will not necessarily help her decide what to say to her adolescent daughter who rings her up at work in floods of tears.

So why have humans adopted Type 1 as the preferred, default thinking strategy? Clearly, the clue is in the effortless nature of such thinking. It is quite simply easier, less tiring and requires less energy. Being able to react quickly to clues from the patient, or to changes in the situation around us, is clearly a helpful thing if we consider it as part of our evolutionary heritage:

better to respond quickly to changing cues or threats, rather than waiting around to see if the creature in the shadows is a leopard or a pussycat.

Imagine if we actually analysed each decision we make in a day, from what to do when the doorbell rings, to which gear to drive to work in, to which patient's records to look at first; we would be slow at assessing things, and inefficient at getting through our diagnostic work. Analysing every response, reaction or decision would be tiring, slow and inefficient. Type 1 thinking is fast!

Type 1 and Type 2 thinking are compared in Table 3.1.

Table 3.1: Comparison of Type 1 and Type 2 thinking

Characteristics	Type 1 thinking – intuitive	Type 2 thinking – analytical
Overall attributes	Associative, concrete, practically based, automatic	Theory based, abstract, rule based, chosen, methodical not automatic
Speed	Fast	Slow
Channels	Multiple, parallel	Single, linear
Effort	Minimal	Considerable
Cost	Low	High
Bias	Easily biased	Less easily biased
Reliability	Low and variable	High and consistent
Errors	Common	Fewer
Affected by emotion	Often	Less often
Scientific rigour	Low	High
Relevance to context	High	Low
Presentation	Visual, conversational	Quantitative, written
Is clinician aware of his thinking?	No	Yes
Guiding methods	Rules of thumb, heuristics, pattern recognition	Rules, protocols, guidelines, algorithms
Effects	Skilled, reflex actions, looks effortless	Deliberate, rule-based actions, takes effort
Predictive power	Low for objective outcomes, higher for emotional/relationship outcomes	High for objective outcomes, low for relationship outcomes
Relationship to Schön's classification of professionalism	'Professional artistry'	'Technical, rational professionalism'

Source: adapted from Dawson,[7] Croskerry,[2,8] Evans[9] and Schön 1993.[3]

How do clinicians develop their diagnostic Type 1 thinking? A deep familiarity with Type 2 thinking is learned early in training, which then becomes 'embedded' in Type 1 thinking in the mind. Learning to take a systems review in medical school is slow and requires effort at first (Type 2 thinking), becoming quicker, more reflex and more intuitive with practice, i.e. becoming more of a Type 1 pattern.

Clinicians can find it difficult to believe that they are often working on 'automatic pilot' and they almost all say that they make deliberate and conscious decisions. However, we underestimate the way that in clinical practice, as we meet more and varied presentations of illness, we build up pictures, mental representations called scripts and schemas, of symptoms, signs and diagnoses.[10] These result in clinicians focusing quickly on what they think are the key features and the most likely diagnoses. We can easily persuade ourselves that we have thought things through, when in fact we have jumped to a Type 1 conclusion. Each clinician's experience is different and thus each clinician's 'collection' of typical illness presentations also varies. As a result, the conclusions of Type 1 thinking are specific to the individual and her past experiences, which makes those conclusions prone to biases of various kinds. When working in areas that are outside their own area of routine expertise, clinicians may not have the same 'bank' of clinical experience to aid pattern recognition and management decisions.

For example, a cardiologist who sees a middle-aged patient with chest pain, high cholesterol and history of hypertension and smoking will put all that information together very quickly (so as to seem 'intuitive') and proceed to evaluate the patient thoroughly for ischaemic heart disease. Simultaneously, he may also be registering subtle cues that the history is atypical and may point towards other diagnoses such as pericarditis (using his Type 1 thinking 'alarm bell', which will pick up deviations from usual patterns). A first-year medical student might struggle even to elicit relevant information such as smoking history, the results of the cholesterol tests or the effects of exercise, and may forget to consider causes of high cholesterol such as hypothyroidism.

If Type 1 thinking has both benefits and weaknesses, how does Type 2 'analytical' thinking impact on the diagnostic process? Analytical thinking finds most use in situations where there is more time, where the outcomes are potentially serious, and where problems are complex, not clearly defined or outside routine practice. In the context of WDYDWYDKWTD situations, choosing the right kind of thinking can assist clinicians in sorting out less straightforward diagnoses. This helps to manage the uncertainties of complex, unexpected or ambiguous presentations in a more structured way. Clinicians develop expertise by seeing many clinical problems, initially working through them using a logical, analytical and methodical approach, i.e. Type 2 thinking. This particularly applies when the presentation is novel, clinicians are inexperienced or the issue is not routine to them. However, Type 2 thinking is more difficult and needs more effort, which may make clinicians reluctant to change their mode of thinking. For example, finding it difficult to change mode from a Type 1 approach to a more analytical approach may mean that a cardiologist will refer a problem of allergic rhinitis to an ENT specialist, where a GP would have expertise to manage it themselves, using her own Type 1 approaches. This does not mean that cardiologists know nothing about allergic rhinitis, but that outside their own sphere they would have to resort to an effortful Type 2 thinking analysis that, in practice, they consider is more efficiently delivered by someone else.

With practice, Type 2 thinking can become rapid enough to seem like Type 1 thinking to the outside observer. This is what learners admire in clinicians who 'just seem to know the diagnosis' or who spot things that other clinicians have missed. This can be because Type 2 thinking is happening rapidly, thus seeming 'intuitive' to observers. Digging deeper into the thinking of these clinicians will often reveal a specific attentiveness, an openness to all types of information that enables them to first notice and then synthesise and analyse *all* the information available to them, using a Type 1 approach, subsequently tested with analysis. Initially, clinicians need to learn their Type 2 thinking and logical analytic structures very carefully so that they actually embed sound reasoning into Type 1 … otherwise they risk not becoming more experienced, but instead 'having the same one year's experience 20 times over' and not really learning or developing.

'Dysfunctional ways out' of uncertainty in the Analysing Quadrant: common pitfalls

> *The mark of a mature, psychologically healthy mind is indeed the ability to live with uncertainty and ambiguity, but only as much as there really is. Uncertainty is no virtue when the facts are clear, and ambiguity is mere obfuscation when more precise terms are applicable.*
>
> Julian Baggini[11]

If a consultation is not yielding a clear-cut diagnosis, clinicians can become stuck and paralysed in their thinking. This creates discomfort in the clinician who may resort to one of several 'dysfunctional ways out'.

Premature reassurance

If the patient doesn't seem especially unwell, and if the clinician cannot formulate a suitable diagnosis, the temptation will often be to reassure – 'This will probably settle' or 'Let's wait and see' – with perhaps some perfunctory safety netting along the lines of 'Come and see me if you don't get better.' This defers the issue and may compound the problem of diagnosis if the patient comes back to someone who may not appreciate all the details from the first consultation.

See a (fe)male GP

If the clinician is unfamiliar with the health issues of the opposite sex, or feels uncomfortable questioning a patient about intimate symptoms such as vaginal bleeding or sexual function, he may mentally opt out of the consultation and defer the issue by suggesting the patient make an appointment to see a GP of the same sex. Although this may alleviate the initial problem, it does not enhance the thinking skills of the clinician opting out, who has implicitly identified an important learning need if he thinks another clinician is the only one who can get a good history or perform a relevant examination. Male GPs risk being deskilled in important areas of women's health if they do this; conversely, male patients are just as likely to see a female clinician about their erectile difficulties. All clinicians have to be able to make safe assessments. Sometimes, the dysfunctional way out is 'See my colleague who knows more about…'. This can be a legitimate strategy, but it can also frustrate patients or sell them short by not taking things forwards in the current consultation. The issues arising from referral are discussed more fully in Chapters 6, 7 and 8.

Investigation

If the diagnosis does not seem clear or if the clinician is reluctant to commit herself to one, a dysfunctional way out is often to 'check a few blood tests' on the assumption that if they are normal there will not be too much to worry about. Although this may help the clinician terminate the consultation, there is a risk of premature or inappropriate reassurance, or of deferring the diagnostic conundrum to the consultation when the patient is seen again with normal results. However, sometimes clinicians hope the follow-up will be with someone else and that too is a dysfunctional way out….

Referral

This is a popular dysfunctional way out that can backfire. If the general differential is accurate (for example rectal bleeding referred to a gastroenterology specialist) it is likely that all will be well. However, if the presenting complaint is insufficiently analysed or evaluated, the risk of referral is that the specialist simply 'rules out' a problem in his own area of expertise, without necessarily 'ruling in' a positive diagnosis. GPs encounter this problem frequently after patients have attended Accident and Emergency departments with chest pain. The diagnosis given is often 'non-cardiac chest pain' because the approach has been simply to rule something serious out. The patient wanting to be given a positive diagnosis will often be unhappy to be told 'it is not a heart attack', with no further diagnosis. Similarly, referral for a patient with tiredness to an endocrinologist may result in there being 'no endocrine dysfunction'; if the true problem is an undiagnosed depression or functional disorder, the correct diagnosis may be missed. Being skilled in the use of referral networks is a skill in itself that is explored more fully in the Networking Quadrant chapters of this book.

Pick your favourite diagnosis

If uncertain, clinicians may try to make the symptoms fit a diagnosis they are familiar with, ignoring information that might indicate otherwise. This selective inattention may mean that important cues or clues from the patient are overlooked. Biases of various kinds contribute to this and are explored more fully later in the chapter, but it isn't hard to see that a cardiologist will look harder for cardiac diagnoses or that a GP or Accident and Emergency clinician may focus more on things that she sees commonly, exploring probability rather than possibility.

Make no diagnosis

In generalist settings (general practice, general psychiatry, Accident and Emergency, general medicine), precise diagnosis isn't always possible. What shall we call an illness with a mild fever, some achy joints and a mild sore throat that gets better after a few days? The chances are that no specific diagnosis can be made if there is no unequivocal 'head cold' or tonsillitis. Searching diligently for viruses in this case will often draw a blank, even in research settings. But we label it 'viral' and wait for nature to do its thing and cure the patient. Many illnesses depend more on management decisions than accurate diagnosis (for example watchful waiting or test and treat). This is a rational approach in cases of self-limiting or minor illness. However, sometimes this approach is taken when the clinician finds himself in a WDYDWYDKWTD situation: he cannot analyse the situation reasonably, so he 'opts out' and hopes that the patient will get better or see someone else.

Stick with a previous diagnosis: 'You had it before, you have got it again!'

Going along with an established diagnosis (which may be from a previous clinician or a senior colleague), ignoring new or inconsistent information that may seem too difficult to incorporate into the clinician's understanding, is a common dysfunctional way out. Junior staff can find it difficult to question seniors, to assimilate new information or stray into areas where they have limited expertise. Older, more experienced, clinicians are also prone to make errors of this type as they stick to what they, and their patients, know and expect. So why do clinicians sometimes persist in following a particular diagnostic path, even if it isn't yielding the expected results, or if they have a small alarm bell ringing in their heads saying, 'This does not really fit'?

Sometimes time pressures, not being clear what the alternatives are, or where to go next, can inhibit thinking. Some diagnoses are costly to make, requiring expensive tests and considerable effort, inconvenience or even danger for the patient. Sometimes clinicians are not aware of alternative diagnoses. However, if the clinician allows herself to recognise and accept the cognitive dissonance implicit in a WDYDWYDKWTD situation, this can be the metacognition that resolves the situation. Recognition and acceptance of uncertainty allow for deeper thinking and prevent 'dysfunctional ways out'. Medical errors often occur when people are *sure* they *do* know what to do, then go ahead without being aware that they are using a Type 1 response that doesn't apply. This usually happens because of various biases in thinking that Type 1 favours. These biases and errors are summarised in Table 3.2.

Focus on only one aspect of the problem

If the situation is complicated, it may seem tempting to focus on the more straightforward aspects. This is also known as 'cognitive anchoring' or 'anchoring bias'. Picking up on the first bit of information that suggests a familiar pathway dissipates the uncomfortable feelings that clinicians get when they are uncertain. The clinician then gets on with assessing a problem he is familiar or comfortable with. This may mean focusing on the chest pain ('let's do an ECG') rather than looking at other aspects that could indicate other diagnoses (poor sleep, anhedonia, weight loss and suicidal thoughts). One effect of this 'dysfunctional way out' is that the patient may not be

Table 3.2: Types of cognitive bias

Type of thinking bias	Effects
Anchoring bias	First bit of information is given more weight than later pieces of information, which are disregarded
Ascertainment bias	Prior expectations colour thinking, 'there is a lot of it about'
Availability bias	Memorable events occurring recently dominate thinking
Omission bias	Omission in case of potential harm (e.g. omitting chemotherapy because the effects of disease are preferred to the risk of side effects of the treatment)
Bandwagon bias	This is what we all do round here (regardless of appropriateness or evidence)
Satisficing bias/premature closure	If one diagnosis/hypothesis is found others are not sought (e.g. a second fracture)
Gambler's bias	A tendency to think a run of things cannot continue rather than taking each case on its merits (e.g. 'This cannot be the fourth case of shingles today')

Source: derived from NPC.[12]

reassured, or not accept the diagnosis (even for apparently minor symptoms), if the clinician does not pay enough attention to the patient's concerns about what might happen, or to the patient's own ideas about what the clinician should do.

Conclusion

It is the task of the clinician to interpret illness narratives from patients, and to assess the nature of the problem and the likelihood of disease. It is no mean feat to do this consistently and accurately. This is especially true when the patient's symptoms do not fall into neat categories or into the typical descriptions of the textbooks, in other words, when things are uncertain. All diagnosis requires judgement: of which symptoms are most important, which signs are the most salient, and which test results are the most important ones to take note of.

The clinician's judgement about diagnosis may be of even more importance when the patient has already done her own first level of interpretation via the internet. The many misconceptions and misunderstandings that follow from the application of information without diagnostic skills highlight the complexity and sophistication of diagnostic thinking, which has not been replicated by any computer program yet. In the complex arena of modern medicine, the evaluation of clinical performance is not simply about avoiding error because there will always be 'honest error'. However, the appropriate response to complexity and uncertainty is not a 'complacent faith in intuitive judgement', but learning and using the right skills to make a deeper and more accurate analysis.

References

1. Baron J. *Thinking and Deciding.* (4th edn). Cambridge: Cambridge University Press, 2007.
2. Croskerry P. Clinical cognition and diagnostic error: applications of a dual process model of reasoning. *Advances in Health Sciences Education: Theory and Practice* 2009; **14(1)**: 27–35. DOI: 10.1007/s10459-009-9182-2.
3. Schön D. *The Reflective Practitioner: how professionals think in action.* London: Temple Smith, 1983.
4. Dowie J, Elstein A (eds). *Professional Judgement: a reader in clinical decision making.* (6th edn). Cambridge: Cambridge University Press, 1993.
5. Stanners M, French HT. *An Empirical Study of the Relationship Between Situation Awareness and Decision Making.* Edinburgh: Australian Government Department of Defense, 2005, www.researchgate.net/profile/Melinda_Stanners/publication/27254567_An_empirical_study_of_the_relationship_between_situation_awareness_and_decision_making/links/00b4952b52229576ad000000.pdf [accessed 25 June 2015].
6. Elstein AS, Schwartz A. Clinical problem solving and diagnostic decision making: selective review of the cognitive literature. *British Medical Journal* 2002; **324(7339)**: 729–32.
7. Dawson NV. Physician judgment in clinical settings: methodological influences and cognitive performance. *Clinical Chemistry* 1993; **39(7)**: 1468–78.
8. Croskerry P. A universal model for diagnostic reasoning. *Academic Medicine* 2009; **84(8)**: 1022–8.
9. Evans JS. Dual-processing accounts of reasoning, judgment, and social cognition. *Annual Review of Psychology* 2008; **59**: 255–78.
10. Schmidt HG, Norman GR, Boshuizen HP. A cognitive perspective on medical expertise: theory and implication. *Academic Medicine* 1990; **65(10)**: 611–21.
11. Baggini J. What is this foolish lust for uncertainty? *Guardian*, 28 October 2011, www.theguardian.com/commentisfree/belief/2011/oct/28/lust-for-uncertainty [accessed 25 June 2015].

12. National Prescribing Centre. Making decisions better. *MeReC Bulletin* 2011; **22(1)**, www.carerightnow.co.uk/wp-content/uploads/2015/08/MAKING-DECISIONS-BETTERmerec_bulletin_vol22_no11.pdf.

Chapter 4

Functional ways through uncertainty in the Analysing Quadrant

There are a number of specific skills that can help to unlock a WDYDWYDKWTD situation when an accurate diagnosis is needed. The clinician may need to 'stand back' mentally and choose the approach that is most relevant, based on the information he has already, cues and clues in the history or examination, and bearing in mind the patient's own thoughts, concerns, worries and expectations of the clinician. This chapter covers:

- examples of common WDYDWYDKWTD situations in the Analysing Quadrant
- clarifying 'functional ways through' common problems by identifying the right skills needed for the right situation.

The key skills needed are:

- hypothetico-deductive reasoning using 'restricted rule out'
- ruling in or ruling out/diagnostic safety netting
- trust and verify
- sharing the clinical reasoning process with the patient
- using clinical guidelines, algorithms, clinical decision tools
- exploring the emotional content of the consultation
- situational awareness skills
- widening the view/explaining functional symptoms.

Hypothetico-deductive reasoning/restricted rule out

> Mr Ruby staggers in to the consulting room complaining that he feels dizzy. He does not say much more than that, repeatedly asking for a tablet to take for the 'damn dizziness! It was all I could do to stagger in here from the taxi and I want to go home and lie down as soon as!!!'
>
> Dr Ash, who is doing his first job in general practice, is a bit flummoxed and feels that he doesn't know what to do. He also feels that he can't ask for help until he has got a bit more information to go on and so feels a bit stuck. Dizziness has always seemed to him like the worst 'heartsink' symptom anyway ... it could mean anything!

Although the doctor here could be perfectly justified in simply calling his senior supervisor to come and help, he wants to learn and knows that the supervisor will appreciate a bit more information than 'my patient is dizzy'. The wide range of possibilities and the rather cut-and-dried request from the patient that 'all I want is a tablet' has raised Dr Ash's anxiety. This is making it hard to think clearly. How can he structure his thoughts and find an effective way to generate some hypotheses about the symptoms, which he can then test with further questions and examinations?

First, he needs to build his relationship with the patient, using time to develop sufficient cooperation to get some more information. So he needs to agree with the patient that a suitable prescription will be forthcoming, and that before doing a prescription he will need to get some more information and examine Mr Ruby to make sure the treatment is the right one.

So what questions should Dr Ash ask? He could go through a full systems review and ask lots of closed questions about everything he can think of and try to make sense of things, but, rightly, he suspects this wouldn't work. One colleague described this approach as like playing the pen-and-paper game of 'battleships'. The doctor might ask a lot of closed questions ('Is it worse when you lie down?') but without a clear structure, this it can be a fairly random process. Inexperienced clinicians may spend much of their thinking time wondering what question to ask next; this interferes with their ability to listen carefully to what the patient is currently saying. This reduces diagnostic accuracy because important information is missed. Remaining quiet and listening to the patient helps to avoid 'premature closure'. Also known as 'search satisficing', this means fixing on a diagnosis too early on in the consultation, before all the information is known. Information that does not fit the initial proposed diagnosis may be wrongly discounted, leading to errors in diagnosis.

So, thinking of a general practice or Accident and Emergency context how can the doctor develop some hypotheses about the cause and then test them rationally?

First, the exact nature of the patient's experience needs to be understood, and the doctor needs to listen hard. Feeling overwhelmed by a vague symptom with many possible causes can mean that the symptom is not fully explored. Is the patient describing a sense of depersonalisation? A sense of rotation, i.e. true vertigo? Is it more like the non-specific dizziness of postural hypotension?

A helpful initial way to order thoughts about a vague symptom can be to use Marshall Marinker's analysis of the roles of the specialist and generalist, and take the generalist route first. The generalist's task, suggested Marinker, is to 'Marginalise danger, explore probability and manage uncertainty.'[1]

Marginalising danger means identifying the key things not to miss; dizziness associated with severe hypotension or postural hypotension, caused by blood loss, sepsis or an intracerebral catastrophe, immediately spring to mind. The popularly named 'red flag' symptoms and signs will help the doctor exclude immediate serious possibilities and orientate the questions asked to those that are most relevant.

Exploring probability means contextualising the patient's complaints. This approach is also called 'restricted rule out',[2] and means that the doctor will attempt to rule out the most significant or serious diseases by checking for symptoms and signs that could point to serious disorder. If such symptoms or signs are absent at the time of the consultation (they may develop later of course) then the significant condition can be considered (temporarily) ruled out.

Managing uncertainty, in this context, means acknowledging that a range of possible outcomes remain, even if serious causes have temporarily been ruled out. Uncertainty needs to be actively managed, usually through effective 'safety net' approaches, discussed in the next section.

How could it go better for Dr Ash and Mr Ruby?

Dr Ash takes a deep breath and thinks about his thinking. What diagnostic approach will help here? Before asking any specific diagnostic questions, Dr Ash encourages Mr Ruby to tell him the story of the dizziness, how it started and what it feels like, initially avoiding interrupting Mr Ruby, and using brief, encouraging phrases like 'go on', 'mmm', 'OK, and then ... ?'

Has Mr Ruby noticed anything else wrong? Dr Ash listens for clues that this might be dizziness caused by hypotension (only when standing up), by brain issues like a cerebellar disorder (intractable, with vomiting, associated with clumsiness or unsteadiness, no ear symptoms) or by ear problems, (with deafness, discharge, pain in the ear).

It emerges that Mr Ruby became suddenly very dizzy two days before. He vomited the first day, but that has stopped now. The dizziness was preceded by some pain and discharge in the left ear, which Mr Ruby has had on and off for a while.

Dr Ash realises that this means the dizziness is probably connected with the ear rather than the brain, but that dizziness after middle-ear symptoms (pain and discharge) may indicate infection spreading into the mastoid. This hypothesis is confirmed by finding that the blood pressure is normal, with no postural drop, that there are no cerebellar signs, and that there is tenderness over the mastoid area with discharge from the ear. Dr Ash now realises that the question for his supervisor is not 'Can you help me, there are 20 causes of dizziness?', but rather 'How do I get the ENT specialist involved?'

Ruling in and ruling out: diagnostic safety netting

There are two WDYDWYDKWTD situations described here that illustrate different approaches.

Mrs Jewel comes complaining of a severe left-sided headache. She is 60, usually well, although has osteoarthritis in both knees and is awaiting a knee replacement. She complains of an odd sensation when she chews, 'like a cramp in my jaw'. Examination shows a slightly tender temporal artery, although the tenderness is mild and spreads across a wide area, not just over the vessel. Dr Beech suspects temporal arteritis and suggests some blood tests and starting a course of steroids as a therapeutic trial.

'Oh no', says Mrs Jewel, 'No steroids for me until I know for sure what's wrong. I had some two years ago for some stiff shoulders. I didn't sleep for a week afterwards and my husband said I went doolally, talking all the time! Can't I wait for some tests?'

Dr Beech suggests referral for a temporal artery biopsy. Mrs Jewel does not want surgery either. The doctor feels he is in a WDYDWYDKWTD moment. If it IS temporal arteritis, it is crucial to get treatment started immediately; Mrs Jewel risks blindness if this condition is untreated, which can happen rapidly. A biopsy will take time to organise, and anyway doesn't temporal arteritis sometime skip part of the artery, meaning it is not a reliable test? Mrs Jewel does allow an erythrocyte sedimentation rate (ESR) test.

Dr Beech agrees to postpone steroids and has a bad night worrying that Mrs Jewel will get complications because of the delay. ESR is done and the result is 30, raised but not dramatic. Surely a biopsy would help? Mrs Jewel is even more reluctant to take steroids now!

Can Dr Beech rule temporal arteritis in or out, while being safe?

Mrs Diamond brings her 2-year-old child Jade who has been unwell for 24 hours with intermittent fever and lethargy. Jade is drinking well and passing a lot of urine, but is off her food. She has a slightly runny nose. The fever responds to usual treatment with paracetamol, recurring a few hours after each dose. Mrs Diamond is diabetic and is concerned that Jade's frequent urination may indicate that she also has diabetes. A child at school has had meningitis recently, and Mrs Diamond is very clear she wants to know for sure if Jade has meningitis too!

Dr Aspen examines Jade who seems only to have signs of a head cold with no 'red flag' signs. Naturally, Dr Aspen shares Mrs Diamond's anxieties about diabetes and meningitis but isn't quite sure what to do. Should the child have a lumbar puncture to be sure?

In textbooks, the symptoms and signs of illnesses are described exhaustively with clear-cut symptoms and signs predominating in the descriptions. In daily practice, things are rarely so clear cut. Diseases may have untypical symptoms, untypical physical signs or test results (as in the first example) or be so non-specific as to be of little direct help (as in the second example where the child's condition could be a cold or the start of meningitis). The 'dysfunctional ways out' of these situations could include referring Mrs Jewel on to the emergency room as a case of 'unexplained headache? Temporal arteritis', thus passing the buck, and also possibly causing delay in treatment. Similarly, if Jade was referred urgently, she might be prematurely reassured if she still seems to have mainly upper respiratory tract infection (URTI) symptoms ('there is a lot of URTI about') or have a premature and possibly hazardous referral (hours in casualty, a lumbar puncture that could be painful and distressing). Dr Aspen and Dr Beech could benefit by understanding their metacognitions ('thinking about thinking') in more detail.

One approach that can help is to consider that there are two different thinking processes. First, there is a need to RULE OUT serious disease: temporal arteritis, diabetes, major sepsis such as meningitis. There are many other causes for a mild febrile illness in a child, such as influenza, urine infection, a gastroenteritis. However, all these are likely to be mild, or self-limiting.

Sometimes, a process referred to as 'restricted rule out' will help to eliminate the most serious problems.[2] In the first example, temporal arteritis could be ruled out if there was no scalp tenderness, if there was a dental abscess that could cause pain on eating, and if the ESR/PV result was normal. A simple dipstick test of the urine could rule out ketosis and glycosuria in the child, making diabetes unlikely. Can the meningitis be ruled out by similar means?

This is, of course, more difficult. Meningitis evolves over time, starts with symptoms similar to most viral illnesses of lesser severity, and is itself a very variable illness. Some viral meningitis is mild and may pass in a day or two with no treatment; meningococcal meningitis is rightly feared for its rapid, relentless and often fatal progression. Could restricted rule out help here? Clearly, it could, but only in a *temporary* way; the key skill is to 'safety net' in the consultation. This means discussing very carefully the encouraging signs that this is a mild viral illness, while also highlighting with the mother the signs she can look for that may indicate deterioration and the need for a further evaluation by the doctor. Being clear that the situation is currently uncertain helps the patient to be more powerfully involved in monitoring what happens next.

A different, yet related, thinking approach to the kinds of problems we are discussing is to consider what can be RULED IN. Mrs Jewel has only some of the features of temporal arteritis. Investigations could help RULE IN temporal arteritis if the ESR/PV was very high, or if the biopsy showed inflammatory changes. These tests can RULE IN, but they cannot RULE OUT. Temporal arteritis can exist with a normal ESR, and biopsy may miss the affected segment, giving a falsely negative result. A trial of steroid therapy is often seen as a helpful RULE IN strategy as the pain of temporal arteritis improves so rapidly and dramatically with steroid treatment. However, other causes of head pain might also improve with steroids, if only because of a strong placebo effect.

In the case of Jade, diabetes could be ruled in, if dip testing the urine showed ketones and glycosuria. However, ruling in meningitis would need blood cultures and possibly a lumbar puncture. Such tests are both unnecessary and distressing if the child has only a bad cold. Moreover, doing too many of such invasive tests is expensive, not just in money, but also in time, staffing and emotional stress on the child and parents while they wait for the results. It is impossible to do those tests on every child that has a cold … services would collapse! Children could develop iatrogenic injuries and complications.

The benefits of a rule in/rule out approach in the WDYDWYDKWTD are amplified if there is adequate diagnostic safety netting. True safety netting is much more than the 'come back if no better' comment at the end of the consultation. This skill aids the diagnostic process, as well as providing a way to safely 'catch' patients as their illnesses develop, the course being unknown and intrinsically unpredictable at the outset. If the doctor shares her clinical reasoning and most likely diagnosis with the patient, they can share planning of what should happen next. The clinician needs to be asking herself, 'If I have made the right diagnosis or assessment, what will I expect to happen? What will tell me that I am wrong? What will happen if I am wrong? What would need to happen in that situation?'

These questions will then inform planning for what might happen next and inform the discussion with the patient about follow-up and safety netting. For example, discussion with the patient could include contacting the service again:

- IF certain things do or do not happen
- UNLESS certain things do or don't happen
- WHEN a certain point is reached that will trigger follow-up.[3]

This helps to increase patients' understanding, empowering them to take the right action in relation to the relevant symptoms and time-frames.[4] This detailed safety netting should also clarify which parts of the healthcare system should be accessed for further assistance.

How might things go better for Mrs Jewel and Mrs Diamond/ Jade?

Although the clinical reasoning is complex, Dr Beech takes Mrs Jewel in detail through her worries about temporal arteritis (the serious diagnosis) and the benefits of a trial of steroids versus various possible tests. She suggests stopping steroids immediately if the side effects are too great or if the tests don't support a diagnosis. Mrs Jewel still opts for delayed steroids. The next day her headache is already almost completely better without any treatment and her repeated ESR is 14. The doctor feels that temporal arteritis has been reasonably ruled out for now, and includes detailed safety-netting advice in the consultation. Mrs Jewel remains well at follow-up and her ESR is still normal a week later. The raised result? Was it accurate? A fluke? Dr Beech will remain uncertain.

Dr Aspen rules out diabetes by dipping the urine, and explains the clinical reasoning behind her view that Jade does not have signs of meningitis at the moment, because she is not especially unwell, has no neck stiffness, is responsive to the paracetamol treatment and has signs of a viral infection in the nose. Detailed safety-netting advice about signs to look out for results in Jade's mother contacting the surgery just a few hours later. The child is clearly worse, less responsive, and more floppy, with increasing fever. Prompt referral results in a firm diagnosis of viral meningitis from which she recovers completely, the mother being impressed by the doctor's clinical acumen in predicting what might happen and giving good instructions about what to do.

Both of these stories illustrate the diagnostic importance of test and treat strategies, and also of the diagnostic importance of watchful waiting. Another important feature of these scenarios is that, in both cases, the clinician will be more effective when accepting and 'staying with' the uncertainty, rather than trying to resolve and dismiss the uncertainty by immediately jumping to a firm (but possibly premature) course of action.

Trust and verify (a Russian military proverb)

It is June, examination season, and 16-year-old Amber presents with intermittent, crampy abdominal pains. She also reports occasional diarrhoea and constipation. She is really stressed out, worrying that she has not done enough to get into the college of her choice; she is eating irregularly and finding it hard to get to sleep because of her worries. She has lost 2 lbs in weight. She has become convinced that there is something seriously wrong with her. There are no identifiable red-flag symptoms and examination is quite normal. Dr Elm, who is seeing her, catches some of this anxiety, worries that she has missed something important and suggests blood tests (full blood count (FBC), plasma viscosity (PV), urea and electrolytes (U and E)), which makes Amber even more anxious and frightened. She rings up twice every day for the results, which are normal. Dr Elm stays behind after work looking up all the causes of abdominal pain in 16-year-olds; could this be the first sign of a serious illness like cancer, connective tissue disease or Crohn's even though the weight loss is very small and may be non-significant? She doesn't know what to do next!

Most clinicians in this situation will rely on fast Type 1 thinking, using 'rules of thumb' (also known by the fancy name of 'heuristics', i.e. practical reasoning). The most likely conclusion is that Amber's symptoms are related to examination stresses and her disordered eating habits, resulting in a functional bowel upset, which could attract a label of irritable bowel syndrome (IBS). Strong reassurance and kindly encouragement about the examinations are the likely approaches to treatment. A helpful way forwards for the clinician is to 'trust and verify' such conclusions. At this age and in a presentation of this type, IBS is most likely. Trusting this diagnostic judgement, the clinician will advise on diet and exercise strategies, and offer an antispasmodic owing to the inconvenient nature of the problem.

However, to 'verify' this judgement the clinician must actively seek and act on any deviations from the expected path; otherwise such deviations may go undetected for too long. The clinician's 'inner alarm bell' needs to be honed and tested through clinical experience. So, what observations could trigger an 'inner alarm bell'? If the diagnosis is correct, things will probably resolve in a few weeks, especially if Amber does well in her examinations. Any red-flag signs, such as continuing weight loss or blood in the stool, would need further assessment. Diagnostic safety netting via a planned review in a few weeks (unless red-flag symptoms occur earlier), monitoring her response to advice and medication, and giving the right emphasis to normal tests may enable the clinician's own anxiety to be held in check. This will also support Amber in keeping her own anxiety about her health at reasonable levels.

Sometimes the 'inner alarm bell' is calibrated to go off too soon (leading to over-investigation), or too late (leading to missed diagnoses). Habitual reflection on the outcomes of diagnostic conclusions helps clinicians to develop clinical expertise. Reflection raises awareness of the situations that may trigger a reaction that is too hasty or too slow. When the alarm bell rings, clinicians need to reflect on what has triggered it. Were there alarming symptoms or signs? Were there clues from the patient that some other diagnosis needs to be considered (emotional disturbance, less common diseases, unusual symptoms?). Or was it the clinician's own need for certainty in an inherently uncertain situation? No one can predict how a mild set of symptoms will develop in the future, but appropriate safety netting will usually reveal those situations that need more detailed attention.

So how might things go better for Amber and Dr Elm?
Dr Elm's initial assessment is that this is most likely to be a form of IBS. She explains to Amber that because the weight loss is so small, and because everything else in the history and examination indicates that she is fundamentally healthy, the abdominal symptoms may be linked to the high-stress situation (leading to too much adrenaline, which affects bowel function) and irregular eating. She gives advice, holds off doing blood tests and arranges to verify her assessment by seeing Amber in four weeks, after most of the exams are over. At that appointment Amber is much calmer. However, she is still losing weight and her bowels are loose all the time. She is finding the hot weather intolerable and feels shaky sometimes. More focused testing reveals normal thyroid tests, a very mild anaemia and a positive coeliac screen. Amber is appropriately referred.

Sharing clinical reasoning

Dr Chestnut is seeing a young man with knee pain; she feels on shaky ground with knees. The anatomy always seems complex, orthopaedics was not her strongest point and the patient is a loud, 6-foot-tall rugby player whom she finds vaguely intimidating.

So the consultation does not start well when Mr Jet says, 'I have got this pain in my right knee, doctor. ...'

Dr Chestnut does her best and establishes that the pain is worse in the mornings, gets worse if he goes running or training, doesn't cause redness or swelling and that he has been able to continue at work and cycling at weekends. It's summer now so the rugby season is over for a few months. Mentally, Dr Chestnut heaves a sigh of relief; there will not be too much pressure to get Mr Jet fit for training. She hopes that the passage of time will cure him (it might at that). So she says that paracetamol, ice and rest should do the trick.

Mr Jet says, 'I have tried all that, it didn't work, what could be wrong with me?!'

Dr Chestnut says that ibuprofen could help and that she will prescribe some with a knee support to use also.

'I have been using those tablets for three weeks now', he insists, 'It is not working. I want to know what is wrong with me and what you are going to do about it!' Internally, Dr Chestnut is beginning to panic, which has the unhelpful effect of making her mind go blank about the main causes of knee pain. Dr Chestnut is facing a WDYDWYDKWTD situation. She reiterates her suggestion about continuing with painkillers and anti-inflammatory tablets using the dysfunctional way out of making no diagnosis, and hoping that watch and wait will work.

Mr Jet gets angry saying, 'This is no good, I want to know what's going on' and he storms out of the room to make a complaint at the desk. Dr Chestnut bursts into tears, tells the practice manager that the patient was 'aggressive' and asks that a message be put on his notes that she should never have to see him again.

Dr Chestnut had perhaps been hoping that Type 1 thinking would make a suitable diagnosis jump into her mind 'intuitively'. Lacking trust in Type 2 thinking, she chooses the dysfunctional ways out of making 'no diagnosis' and ensuring that a colleague will see him at a future date if things don't improve.

Her hopes that the patient will go away have not worked; Dr Chestnut is facing a frustrated patient. In a way, this covers up her need to face her own WDYDWYDKWTD situation; it all gets wrapped up in her feeling that he has been 'aggressive' and 'difficult', and that she is somehow the victim of this. She is not facing up to her own role in the débâcle.

When in doubt and even if you can't remember all the details about a clinical topic that is not in your field of expertise, or just not your favourite area, go back to basics and share your clinical reasoning with the patient.

'When it's a mystery, go back to the history' is a useful aphorism here. Dr Chestnut could help the patient to feel more understood by taking a fuller history and trying to understand how the problem started, what makes it worse or better, what indications there may be of serious disease (see hypothesis testing above) and understanding what the patient has tried already. If Dr Chestnut had examined the knee using first principles (inspection, palpation, mobility), she could explain her observations. Dr Chestnut can also 'think about her thinking' and remember to be curious about and explore the patient's own concerns, worries and ideas about what he needs from the discussion. A diagnosis? A sick note? Advice about whether or not to pay for some physiotherapy at his rugby club?

Then Dr Chestnut will be in a position to share her more informed clinical reasoning, going through her Type 2 thoughts with the patient and plan the way forwards. Again we can see that 'thinking about thinking' (metacognition) will help the clinician here. Dr Chestnut has observed orthopaedic doctors examining knees and they seem to 'just know' what is wrong. She is aware that her intuitions may not be reliable. If she herself was more aware of her initial unease, she could deliberately employ a systematic approach using Type 2 thinking, working from first principles, using the 'surgical sieve' to work through the possibilities. (Is the problem congenital or acquired? Inflammatory, malignant, mechanical? This is medical student thinking, which will be of use to Dr Chestnut forever.) This would take the anxiety out of the consultation for clinician and patient alike.

How might things go better for Dr Chestnut and Mr Jet the rugby player?

When Mr Jet asks for the second time, 'What is actually wrong with me?', Dr Chestnut could start to share her clinical reasoning with him.

'From what you have told me this is not interfering in many functions of your life as you are able to sleep, work and cycle. The examination findings confirm that the knee seems fundamentally healthy with no redness, swelling or deformity that might indicate infection or damage. The movements are complete, which is reassuring that no tendon or cartilage damage is present. I think this would usually settle with the tablets you have been taking, but as it hasn't I am thinking that some active treatment from the physiotherapist could be a useful next step ... what is your response to that?'

The rugby player is keen to see a physiotherapist. This appropriate referral means that a more experienced eye will look at the knee and gives Dr Chestnut time to look up knee problems and discuss her approach with her supervisor.

Clinical decision tools, algorithms and guidelines

The 'winter pressures team' has sent a message to all GPs saying, 'Casualty is overloaded and there are no empty beds at the hospital. Please only refer if essential.' Mr Sapphire comes to the GP at 6 p.m. complaining of pain in his left leg. It hurts when he walks on it and he would like an X-ray to see 'if there is anything broken'. He remembers tripping up when he was on the beach recently and thinks he may have torn something near his ankle. Dr Rowan finds some slight tenderness in the calf but isn't sure if there is any swelling. The mention of a beach makes her ask where Mr Sapphire has been; he drove to the north of Scotland to visit his brother. It crosses Dr Rowan's mind that this might be a deep-vein thrombosis (DVT) but the signs are not clear cut and she is hesitant to refer on because of the strong message that Casualty is overloaded already.

Many conditions begin with relatively 'soft' signs and symptoms, and external pressures inevitably affect our thinking, however much we would like to believe we are only thinking about the patient in front of us. Dr Rowan feels stuck, so what could she do?

This is a situation where using a clinical decision tool or algorithm can help to clarify thoughts and inform decision making. Dr Rowan may well not know all the details of the Wells score off by heart. However, in our twenty-first-century consultations, the power of the internet is always at hand. Clinicians can look things up and use the guidance to help make a decision. Sharing her reasoning process with the patient will help to explain the situation clearly and enable clinician and patient to share the decision-making process.

Saying, 'I have not got a clue what is wrong with you' doesn't inspire confidence in most patients. However, saying, 'There is a special process for working this out. Will you excuse me while I load us the right information on the computer and we can go through it together?' demonstrates competence. You know the patient has a condition that needs particularly careful assessment, you know where to find the questionnaire/tool, and you are prepared to share your reasoning and explain things. All this makes for the kind of clinician that patients are keen to interact with.

Going through a decision rule can apply in many different circumstances. DVT, decisions about anticoagulation, assessing febrile children, prostatic symptoms and many other conditions have similar decision guides. There are many guidelines … don't try to remember them. Just ask yourself, 'Is it likely someone will have looked at this type of problem and is there some information I could use?' Use your information resources and discuss them with your patient.

How might it go better for Mr Sapphire?

Dr Rowan remembers that there is a tool for assessing DVT but can't remember all the terms. She gets it up on the computer and scores Mr Sapphire.

The long road trip and a painful calf both give Mr Sapphire a relatively high score. Measuring the calf with a tape measure also reveals some mild swelling not easily seen with the naked eye. This makes the decision to refer easier and better informed. Mr Sapphire is referred and a DVT later confirmed. He comes back the next week to get his heparin and warfarin prescription saying, 'Thanks, doc … you were on the ball there.'

Exploring the emotional context of the consultation

Mrs Sandstone is a middle-aged social worker, with shoulder pain and difficulty in raising her arm for a few weeks. She found it difficult to drive and has been off work. She comes to see Dr Willow today to get 'another sick note' and the results of an ultrasound scan and blood tests ordered by a colleague, who is now on holiday.

Dr Willow is pleased to relate that the scan is normal. Mrs Sandstone agrees that the arm movements are a little better. Dr Willow raises the issue of returning to work. Mrs Sandstone looks away and says, 'I have been referred to Occupational Health because I was off a few months ago when my periods were bad.' Dr Willow agrees that Occupational Health referral is often routine in these circumstances. Mrs Sandstone sighs again and looks away. She bites her lip and seems on the verge of tears. Dr Willow doesn't notice, being busy looking at the blood results on the computer. He announces that they too are normal. Mrs Sandstone asks for another sick note and says she really can't go back to work while her shoulder is so stiff. Dr Willow reiterates the normal findings and the expectation that Occupational Health should be involved and are likely to encourage return to work. The conversation goes round in circles for a bit and then Dr Willow gives a sick note because he can't think of anything else to do.

Interactions like these between clinicians and patients are common. In a secondary care setting the clinician may simply note all the normal results and the slight improvement, and refer Mrs Sandstone back to her GP's care. GPs don't have this option of discharging the patient. Dr Willow thinks that his patient could return to work. However, she clearly doesn't want to. He hopes that Occupational Health will somehow sort out the return to work without him having to push his patient too hard. He reasons that if he did that he may damage his longer-term relationship with her.

At the same time he feels uncomfortable: the consultation seemed to go round in circles and get nowhere except for 'another sick note'.

In this situation there is often a mismatch between what the clinician is focusing on (the facts, the signs, the blood tests, his attempt to make a physical diagnosis) and what is going on for the patient. Her sighs, reluctance to return to work and evident discomfort point to a more emotional side to the consultation. Making a diagnosis (or even excluding one) means paying attention to the patient as a whole, and picking up clues and cues about the whole picture. Clinicians readily do this for physical disturbances. If Mrs Sandstone had a bad limp, or winced when he touched an inflamed red area of skin, he would take that as a 'clue or cue' that the affected part was the leg or the painful limb.

However, sometimes we overlook clues and cues about emotional components of the consultation. When a consultation goes round and round in circles, especially where no clear diagnosis has been reached, it is often because the patient doesn't feel that he has been heard, or that he has not voiced an important concern. Why could that be when the clinician thinks she has attended to the patient's pain, organised investigations and even given a sick note she was not that keen to issue?

It is the emotional component that has been ignored. Patients give us all sorts of clues that their psychological or social situation is not satisfactory; clinicians ignore these aspects of the consultation at their peril.

So what cues were present here?

Mrs Sandstone looks away, bites her lip, tears are in her eyes. Perhaps a more attentive listener may note that she talks in a flat, quiet voice, sighs a lot and doesn't smile much. Perhaps the words she uses about the Occupational Health referral may betray a sense of resentment or anger towards her boss. Paying attention to cues and clues will pay dividends. But what does it mean to pick up a cue in the consultation? What should the clinician do next? Clues can be handled in three ways:

- **pick them up** immediately ... and explore with the patient
- **park them** in your mind to refer back to later on in the consultation
- **put them in the whole context** of the consultation, using them to build up a full picture.

In this situation picking up a cue may mean mentioning that Mrs Sandstone seems unhappy. Parking the cue may mean noticing a cue and waiting until later to mention it, when the time seems right. Putting it in the whole picture can allow the clinician to summarise a whole series of cues by making an interpretation: 'So it seems overall you are pretty unhappy about work and the Occupational Health referral' and then taking that forwards with 'I am wondering what effect all this is having on you.'

If clinicians see themselves as only having a role in diagnosing and treating physical disease they may see these clues about the patient's emotional and social status as irrelevant. However, making an accurate assessment of these other issues will facilitate the treatment of any disease that may be present, will direct the clinician's attention to psychological disturbances such as anxiety or depression, and will help the clinician build an effective therapeutic relationship with the patient. All aspects of their care can then be negotiated effectively. The skills for this are discussed in more detail in Chapter 10.

How might things go better for Mrs Sandstone?

Dr Willow pauses after looking at the computer and gives his whole attention to Mrs Sandstone. He notes her downcast eyes with tears just forming and the tone of voice that gives away her unease and resentment about her workplace.

'It seems like the situation at work is difficult for you', he tentatively says. 'You seem upset.' Mrs Sandstone gulps and weeps. She blurts out that she can't face work any more. Hers is an understaffed, yet demanding, branch of social services. Half her colleagues have left and her boss has been hinting that her records aren't good enough and she may be disciplined. She is scared of losing her job, because as a single parent she needs the money. She finds work so stressful she isn't sure she can do it any more. Although Dr Willow can't fix this whole problem, he helps her work out the next steps, including sharing some of her workplace stress with the Occupational Health team and assessing her for depression and anxiety. He starts to mobilise Mrs Sandstone's own problem-solving skills. The consultation is no longer going round in circles and Dr Willow can follow her up with a clearer idea of what the issues are.

Situational awareness

It's 4 p.m. on Christmas Day, snow is thick on the ground and the out-of-hours GP service is quieter than usual. Dr Holly is passing through the waiting room to meet with the nurse to arrange a nebuliser for a very wheezy patient with asthma. She sees a young man, Peter, pacing up and down and recognises him from a shift before Christmas when he had been put on antibiotics for a 'chest infection'. A woman with him asks him to sit down and wait for the doctor, but he takes little notice and keeps wandering around.

Seeing the doctor, the woman comes over and says, 'Please can you see Peter as soon as possible. It was hard getting him here and he is so restless.'

There are several unwell children, who have been waiting longer than Peter, and Dr Holly can see their parents glaring at him. She has clear targets about how long people are supposed to wait before being seen and that usually means people being seen strictly in turn. Her wheezy patient needs a nebuliser as soon as possible too.

Dr Holly does not know what to do for the best.

Working as a clinician is rarely about looking after one patient at a time, or dealing with one problem at a time. We all have to work in clinics where there are routinely more patients than we can comfortably see. We work in hospital wards or in nursing homes where there are many patients who need attention. Even when we are doing planned elective work, emergencies or unexpected occurrences can derail the plans we have for our time.

The skills that can help this are collectively referred to as 'situational awareness' and the outcomes from the skills lead to 'situational judgements'.[5] These skills are routinely tested in many medical recruitment programmes. This is because the ability to bring together disparate information about a situation, and to use it to make a sensible judgment about what to do, reveals much about a clinician's assessment, prioritising and thinking skills. So what skills could help in this situation?

These can be summarised as monitoring the baseline, being aware of our bias towards normality and avoiding 'focus lock'.

Monitoring the baseline

This skill uses the Type 1 thinking that was described earlier in this chapter. We need to allow ourselves to briefly scan the whole environment regularly, asking ourselves, 'Is everything generally OK?' and 'Is there anything anomalous, unusual or threatening happening here?' This is a kind of scan for alarm signals of any kind. What these alarm signals might be depends on the situation. Doing a home visit may reveal alarm signals such as a large dog blocking the path or a mugger waiting to steal your doctor's bag. In a nursing home, a flurry of activity at the other end of the corridor and nurses leaving the drug round may indicate that a resident is in distress or collapsed. In theatre, subtle signs of consternation on the part of the anaesthetist or other colleagues may indicate to the surgeon that something is going wrong. In all settings, clinicians need to have some way of mentally 'sweeping' their environment and assessing the overall situation. This may include being aware of all the current tasks (acutely ill patients, problems from yesterday), which staff are around ('Who is off sick, struggling with their own workload or preoccupied?') and what the associated services are coping with ('Are there any available appointment slots, beds, trolleys, pharmacies open …?').

Being aware of bias towards normality

Although we do scan our environments for interesting or alarming changes, we would prefer everything to be 'business as usual'. We can easily have a tendency to ignore signs of change or impending difficulty that may be threatening, difficult to deal with or outside our comfort zones. We want things to be OK so we look selectively for evidence that things *are* OK, and this may obscure other signals. If we are aware of this we can avoid this bias, and actively scan for problems at an early stage.

Avoiding focus lock

All clinical work needs concentration and focus. However, if the focus gets too narrow, there is a risk of ignoring other aspects of the problem or things going on elsewhere in the environment. A clinician focusing on a particular element of the history may not notice hints in what the patient is saying about his suicidal risk. After asking a question a doctor may not notice a hesitation in the patient's reply indicating that there is more information forthcoming. This requires a pause, rather than a rapid change of subject, by the doctor. Focus lock can easily cause errors because of anchoring bias (a human tendency to rely heavily on the first bit of information that we obtain, which 'anchors' thinking to a particular issue and makes information arising later get less weight) and ascertainment bias (when we are more likely to choose a diagnosis that we have seen a lot of recently). If focus lock is combined with a bias towards normality, situations may develop in seemingly unexpected ways. In fact, the signs were there, but not acted on.

There are several clues for Dr Holly that all is not well. Peter is a young patient, usually fit and well, who has come twice over a short time, over Christmas too, when most families will absorb problems until a more convenient day. He has come with his mother who is clearly concerned, saying 'he is so restless', which is an unusual symptom to complain of in a waiting room. She also mentioned it was hard to get him there. What could these odd comments mean? How is Dr Holly going to manage the competing requirements of effectiveness (doing the right thing), efficiency (doing the right things in the right way with the least effort or expense), fairness to all of her patients (addressing needs not just wants) and meeting her waiting targets?

How could it go better for Dr Holly and Peter?
Dr Holly's current baseline is that there is an important issue with the wheezy patient, there are only a few children waiting and she is doing things in order. Dr Holly notes her initial impulse to continue 'more of the same', but also picks up clues that not all is well with Peter. His mother is clearly worried and has struggled to get him to the clinic. A few days before Dr Holly remembered him as a pleasant, relaxed young man looking forwards to playing football at New Year. His restless pacing has an odd quality to it and Peter is not very responsive to others around him. Dr Holly is using her Type 1 alarm bells that indicate there night be a problem. She avoids 'locking in' on the waiting time issue alone and thinks more broadly.

Dr Holly apologises to the parents waiting in the room and says there will be a short delay. She asks a nursing colleague to take over the care of the wheezy patient until the nebuliser is complete and ushers Peter gently to a clinical room. Peter is a bit confused and vague in his replies to questions. He has a very high fever, and is breathless at rest with a fast pulse. He is confused and his lips are bluish. His SATS are confirmed to be low. The whole of the left side of his chest is dull to percussion. Clearly, Peter is severely septic and Dr Holly sends him to hospital by ambulance. His mother phoned later to say he had collapsed on arrival at the hospital and had needed to be ventilated and thanked the doctor for seeing him so promptly.

Widening the view/explaining functional symptoms

Mrs Beryll is seeing her clinicians about longstanding troublesome abdominal pains. The gynaecologists have ruled out problems in their area of expertise and the gastroenterologist has discharged her from the clinic with a diagnosis of IBS. Mrs Beryll comes back to her GP, Dr Alder, again complaining about abdominal pains. As she is otherwise well, and has been fairly thoroughly investigated, Dr Alder feels a bit stuck when Mrs Beryll says, 'I do not like those IBS tablets, and anyway, there is nothing wrong with my bowels. Can't you help me, Dr Alder?'

In general practice it is quite common to be looking after patients who are 'post specialist', in other words, who have been seen in one or more specialist clinics and who are now discharged, the specialist having done all she can. This does not mean that the patient is cured, healed or even diagnosed. Patients who have completed psychotherapy, or who have symptoms sometimes referred to as 'medically unexplained', also come back to the GP for ongoing care. This can be challenging, and, if the patient's symptoms do not resolve, the option of referral onwards may now be closed off, especially if services such as psychotherapy offer only a limited number of therapeutic sessions, in attempts to enable more patients to benefit and shorten waiting lists. There are two specific skills that can help here: building the relationship and being able to explain the physiological origin of symptoms.

Building the relationship

Concentrating on relationship building and listening skills in the consultation can widen the view that the clinician has of the patient. Seeing the patient as more than a set of symptoms, or more than a puzzle to be explored, and seeking a more holistic understanding of the patient builds an effective therapeutic relationship in any clinical sphere. This means exploring what the patient's life is actually like, what impact his symptoms have, and what he himself wants from his care. This is discussed further under 'shared decision making' in Chapter 10. Whatever the underlying reasons for the patient's symptoms, developing a therapeutic alliance with the patient, getting to know him and offering support will enable greater clarity about the 'functional ways through'.

Explaining the physiological origin of symptoms

All clinicians will care for patients whose symptoms are functional, rather than caused by damage to the structure or physiology of the body. This does not mean that these are 'medically unexplained' symptoms, although that is the terminology often used. Rather, these are disorders of how the body functions, distortions of normal physiology. These can be explained in ways that are helpful to patients struggling with the impact of their symptoms on daily life. Using physiological explanations can help patients manage functional symptoms by avoiding what many patients perceive as 'blaming' or 'shaming' psychological explanations, and also lead to useful strategies for pain management. Some examples of helpful explanations are given in Box 4.1.

Box 4.1: Useful explanatory phrases to help patients understand functional descriptions of their symptoms

- For abdominal pains: 'intestines/guts are overly sensitive to stimuli', 'spasm and relaxation'.
- For headache: 'tension-type headache', 'medication overuse headache', 'increased sensitivity in the neck muscles'.
- For joint pains: 'wear and repair processes', 'irritation of the nerve endings causing pain'.

This subject is covered in much more detail in the *ABC of Medically Unexplained Symptoms*.[6]

How might things go better for Mrs Beryll and Dr Alder?

Dr Alder feels fairly sure that serious disease has probably been ruled out (by all the specialist tests and by a 'test of time'). Her symptoms persist, but overall Mrs Beryll remains well and able to function in her daily life. Dr Alder explains the pain in terms of variable spasms and tightness of the bowel, agreeing with Mrs Beryll that her bowels are not diseased, only not working in a smooth way.

Dr Alder also attends closely to the cues and clues that Mrs Beryll gives about her life, and how the abdominal pain annoys her husband who is pressurising her to 'get it sorted'. Picking up this cue that all may not be well at home, Dr Alder gently enquires about the marital relationship, finally asking if Mrs Beryll has ever felt unsafe at home.

After a pause, she blurts out that her husband does get very angry, that he drinks too much and sometimes gets 'a bit aggressive'. A history of domestic abuse emerges, and Dr Alder recognises, to his chagrin, that unexplained abdominal pain is common in those who are being abused.

Mrs Beryll is relieved to talk about this problem, although keen that her husband should not know she has told anyone. Dr Alder refers to local services to support victims of this type of crime and Mrs Beryll uses the support offered to make decisions about her marriage.

References

1. Marinker M. Standards. In: M. Marinker (ed.). *Medical Audit and General Practice*. London: The MSD Foundation, 1990, pp. 12–13.
2. Heneghan C, Glasziou P, Thompson M, *et al.* Diagnostic strategies used in primary care. *British Medical Journal* 2009; **338**: b946.
3. Neighbour R. *The Inner Consultation*. Lancaster: MTP Press Ltd, 1987.
4. Almond S, Mant D, Thompson M. Diagnostic safety-netting. *British Journal of General Practice* 2009; **59(568)**: 872–4.
5. Stanners M, French HT. *An Empirical Study of the Relationship Between Situation Awareness and Decision Making*. Edinburgh: Australian Government Department of Defense, 2005, www.researchgate.net/profile/Melinda_Stanners/publication/27254567_An_empirical_study_of_the_relationship_between_situation_awareness_and_decision_making/links/00b4952b52229576ad000000.pdf [accessed 25 June 2015].
6. Burton C. *ABC of Medically Unexplained Symptoms*. London: Wiley-Blackwell and BMJ Publishing, 2013.

Chapter 5

The clinical setting, assessment and teaching methods for uncertainty in the Analysing Quadrant

Clinical decision making, including diagnostic thinking, is strongly influenced by context: the differential diagnoses considered will be different in an emergency department, a nursing home or a routine follow-up clinic. Can the setting we work in be set up to help to avoid WDYDWYDKWTD moments in the Analysing Quadrant? What methods of teaching help? This chapter covers:

- how clinical settings can help the management of uncertainty in the Analysing Quadrant
- assessment and teaching methods for uncertainty in the Analysing Quadrant.

How clinical settings can help the management of uncertainty in the Analysing Quadrant

Developing a diagnosis is often an iterative process, with test results casting light on what may need to be done next. Can the clinical setting help or hinder uncertainty in the Analysing Quadrant? Accurate diagnosis is likely to be greater if the setting both permits and encourages follow-up, and supports overall continuity of care, including the assessment of test results or clinic letters that may elucidate the problem. The availability of appropriate investigations, especially in generalist settings, can assist only if learners are coached in the appropriate use of diagnostic networks (see Chapter 7). Safety netting works best with continuity of care, which appointment systems can help to promote (for example, by GPs booking their own follow-up appointments with the patient). Where safety netting may involve more than one service (for example out-of-hours care), then organisations should ensure that they have robust methods for transmitting relevant information between providers to inform subsequent decision making. This is likely to become even more important in the future as services change configuration.

Other elements of the workplace can help to mitigate WDYDWYDKWTD situations. When designing instrument panels in cars or aircraft, designers consider how they can arrange things to promote appropriate situational judgements, including warning lights, the arrangement of information and so on. In complex settings like Accident and Emergency or primary care, where there will be many competing priorities at any one time, clinicians can be encouraged to develop a 'dashboard' approach to develop situational judgement, which will help to facilitate prompt diagnosis, especially in acute care. Who is waiting? Do we have enough information to prioritise? What early warning systems are in place to pick up problems earlier?

Helping juniors to develop systematic approaches to difficult situations, including prioritising and delegating to others appropriately, will help many WDYDWYDKWTD situations and is further discussed in Chapter 13. Acute care has some automated systems for this: GP computer systems can highlight available appointments, who is in the waiting area, available staff and other information. Learners could look at the tasks for the day with a trainer's supervision and plan how they will assess urgency, importance, priorities and sequencing of work. Suffice to say, organised settings with appropriate time allocations are more likely to yield accurate diagnoses. The task of 'sweeping' the environment for impending problems may need to be shared or delegated.

Modern medical practice is very complex. However, there are many algorithms, guidelines and protocols than can help in the Analysing Quadrant, the Wells score for DVT being just one such example. Such guidance should be freely available in clinical settings whether via the internet, mobile phone applications or information in departments. Induction and training can address the availability and use of such aids, and senior clinicians can model using them for reference.

Assessment and teaching methods for uncertainty in the Analysing Quadrant

Many issues in the Analysing Quadrant will come to light when the adverse effects of dysfunctional 'ways out' become apparent, including delays in diagnosis, new information being ignored, or failure to appreciate complex or multiple diagnoses. Trainers and supervisors need to identify 'ways out' and clarify what makes them dysfunctional. Otherwise, learners, finding them easier, may continue to use 'dysfunctional ways out' rather than working to achieve 'functional ways through'. Developing 'cognitive forcing functions' in systems helps to avoid this.[1] Examples could include always checking all bones for fractures after trauma, even when the first fracture (or two, or three) is identified. Using computer systems to prevent prescriptions of drugs that interact, or that the patient is allergic to, is another example of a cognitive forcing function that nudges clinicians to do the right thing.

Some difficulties in the Analysing Quadrant arise when the clinician is inexperienced or when the situation is complicated or untypical. Supervision must be reliably available. All clinicians, especially those in training, need opportunities to discuss diagnosis with more experienced colleagues and to share their diagnostic difficulties. This is also true of experienced clinicians, however, because they are likely to be responsible for more difficult diagnostic challenges. Multidisciplinary team meetings and regular opportunities to discuss diagnoses are the key to effectiveness and continuing learning in this Quadrant.

Are experts uncertain less often than novices? Actually, all clinicians recognise the WDYDWYDKWTD moment, although more expert practitioners may have different thresholds for their sense of difficulty. What makes for expertise in WDYDWYDKWTD situations is the ability to step aside from a fixed mode of thinking and examine alternatives, to change tack if the information does not support the proposed diagnosis, to recognise if a diagnosis doesn't 'fit'. Less expert thinkers can find it hard to change direction; it requires effort and may involve exchanging a comfortable (although wrong) place for an exposed and uncomfortable uncertainty. Clinicians need to provide psychological, cognitive and practical support to each other in these situations.

A change of tack may be resisted for other reasons too: perhaps a more senior colleague has made a particular diagnosis (which becomes accepted without review) or perhaps the clinician doesn't know how to generate new ideas, or fears picking a diagnosis that she will not know how to handle. There may be time pressure to act, and alternative diagnoses may be more expensive to the health system (the costs of investigations are considerable and clinicians have a responsibility to manage resources wisely). Changing tack may mean that the possible tests carry hazards to patients (all diagnostic tests have a cost to patients' wellbeing and some are potentially lethal). Educators need to discuss all these issues with their learners in the context of accurate diagnosis, and senior staff need to model being open to feedback and being challenged to explain their thought processes.

Diagnostic methods can be formally taught and assessed. Trainers and supervisors can encourage clinical 'ownership' of an individual patient's care; feedback and follow-up on their diagnoses and outcomes will follow and speed up learning. Using Random Case Analysis and Problem Case Analysis can highlight diagnostic reasoning skills and allow review of the history, test results and referral outcomes, by asking learners to:

- articulate and explain their thinking methods, their clinical reasoning
- articulate how they made their judgements
- receive feedback from seniors about their diagnostic processes.

Reflection-on-action in case-based discussions, case reviews and learning logs in ePortfolios can focus on whether or not the clinical reasoning and diagnostic outcomes are appropriate. When clinical information does not support the trainee's proposed diagnosis, he will benefit from challenges to his thinking, provided that he has adequate support to think through the alternatives. Asking the 'deeper question' about how a situation has come about will facilitate improved situational judgement and encourage flexible, reflective thought.

Medical educators need to be familiar with the concepts and thinking strategies outlined in this chapter. Metacognition, by which one steps back from the immediate anchoring situation to reflect on the thinking process, should include:

- reminding oneself of the limitations of memory
- checking the wider clinical perspective, not just the immediate presenting complaint (representativeness error). What doesn't fit? What else could this be?
- checking for known pitfalls or problems, also known as cognitive forcing strategies.

These strategies are usually addressed to processes, for example having found one fracture keep on searching for the next one.

Learners should rehearse these issues regularly in discussion, to ensure that they are thinking both widely and deeply about the clinical situations they face. Learners should be encouraged to make the most of any opportunity to see, diagnose and check the outcome of patients under their care.

To reduce errors, all clinicians need to be asking themselves 'How do I know it's this diagnosis?' and 'What else could it be?'. They should be mindful of how to exclude the rare but serious problem as well as including the most likely. Ask 'the deeper question' about how the current problem arose, how it fits in with other information about the patient's condition, and whether or not a diagnosis makes sense in the overall context.

In group teaching in study release settings, educators can explore 'what you do when you don't know what to do'. Creating opportunities to work through diagnostic pathways in a variety of clinical contexts will help learners relate them to theories of diagnostic thinking. Understanding bias and metacognition will be more readily achieved with regular case review and analysis. Helping learners to think through how 'red flag' signs can contribute to ruling in or ruling out significant conditions can help more flexible thinking to develop. Trainers should also explicitly address the question of diagnostic biases and uncertainties. Symptoms and signs of different disease states overlap and mimic each other; diagnostic tests are not perfect.

Training and discussion with colleagues also needs to cover the thorny question of when a diagnosis is 'good enough'. Thinking about the worst-case scenario is important and can help direct progress down diagnostic algorithms. However, many important diagnoses will be excluded simply by a test of time or by a test of treatment. It isn't necessary to do immediate MRI scans on every swelling or carry out tests for temporal arteritis for every patient with a headache. Teaching and modelling effective safety-netting strategies will ensure that, when things do not go to plan, there is a robust arrangement in place for an iterative approach to diagnosis. Information can be reviewed and revisited in the light of changing or evolving symptoms. The usefulness and importance of these 'holding strategies' should be particularly emphasised in generalist settings such as primary care. Learners can be supported in appropriate 'watchful waiting', while also being challenged to justify their choice of strategy. Uncertainty can be understood as a normal experience for clinicians, which should be embraced as interesting and a trigger to deeper thought.

Donald Schön sums it up when he says:

> *Because of troubling, interesting phenomena, a physician expresses uncertainty, takes the time to reflect and allows himself to be vulnerable. Then he restructures the problem. This is the key to the art of dealing with situations of uncertainty, instability, uniqueness and conflict.*[2]

References

1. Croskerry P. Cognitive forcing strategies in clinical decisionmaking. *Annals of Emergency Medicine* 2003; **41(1)**: 110–20.
2. Schön D. *The Reflective Practitioner: how professionals think in action*. London: Temple Smith, 1983.

Resources for the Analysing Quadrant

Burton C. *ABC of Medically Unexplained Symptoms*. London: Wiley-Blackwell and BMJ Publishing, 2013.

Dowie J, Elstein A. *Professional Judgement: a reader in clinical decision making*. (6th edn). Cambridge: Cambridge University Press, 1993.

Groopman J. *How Doctors Think*. New York: Mariner Books, 2007.

THE NETWORKING QUADRANT

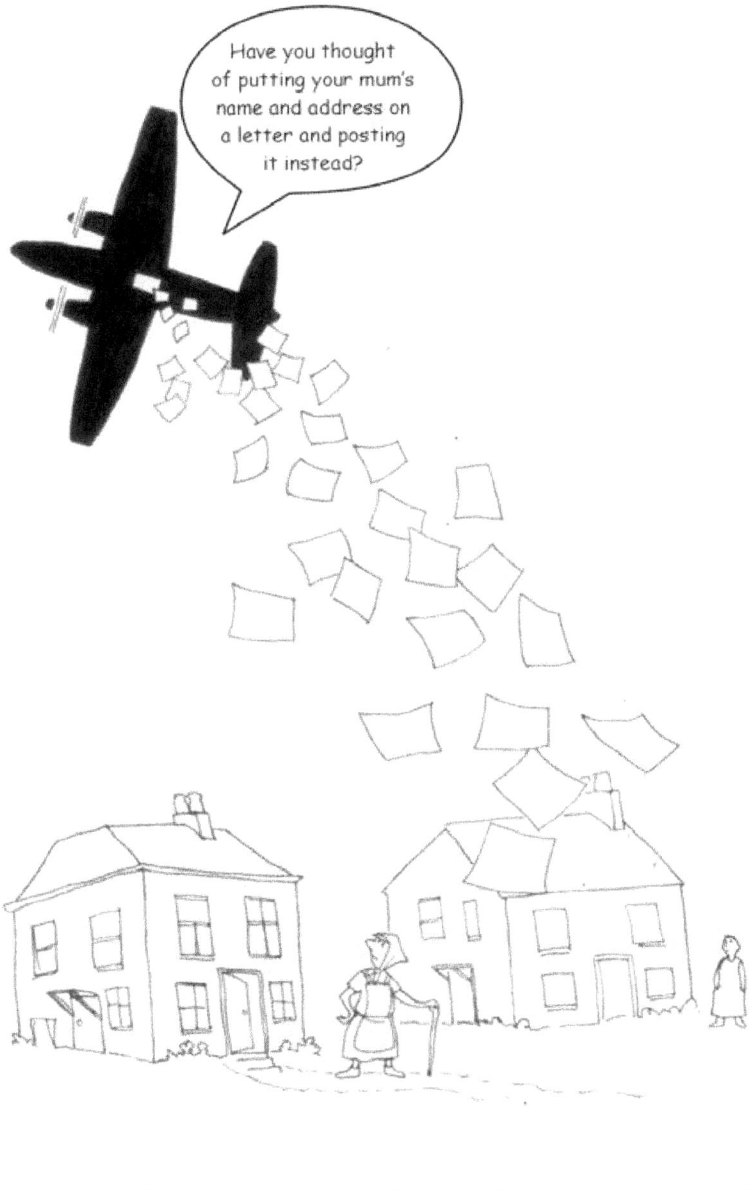
Have you thought of putting your mum's name and address on a letter and posting it instead?

The Networking Quadrant is concerned with diagnosis, just as the Analysing Quadrant is. However, in the Networking Quadrant a wider diagnostic network is involved.

Chapter 6 is an introduction to uncertainty in the Networking Quadrant and also discusses 'dysfunctional ways out'. **Chapter 7** works though examples of common WDYDWYDKWTD situations in the Networking Quadrant, identifying 'functional ways through' common problems, and the right skills needed for the right situation. **Chapter 8** explores how the clinical setting can help to deal with uncertainty in the Networking Quadrant, and suggests assessment and teaching methods

The key skills are:

- holding skills
- managing expectations of referrals or investigations before they take place
- understanding the referral network
- breaking good news
- dealing with exceptional circumstances
- continuing care after referral.

Chapter 6

Introduction to uncertainty in the Networking Quadrant

'Doctor X is marvellous', a patient said to a junior doctor, who was struggling to manage a huge 'take' of emergency patients. 'If she is in any doubt at all she always sends you straight up to the hospital to get it sorted out.'

Needless to say, this doctor sent patients to the emergency department every single day, sometimes several patients per day. The patients who came were not usually that unwell, didn't need admission and rarely needed much investigation. Referral was a way of resolving the doctor's doubt, unwillingness to dig deeper, to 'hold' any uncertainty or to get the patient involved in that process. Doubtless the secondary care services heaved a sigh of relief when she retired. These days when everyone's referrals are under scrutiny, perhaps this would happen less, and certainly Primary Care Organisations and other regulators are looking at 'outliers' in referral frequencies to try to standardise care. So is there really a problem in the Networking Quadrant?

This chapter covers:

- an introduction to the Networking Quadrant
- 'dysfunctional ways out' of uncertainty in the Networking Quadrant: common pitfalls.

Introduction to the Networking Quadrant

The Networking Quadrant is concerned with how doctors try to make diagnoses, just as the Analysing Quadrant is. However, although the Analysing Quadrant is concerned with what happens when one doctor–patient dyad are working together, the Networking Quadrant is concerned with what happens when the wider diagnostic network becomes involved.

Most of the time, a good history and appropriate examination will yield a working diagnosis or set of differentials, which mean the doctor and patient can move forward. Resolving a clear differential, such as 'Is this rectal bleeding caused by cancer?' that results in referral for endoscopy is not a WDYDWYDKWTD issue. This situation is like roulette: risky but not uncertain. Not all patients with rectal bleeding have cancer. Until we investigate, we don't know which ones will turn out to just have piles or an anal fissure. Problems arise in the Networking Quadrant when referral for tests or investigations is not really necessary, or where the referral goes to the wrong place, provides results that do not help the patient or doctor, or even result in a cascade of inappropriate or even dangerous investigations.

The array of diagnostic services that we have access to is unprecedented and expanding all the time: laboratory tests, ultrasound, radiology of all kinds, endoscopy. This can create a paralysing sense of not knowing what to do. Which service or test is most appropriate? How many tests could, should or need to be done before referral? What degree of uncertainty can we accept before referral is triggered? How much risk is acceptable … for the patient? Or the doctor? The use of time as a diagnostic strategy is often discussed in the context of general practice,[1] but can be difficult for inexperienced clinicians to use confidently.

If problems don't seem to be resolvable within their own sphere of expertise, referral to a different specialist (if you are working in hospital practice) or referral back to the GP, or admission to hospital if the patient is acutely ill, seems a comforting strategy. After all, if the clinician doesn't know what the problem is, how can it be harmful for a doctor to do investigations, or refer to someone else who will know the answer? Conversely, when specialist services are stumped they say, 'Just ask your GP about that' or more controversially, 'Tell your GP to refer you to service x.' Difficulties soon start if the receiving GP does not have access to such a service, or believes that service x is not the correct one for this particular patient. All those receiving referrals, including GPs, are aware of referrals that go wrong or don't have the hoped for clarifying effect, with no usable diagnosis yielded from the tests and opinions. The Networking Quadrant explores these issues in more detail.

Patients are at greatest risk at times of handover: perhaps between colleagues in the same location, certainly when being referred between institutions or between services. Patients can easily fall 'between the cracks'. Developing efficient and effective relationships and interactions in the Networking Quadrant is a major professional responsibility; it means having systems in place to maintain continuity and a sense of ownership for the patient's wellbeing as she travels through the system, as well as the skills to refer appropriately and manage scarce resources wisely.

Too little, or inappropriate, referral risks compromising high standards of care. However, excess referral or investigation wastes resources, creates expectations that may not be fulfilled and over-medicalises many problems. There are clearly ethical issues here too: balancing the use of resources for different patients, the potential to do harm and uncertainty about which course of action will enable the patient's autonomy to flourish the most. Managing uncertainty requires the skills to analyse ethical issues quickly.

There are two aspects to the skills needed for the Networking Quadrant. First, the clinician needs to understand and manage his own thoughts and feelings when he is having a WDYDWYDKWTD moment that is connected with making a diagnosis. This is 'metacognition' again. Commonly, clinicians feel uncomfortable when they cannot make a diagnosis, or if they have a niggling doubt that the diagnosis that seems correct is not the right one. What if the true diagnosis is something rare? Or that needs some special tests to rule it out? Second, the clinician needs the skills to discuss these issues with the patient, in such a way that the patient is involved in the decision making. It may not be easy to find the 'sweet spot' between referring too little, which risks missing important diagnoses or therapeutic options, and referring too much, which causes iatrogenic harm and wastes resources.

Although clinicians aim to be systematic and rational about their work, as we have seen in the Analysing Quadrant, quite a lot of decisions are made using intuitive Type 1 thinking, in which the reasoning behind a decision is not articulated and may be strongly influenced by non-rational factors, including the emotions of the clinician or patient. This can often happen where there is uncertainty, as clinicians make rapid, intuitive decisions so that uncertainty is replaced with a firm decision. Such responses to uncertainty probably underlie some referrals to the wider diagnostic network.

These responses to uncertainty, and how they influence clinicians, are discussed in more detail in Part III 'Mapping the psychology of uncertainty'.

'Dysfunctional ways out' of uncertainty in the Networking Quadrant: common pitfalls

Referral for investigation usually occurs in situations of diagnostic doubt, so the most important thing that the doctor and patient hope for is a clear-cut diagnosis. Sometimes a clear-cut 'ruling out' of a condition is aspired to, but that doesn't tend to cause the WDYDWYDKWTD question. The resolution of straightforward differentials is not the subject of this chapter.

So what pitfalls are there in this apparently innocuous process?

Mismatch between the doctor's understanding of the purpose of the tests and the patient's understanding

Tests and investigations can be performed to 'rule out' certain conditions. For the doctor, *ruling out* serious things may be sufficient. However, the patient has other questions. She wants to know what is wrong and why. She wants tests that will '*rule in*' a specific diagnosis so that she can understand her condition and hopefully find a cure or treatment for it. If the doctor and patient are at cross-purposes about why tests are being done, then their response to normal tests may also be at odds. If all the tests come back normal (reassuring and satisfying the doctor that the risk of serious disease is low), the patient becomes even more worried. Why can't the doctor find the answer? This can trigger further rounds of fruitless and sometimes risky testing. For example, if the investigation for chest pain is pursued in spite of normal initial investigations the patient may end up undergoing angiography, which has a morbidity and even mortality attached.[2]

Over-reliance on tests and investigations to create a diagnosis

Diagnosis is not a fixed concept: it evolves during the assessment of the patient. Investigations can only rule in/rule out to the extent that a rational differential is arrived at in the Analysing Quadrant. Random, scattergun or sets of 'routine' investigations are no substitute for a properly thought-through differential, so one of the dysfunctional ways out of the Analysing Quadrant is prematurely moving to the Networking Quadrant and investigating in an unstructured way.

Under-appreciation of the frequency of 'functional' conditions

About 30% (and possibly up to 60%) of patients in general practice have functional disorders, which also occur frequently in every specialty (e.g. IBS, atypical facial pain, trochanteric pain syndrome are all disorders of function rather than structure). When all the 'basic tests' are done, referral to a specialist or to get 'more tests' or 'an X-ray to be sure' can set off a cycle of non-contributory investigations that leave doctor and patient rather frustrated. Not having the skill to explain and manage these types of syndromes is a common reason for referral. However, this can be very dysfunctional because many specialty doctors also lack these skills.

Increasing anxiety in both doctor and patient

If we are honest with ourselves, sometimes the purpose of investigating or referring a patient can really be 'to get this person out of my consulting room', because the way forwards is unclear, and the patient's anxiety, and sometimes the doctor's, is escalating to the point where it is becoming intolerable for both parties. The complexities of the doctor–patient consultation have been well described as stable complex systems, with creative or novel events happening 'on the edge of chaos'.[3] This can mean that unexpected outcomes, including referrals, may happen somewhat unexpectedly as many factors come into play. However, we do not usually write 'must get this patient out of my hair for a bit' on the referral form. This means referrals sometimes do not achieve their aim from the patient's view-point. Patients are more likely to be asking, 'What is the matter with me? Who is going to cure me?' Furthermore, doing tests and investigations to end the consultation is wasteful. There are practical, ethical and financial reasons why referring for diagnostic tests needs skilful handling; being able to analyse the possible ethical constraints quickly in a consultation is a key skill for generalists.

Sometimes reflex or poorly thought-through diagnostic referral has a more sinister effect. The investigations may reveal unexpected abnormalities that result in a cascade of investigations, further removing the patient from the effective analysis that should precede this. If cues from the patient have been missed (e.g. a travel history or important psychosocial issues) then merely doing more tests is a 'dysfunctional way out'. It can lead to over-medicalising of the patient's experiences, and weaken the doctor's analysing skills through atrophy and disuse.

Emotional difficulties in the consultation

Sometimes referral is a way of trying to resolve an emotional or relationship difficulty in the consultation. The communication style of the clinician affects relationships; patients prefer an affiliative to a dominant style.[4] If there is a dominant style of communicating and patients are not satisfied, referral onwards is a rapid way to resolve the situation. For example, if all the gastroenterological investigations are normal and the gastroenterology clinician is making a diagnosis of IBS, the doctor may find the patient's distress difficult to cope with, and not know how to deal with it. So he says something like 'I am sure the GP could refer to Z hospital' for some new therapy he is trying (adding acupuncture, hypnotherapy or whatever it might be). This gets the patients off the specialist's list, but that treatment may not in fact be available. Many patients with painful conditions are discharged from specialty clinics when investigations are complete, and the letter to the GP says, 'I have told the patient she should be referred to a Pain Clinic.' Pain Clinics are overstretched, with long waiting lists, yet this message means that patients get the impression that the Pain Clinic will 'cure' them of their pain. However, the complex bio-psycho-social approach of Pain Clinics is orientated towards coping with and managing pain, rather than 'curing it'. If patients are not ready for this approach another cycle of failed referral and frustration may result.

All these difficulties can be compounded by the increasing fragmentation of health services. Referral networks are constantly changing, with contracts being moved between different providers and having different criteria for referral. This is a particular problem for GPs; navigating a complex service has always been part of a GP's role, and requires particular attention when resources are limited. Being able to maintain a good database of appropriate diagnostic facilities to refer to and being aware of what they can and can't deliver is a crucial skill.

References

1. Irvine G, Holden J. The time-efficiency principle: time as the key diagnostic strategy in primary care. *Family Practice* 2013; **30**: 386–9.
2. Mold JW, Stein HF. The cascade effect in the clinical care of patients. *New England Journal of Medicine* 1986; **314(8)**: 512–14.
3. Innes AD, Campion PD, Griffiths FE. Complex consultations and the 'edge of chaos'. *British Journal of General Practice* 2005; **55(510)**: 47–52.
4. Buller M, Buller D. Physicians' communication style and patient satisfaction. *Journal of Health and Social Behavior* 1987; **28(4)**: 375–88.

Chapter 7

Functional ways through uncertainty in the Networking Quadrant

Clearly, a fully thought-through Analysing Quadrant will prevent many problems in networking: 'If it is a mystery, then go back to the history', as US doctors say. If parties other than a single doctor–patient dyad need to be involved to reach a working diagnosis, negotiation of the purpose and meaning of referral or investigation must address the expectations of both parties, and clarify what is likely to be achieved. At times, better negotiation and explanation will obviate the need for referral or investigation completely in general practice and this will greatly reduce the likelihood of unexpected or irrelevant findings clouding the picture. Nowadays, information about the criteria for referral and what should be done in primary care first are very easily obtainable on every desktop. This chapter focuses on:

- examples of common WDYDWYDKWTD situations in the Networking Quadrant
- clarifying 'functional ways through' common problems by identifying the right skills needed for the right situation.

The skills needed are:

- holding skills
- managing expectations of referrals or investigations before they take place
- understanding the referral network
- breaking good news
- dealing with exceptional circumstances
- continuing care after referral.

Holding skills

Following a diagnosis of coeliac disease, Amber gets much better when she is on a gluten-free diet. However, her mother becomes extremely anxious, bringing Amber to the doctors all the time for minor issues, ringing up about prescriptions, asking if Amber's symptoms are due to cancer and insisting on a referral to a cancer specialist, which is not clinically warranted at all. Dr Elm does give in and refers the child to a paediatric oncology unit, but the referral is returned because it does not meet the criteria for a two-week wait referral. This makes Amber's mother even more upset. The doctor gives Amber's mother some leaflets, refers her to a counselling service and gives her some antidepressants. Amber's mother writes a letter of complaint that she has been sent to mental health services, as she sees such a referral as stigmatising: 'I am not mental', she says to the Practice Manager.

As we have seen, referral to some other part of the NHS network to make a diagnosis can be a response to uncertainty, and can bring its own difficulties and even harms. Doctors and their patients feel uncertain when situations are unclear, which can often arise when symptoms are ambiguous, confusing, give rise to conflicting feelings or where there is a faint (but worrying) possibility of serious disease. In the latter situation patients worry that something will be missed; doctors know if they do miss something they will feel guilty, face possible censure and lose their professional confidence. The kinds of symptoms that cause uncertainty and may lead to difficulties in the Networking Quadrant are summarised in Box 7.1.

At first sight, it may appear that the possibility of serious outcomes in the above cases should always warrant referral. The early stages of many conditions are undifferentiated: a flu that will be better in a week may look the same as malaria that may kill. However, doctors need to calibrate their 'signal to noise ratio' according to the setting they are in. This will help them to hold a degree of uncertainty confidently, if they have systems in place to pick up changing situations and change the management accordingly.

These concepts will help.

Box 7.1: Examples of symptoms likely to cause uncertainty

AMBIGUOUS symptoms

Weight loss in an overweight diabetic ... is this because he is sticking to his diet or has he developed another disease like cancer or hyperthyroidism?

CONFUSING symptoms

A patient who says she feels suicidal, but who is well dressed and full of plans for the future including upcoming holidays and applying for new jobs.

UNDIFFERENTIATED early symptoms

The onset of influenza can be the same as that of malaria, meningitis or chronic fatigue syndrome.

Understanding that primary care and secondary care have different conceptual approaches to diagnosis

In 1994 Marshall Marinker in a Bayliss Lecture for the RCGP[1,2] commented that 'Specialists aim to reduce uncertainty, explore possibility and marginalise error. Generalists aim to accept uncertainty, explore probability and marginalise danger.'

Marginalising danger in primary care doesn't mean doing a lumbar puncture on every child with a fever 'in case' it is meningitis. It does mean understanding the way to differentiate possibility from probability, by thinking through the symptoms and signs carefully (a successful Analysing Quadrant), followed by safety netting and arranging appropriate follow-up. Accepting uncertainty in primary care settings doesn't mean shrugging your shoulders because 'it's impossible to know'. Uncertainty needs to be managed using appropriate follow-up safety netting and understanding of risk.

Understanding how time will resolve many ambiguities

The child with a cold will gradually improve; the child with meningitis will deteriorate. So having good 'safety-netting' arrangements in place, with regular review available for those at risk of deterioration, will allow some ambiguities to resolve themselves.[3]

Anxiety is 'catching'

Patients can transfer their anxieties to clinicians, and, as in the example quoted at the beginning of this chapter, clinicians then transfer anxiety to other clinicians.

Clinicians need to learn to identify what the patient's anxiety is really about, make a proportionate response to it, and use the skills of explanation and negotiation to 'hold' anxiety while time, nature or referral do their clarifying work. Picking up cues, being willing and able to explore and accept anxiety, does not always come naturally to doctors, who may prefer to stay in a 'problem solving' mode. Training issues for the Networking Quadrant are discussed in Chapter 8.

How might it go better for Amber's mother?

Dr Elm always takes Amber's mother seriously when examining Amber, and remains calm about the extremely low risk of malignant disease, making an appointment to see Amber's mother alone, to discuss her thoughts more deeply. Exploring her concerns it seems that there is guilt there (should she have brought Amber to the doctor earlier?), worry about what she has read on the internet (some people with coeliac disease go on to develop cancer, are we missing that in Amber?) and frustration that her husband does not share her concern and even lets Amber have biscuits that contain gluten sometimes, which makes her angry and worried for Amber.

Dr Elm empathises and works through these worries, explaining how coping with the loss of health in a child can feel almost as upsetting as a bereavement. There are several follow-up appointments that enable Dr Elm to normalise these responses to illness in a child. Neither the oncology nor the mental health referrals are needed in the end.

Managing expectations of referrals or investigations before they take place

Ms Gemstone is aged 35. She complains of tiredness and unrefreshing sleep. She thinks her hair is getting thinner and that her skin is dry. She is clinically euthyroid, of normal weight and her hair seems normal on examination. Dr Birch sends a thyroid function test (TFT), FBC, PV, C-reactive protein (CRP), U and E and glycated haemoglobin (HbA1c). All come back normal, which reassures Dr Birch that serious illness is unlikely. She asks about stress in Ms Gemstone's life, which irritates Ms Gemstone, who says that she is not under that much stress and asks for a 'scan' or some 'X-rays'. Dr Birch wants to avoid the 'dysfunctional way out' of lots of pointless tests, but still is not sure what to do.

If the doctor or patient does not understand and accept the purpose of tests, crossed wires, frustration and WDYDWYDKWTD situations can develop. If the doctor is referring for tests for reassurance that 'there is nothing serious', the doctor may be happy with normal results. If the patient is expecting the test to yield a formal diagnosis, he may be disappointed, and take this to mean that the doctor 'still does not know what is the matter with me'. If the doctor picks up on the patient's expectation for a single diagnosis, rather than explaining the concept of 'ruling out' something, the doctor can end up saying things like 'unfortunately your ultrasound was normal'. This negative view of what is actually good news can leave doctor and patient frustrated and confused.

There will always be symptoms that doctors can't explain. Some 30–60% of consultations in primary care settings may include some 'Medically Unexplained Symptoms'. Using appropriate 'analysing' strategies to 'marginalise danger' may indicate which symptoms are likely to not have a (currently) medically explainable cause. This is NOT to say that the symptoms are in some way 'not true'. The symptoms are real, distressing to patients and require diligent attention from the doctor. The language that is used in the consultation, and effective use of explanation and planning skills, will often go some way to preventing the impasse reached with Ms Gemstone, by preparing the patient for the range of possibilities before the tests are done. This process is explained in detail in the book *Skills for Communicating with Patients* (see Resources, p. 94). In summary, before the tests are done, the purpose of the investigation needs to be clearly thought through and discussed with the patient, the value of the tests explained (for example, to provide reassurance if they are normal) and the patient's thoughts, anxieties and expectations of the tests should also be explored. This will anticipate and correct misconceptions such as the patient hoping that all her symptoms will be due to a single disease process, or that a normal test means further tests need to be done in the search for an 'explanation'.

Using the patient's exact words and concerns during explanations works better than jargon. Have explanations that accept distress, and also encourage expectations of healing and improvement ('wear and repair' and 'spasm and relaxation' are useful phrases). If anticipating normal tests (e.g. to rule things out) explain this as 'We need to rule out something serious. If the tests are normal as we anticipate, we will both be reassured. Then we can concentrate on what we need to do to help relieve your symptoms.' Using the strategies in this chapter in ALL consultations can prevent some of the conflict or impasse that sometimes occurs when the doctor's and patient's expectations are different.

Clearly, this planning of tests with the patient may take a little time and is the opposite of the 'dysfunctional way out' of dismissing the patient by 'arranging some tests and seeing what comes up'. However, in the longer term, more time will be saved, as both patient and doctor are clear about what is being asked of the tests, and are prepared for the next stage of the process of treatment.

Anticipating results can take place even earlier in the consultation. When examining patients, using positive statements like 'the chest sounds healthy', rather than negative ones like 'there does not seem to be anything wrong', is reassuring. What patients will remember from the last example are the words 'not', 'seem' and 'wrong', which will not inspire confidence. The phrase 'I can't find anything wrong' may lead the patient to believe that the problem is a hidden, more sinister one, whereas what the doctor really means is 'things are normal'.

How might things go better for Ms Gemstone and Dr Birch?

In the Analysing Quadrant, before ordering any tests, Dr Birch went further in establishing the possible causes of tiredness and will have also explored the impact of the tiredness on Ms Gemstone and the worries that she has. Having explained the examination findings fully and in positive language, Dr Birch could also relate the tiredness to Ms Gemstone's heavy workload and the energy-sapping effects of covering for a sick colleague at work. Finding out about, understanding and accepting her worries about cancer, Dr Birch carefully explains what the tests are for and how likely they are to be normal, and why that would be reassuring. In the presence of cancer, the blood count, PV or CRP would be very likely to be abnormal. If the tiredness persists they can look at ways to increase her resilience and build up her strength. This may be as much about lifestyle changes as any medication, if Ms Gemstone has no symptoms of depression. All this can be signalled at the first consultation as part of the work that doctor and patient need to do between them to improve Ms Gemstone's health overall.

Understanding the referral network

Dr Alder is seeing Mrs Beryll again. After a long and emotional consultation it appears that Mrs Beryll is quite low, but does not really fit all the criteria for a major depression. Mrs Beryll says that she is finding her life difficult. Her husband is less aggressive than he used to be, but they still have problems and she would like someone to talk to. Relieved to have got closer to the problem, but still not quite sure how to proceed, Dr Alder agrees to refer her, only to find that there is a plethora of different types of mental health service available. How will they work out which one to use? Dr Alder refers to a psychiatrist for advice about whether Mrs Beryll does truly have depression, only to have the referral bounced back with a comment from the Referral Management Service Doctor saying, 'There is insufficient information on this referral. Please complete the full assessment on the attached pro forma.' Dr Alder feels a bit stuck and Mrs Beryll is cross because the referral is delayed.

Changes in the NHS have resulted in fragmentation and separation of providers, and this makes it even more difficult to use referral networks effectively. In some areas there are Referral Management Services that triage or assess referrals and guide them to the 'right' place. Complex services such as mental health may have a single point of access where referrals are screened. However, in most places there will also be a variety of non-statutory services, wellbeing services of various kinds, voluntary-sector services, helplines, drop-in centres and so on, which can be very difficult to navigate. Knowing your network is a crucial skill.

An effective referral means thinking about the *reason* for referral (in Mrs Beryll's case mood disturbance because of marital difficulties), which is something we can usually assess fairly quickly. But it also means being very clear about the *purpose* of referral, which is a different thing all together. A well-written referral letter should clarify both of these points (i.e. the reason and purpose of the referral). If the question being asked is lucidly expressed, the referrer, the patient and the recipient will all be better served. Vague referrals without clear questions may give vague and unsatisfactory outcomes.

Referrals may be for some or all of the following purposes:

- for a wiser head to establish a diagnosis
- for **investigations not available** to the clinician's own practice/department/setting

- when the diagnosis is made, for **treatment** that can't be given in the referrer's setting
- **for a second opinion** to confirm or refute the referrer's ideas, especially when the patient is not too happy
- **to reassure a clinician** who has had a previous bad experience with a particular symptom complex (for example, a headache that turned out to be a subarachnoid may lower his threshold for subsequent referrals)
- **to compensate for a clinician's lack of confidence** in a particular area (everyone thinks of GPs here, but secondary care doctors often say 'refer to dermatology' in situations that GPs would happily manage themselves)
- **to forestall any criticism** of difficult decisions like 'is this patient fit to fly?'

The purpose of a referral can usually be summed up in one line. Discussing and establishing the exact purpose of a referral with the patient before referral will make for better outcomes. See also the **S**ituation **B**ackground **A**ssessment **R**ecommendation (SBAR) 'handing over skills' section in Chapter 13.

Effective referral is also *timely*, getting the right advice at the right time. This means knowing what the local referral criteria are for certain clinics, using a clinic pro forma correctly and also knowing what informal or virtual sources of information are available. Many referrals can be given the right priority if there is a conversation (by email or phone) with colleagues in the relevant department. Discussing expectations before referral can save difficulties afterwards, if referral has failed to deliver the hoped for outcome (see Box 7.2).

Box 7.2: Effective informal strategies to assist effective referrals

- Referral meetings, discussing options for referral beforehand.
- Having 'reason for referral' and 'purpose of referral' on every letter/referral sent.
- Getting to know colleagues on both sides of the primary–secondary care divide.
- Telephoning or emailing for advice.
- Developing a culture of writing the purpose of tests/referrals in the notes.
- Maintaining a culture of continuity so that test follow-up is done by the referring doctor.

Informal approaches can supplement a well-written referral letter to good effect in more complex situations. For example, many methadone or heroin users avoid seeking care because they think their drugs will be stopped in hospital (often they are correct). A hernia ignored for some time because of such fears may end up being incarcerated or obstructed with serious results. If the GP talks to the surgeon in advance and helps to make anticipatory plans for appropriate prescribing when in hospital, such problems may be pre-empted. Having informal discussions at the time of referral can also smooth the path for patients with multiple morbidity, who may be using difficult medications such as steroids or immunosuppressants, or whose frailty requires nuanced decision-making.

Part of the doctor's job in helping patients use the NHS network appropriately is to inject a kindly note of realism about the limitations of diagnosis and treatment. For example, when referring for *in vitro* fertilisation (IVF) it can be useful to discuss the 80% *failure* rate and the limits of NHS expenditure for this treatment, and to help patients to think about how much of their own money they can afford to spend *in advance*. If this isn't discussed before, then some couples will get themselves in a futile cycle of spending on IVF that is not likely to work and they can get into serious financial trouble. Helping patients join in the discussion about the limitations of any referral can help them retain a sense of control over the process.

How might it go better for Mrs Beryll, with a shorter delay?

Dr Alder and Mrs Beryll decide together that, although the reason for the referral is that she is feeling low, the purpose of the referral is to clarify her approach to her marital problems and provide her with some assistance in thinking through and solving her problems. She is not mentally ill as such, and does not need a psychiatrist.

Dr Alder takes advice from peers about which parts of the mental health services may be of greatest benefit for Mrs Beryll and learns the difference between psychiatry, psychology, psychotherapy and various assisted self-help services. After the referral, Dr Alder gets a letter from a graduate worker at the psychology service (Improving Access to Psychological Therapies (IAPT)) saying that Mrs Beryll has taken a number of steps to improve things at home and at work, and is now going to marital therapy at Relate (an organisation that supports and counsels couples) with her husband.

Breaking good news

When Mr Crystal develops chest pain he goes to Accident and Emergency immediately because he has seen all the posters saying this could be a heart attack. He is told that all the tests are normal and is sent home, still with some chest pain. He requests an immediate emergency appointment with his GP Dr Oak, and is now very scared.

'Perhaps my heart attack is not showing upon the tests? What is the matter with me? Why can't those doctors at the hospital find out what is wrong?' He gets angry and shouts at Dr Oak, saying that he 'should have been admitted' and that he 'needs more tests', and has he got to 'collapse and die before anyone does anything to help me?'

Outcomes of the Networking Quadrant may lead to the doctor having to give good news to the patient, perhaps that investigations are normal. This is often more reassuring to doctors than it is to patients. We think of good news as something that will be greeted with relief or even gratitude. This doesn't always happen: the news of normal investigations can be disheartening to patients who were hoping for a diagnosis or explanation of their problems. Doctors may be surprised to discover that some patients are almost relieved to hear bad news: 'I thought there was something wrong. Now I know what I am dealing with.' If we go back to one definition of bad news as 'any information that ... drastically alters the patient's view of his or her future',[4] then it becomes clear that some 'good news' may be experienced as 'bad news' by the patient.

Mr Crystal is expecting to be told there is something wrong with his heart. This would be bad news, but he is anticipating that and it is a type of disease he understands. He has not been given an alternative diagnosis, only that it is NOT his heart. So he now believes he may have a mysterious disease, or that the doctors were not competent to diagnose his heart condition, and so is very frightened indeed, hence his rather assertive manner.

The effect of information will depend on prior expectations and what personal impact is anticipated for the individual. If a patient with back pain has been expecting two weeks off work with a sick note, she may have been really hoping for an opportunity to get away from a stressful office or a bullying colleague at the same time. The respite may have seemed very attractive. Hearing that her back examination shows only muscular dysfunction, and that normal activity and continued work are the best thing, may be experienced as a big disappointment and will need handling as such. In other words, even good news can drastically alter someone's view of his future.

To increase the patient's satisfaction with the 'breaking of good news', we need to attend to the gap between expectation and what patients actually receive. Understanding more precisely where the patient is coming from *before* arranging the investigation or referral and tailoring our advice to that exact place can transform the post-test discussions.

First, there are two kinds of 'good news'. There is news that both doctor and patient recognise and receive as such. For example, if the histology on a mole comes back as benign when patient or doctor have feared a malignancy, then both will be relieved. This does not normally give rise to the WDYDWYDKWTD question of course!

However, many patients have unpleasant or worrying symptoms that are not serious medically, and may not be explained by conventional diagnoses. Examinations, tests and investigations are often normal in patients with pain, itching or other symptoms. However, a patient whose symptoms are unpleasant and who is told they are 'not serious', and that there is no established diagnosis or treatment, is still stuck with her symptoms and may not regard this formulation as good news at all. For many patients who have uncomfortable or irritating symptoms, being told that they are 'normal' feels insulting, lacking recognition of their real suffering and missing the point. If we approach things more systematically we can alleviate many of these difficulties (see Box 7.3).

First, plan ahead

Clarifying the exact purpose of the tests (to rule out or rule in?) and relating this to the patient's own ideas and concerns will enable the meaning of the tests to be discussed before the results arrive. For example, saying clearly, 'If the test is normal then it means this, and if it is abnormal we will need to do that' prepares the patient for the possibility (even likelihood) of normal test results. The conversation needs to pre-empt questions like 'So what is actually wrong with me?' by indicating the possibilities beforehand. Expressing empathy and understanding about the symptoms is important.

Signal good news

When the results are available, it must be signalled as helpful news. Saying 'Unfortunately your ultrasound result is normal' gives the wrong message! Start by saying that the tests show helpful or good news. Use words like 'healthy, normal, great for your age', rather than 'not abnormal'. Using accurate, positive language can be reassuring in its own right, and is easily done as a commentary, during the examination, for example.

Then interpret the results in the light of the previously expressed concerns

'So then, as we thought, the tests show you have healthy blood, enough iron and no anaemia. The tests for inflammation are normal. This tells us it's what we thought, that this pain is largely in the muscles, mainly due to tightness and spasm, and it should settle with time if we do the following things….' Pick up the patient's responses and aim for a dialogue about the issues coming up.

Box 7.3: Breaking 'good news'

- PLAN AHEAD: clarify the reasons and purpose of tests beforehand, and what the likely outcomes are.
- EMPATHISE with the impact that symptoms are having on the patient.
- SIGNAL that GOOD NEWS is coming.
- Use POSITIVE LANGUAGE, words like healthy, normal, great for your age rather than negative terms like 'not abnormal'.
- INTERPRET results in the light of the patient's own concerns and use these to lead into plans for his care that relate to the patient's own concerns.
- Aim for a DIALOGUE, picking up on the patient's responses to your information.

Clearly, many investigations result in bad news that must be broken tactfully and honestly to patients too. Although this is taxing for both parties, it is more unusual for this to lead to the WDYDWYDKWTD question, perhaps because it is more predictable territory for clinicians. All clinicians need to learn about and practise the skills of breaking news, both good and bad.

How things could have gone better for Mr Crystal

In the Accident and Emergency department the assessing doctor thinks the likelihood of a heart attack is low. She explains that chest pain is often caused by spasm in the muscles across the chest and this settles with time and painkillers. She explains that the tests they are about to do (ECG, troponins) are to make double sure that there is no heart issue and that, if they are normal (as expected), he will be able to go home quite soon. She uses her explanation skills (see the Negotiating Quadrant) to explore Mr Crystal's specific concerns; his father died of an untreated heart attack at the age Mr Crystal is now, so he fears the same thing happening to him. The Accident and Emergency doctor recommends a health check at the GP to assess his overall risk and to make a plan for maintaining his health in the future, to reduce the risk of heart attack. When the results are normal, Mr Crystal is relieved, rather than being left in doubt, and is able to make an appropriate appointment for a check-up with his GP. His concerns about his heart are picked up and followed through with a full risk assessment, advice about reducing his risk and regular annual follow-up.

Dealing with exceptional circumstances/ethical skills

Ms Emerald is 28 years old and has consulted an aesthetic breast surgeon who says that her breasts are abnormal and that she could probably obtain breast reduction and correction of her inverted nipples via NHS treatment. She has seen a GP who indicated that such surgery is not available via the NHS. She was not happy with this and keeps coming back to see different doctors in the practice wanting a referral. She now comes to see Dr Hawthorne saying that her 'weird nipples' are causing her terrible psychological distress and that she wants a request for special funding for her to have surgery. Examination shows normal, although inverted, nipples and normal-sized breasts.

Mrs Pearl attends in great distress. She was referred for IVF treatment locally, having had three failed cycles of IVF privately in another country. She completed an NHS-funded cycle six months ago that worked, but sadly the foetus had anencephaly and died *in utero* at a very early stage. The local commissioning guidelines offer only one cycle of NHS IVF treatment (although in a neighbouring district two cycles will be funded). She is desperate to get pregnant as she thinks her husband will divorce her if she doesn't have a baby soon. Dr Hawthorne knows the local guidelines and is not sure what to do next.

Complex ethical issues are at play in every consultation, especially those where clinicians recognise the WDYDWYDKWTD moment, as these are most likely to involve some kind of competing benefit, equipoise or lack of clarity about the best way forwards. Familiarity with basic ethical thinking skills will enable many difficult situations to be 'unpicked'. Practising these skills until they become second nature will mean that doctors can also discuss these issues openly with patients, who are often quite good at ethical reasoning themselves. Before any investigation or referral, the following issues need to be explored and clarified in the particular situation, and preferably discussed with the patient.

Non-maleficence: first do no harm

In the Networking Quadrant, consider how testing or referral might result in harm to the patient. Harms from the test itself (bruising? allergic reactions to contrast, X-ray exposure?), false positives or false negatives, the risks of finding irrelevant incidental findings all need to be factored in. Remember, 1/20 tests will fall outside two standard deviations, even if the patient is normal. Explaining this can be difficult, even when you are talking to other professionals. Many patients find it hard to understand why a cholesterol level of 5.5, although outside the usual 'normal' range, may require no action, and be considered 'normal for that individual' when the overall cardiovascular risk is low. Unless you are clear about how your results will impact on the patient, don't do the tests. Beware of triggering a cascade of interventions that may be irrelevant.

Beneficence: make sure that the referral is to benefit the patient (not simply treat the doctor's anxiety)

This means remaining aware of our tendency to bias of one kind or another (discussed in more detail in the Analysing Quadrant). Clinicians who have made a diagnosis of serious disease later than they would have liked can easily develop a tendency to lower their thresholds for investigating for that condition, even where that may increase the potential harm to the individual patient. Missing a subarachnoid haemorrhage or meningitis may not be preventable by over-referring many patients for unnecessary scans or invasive, risky tests. Clinicians are usually acutely aware of the opinions of others and seek to be seen to be doing the right thing. We feel that action is preferred to inaction, however, and clinicians should remain aware that most referrals have a cost/hazard of some kind, whether it is a sharp needle for a blood test, inconvenience or an escalating round of tests, some of which have real potential harms attached (e.g. perforation when doing an endoscopy).

Autonomy: how will this action increase the patient's autonomy?

Converting a well woman, with regular periods and a few spots, into someone who has a diagnosis of polycystic ovarian syndrome that doesn't require treatment is not necessarily doing her a service. Many screening tests, such as mammograms, prostate-specific antigen (PSA) screening and cervical cytology, have the potential to diagnose early irrelevant and non-progressive conditions. This may give rise to much anxiety and potentially unnecessary treatment, and therefore compromise the patient's ability to be healthy and autonomous.

Justice and fairness

However much we would prefer to treat all patients with the maximum that medical science allows, the fact is that resources are limited. NHS resources are finite and dictated by what parliament, elected in a democracy, is willing to allocate to the Department of Health. The allocation of resources is the business of the commissioning organisations of the NHS, which are currently Clinical Commissioning Groups, but which have been Primary Care Trusts, Commissioning Groups and other organisations in the past, and it is likely that commissioning will be undertaken by new bodies in the future. To be fair to everyone, there are guidelines about the nature and duration of many types of treatment, especially cosmetic or expensive treatments or those that have limited success rates, for example some third-line oncology treatments, IVF and so on.

Managing situations such as those described above can give rise to the feeling of WDYDWYDKWTD because patients' emotions run high, they may be very persistent and not take 'no' for an answer. Clinicians will often feel sympathetic to the patient's predicament.

In this situation clinicians must be clear about what their options are. All districts will have a process for dealing with 'Individual Funding Requests' (IFRs). These have been called Exceptional Funding Requests, Effective Use of Resources requests or Extra Contractual Referrals in the past and will doubtless change their name again in the future. Doctors should be able to weigh up the ethics of such situations quickly, working through the main ethical principles of beneficence, non-maleficence, justice and autonomy, and consider how they may apply to the patient concerned. Referring the patient onwards (hoping someone else will make the decision and break the bad news) without discussing the likely outcome beforehand is a 'dysfunctional way out' that may harm the doctor–patient relationship.

When in such a WDYDWYDKWTD situation, combine advocacy for the patient, tempered with realism about what is actually likely to be funded by the local health economy. In the NHS we face these issues very directly as all patients have free access, and are subject to the same constraints. In health services where patients pay, the fee payers and doctors tend not to be directly concerned about the patients who are deprived of treatment due to poverty, and who therefore are not even in the clinic at all.

Clinicians should be familiar with the local processes and guidelines to be able to give accurate information to patients. Letting a patient enter an IFR process with the impression that this will automatically get her the funding can risk harming her; all too often funding will be refused.

So what should the clinician do now? First, the skills of the Negotiating Quadrant will help here, to clarify the patient's views and what he hopes for, and to inject a note of realism. Second, every doctor should be aware of the processes for applying for such funds in her area and fill in the form with as much detail as possible if requested to. Psychological distress is not deemed a reason for allocating funding in most situations.

How might things go better for Ms Emerald and Mrs Pearl?

Dr Hawthorne explains to Ms Emerald that the aesthetic surgeon was in error in thinking that the NHS will pay for breast reduction and nipple surgery. The breasts are normal and operating on normal tissue means the risks will outweigh the benefits. A request for exceptional funding will be refused. If Ms Emerald insists the doctor could complete a request form for funding, including the information that he has counselled her against having surgery to normal organs.

Mrs Pearl has got exceptional circumstances and a request for exceptional funding may result in funding for another round of IVF. However, most funding panels will take into account how many private cycles of IVF have been tried because success rates will diminish with subsequent cycles anyway. Mrs Pearl will have to wait and see. Meanwhile Dr Hawthorne can help her to start to prepare for a life without children of her own; will she consider adoption or accept things as they are?

Other exceptional circumstances relate to the vulnerability of certain groups in society. Clinicians facing the care of those addicted to drugs or alcohol, homeless people, especially young people who 'sofa surf', or unkempt street dwellers may 'not know what to do'. Simply being aware that asylum seekers, Travellers, ex-prisoners or those with intellectual disability have special needs and knowing where to access the appropriate information will be helpful. Doctors often see health and medicine in isolation, whereas there are extensive networks beyond health that can give advice about many of these issues. A useful starting point can be found in the book *Working with Vulnerable Groups*, details of which can be found in the resources list at the end of the Networking section (see p. 98).

Continuing care after referral

Mrs Silver comes to see Dr Hawthorne, whom she knows well. A few weeks ago she was referred for a cholecystectomy after a scan showed gallstones.

'How did the gallstone op go?' asks Dr Hawthorne cheerfully. 'I thought you would know', replies Mrs Silver. 'They found an inoperable cancer at the time of the operation. The surgeon told me to come and see you to organise some palliative care.' Ouch. It is hard to recover from this situation in a consultation, although if the patient knows and trusts her doctor already it might be easier.

Dr Willow referred Mr Topaz into hospital urgently, suspecting urinary sepsis. Mr Topaz has insulin-dependent diabetes and was febrile, confused, hypotensive and generally weak when he went in. His daughter telephones Dr Willow saying, 'Please will you tell the ward staff to give him his insulin! Its 3 p.m. now and he has not had any insulin since yesterday. The ward staff will not listen to me because they say he has not given them permission to talk to me about his condition.'

Our care for our patients does not come to an end when we refer them to others; this is especially so in general practice. However, even in hospital work it must be clear who has responsibility for the patient. Is the referral for an opinion only or to take over the patient's management? Failure to consider these issues can lead to problems like the above or worse. Develop a system for tracking where your patients are, whether this is electronic or a notebook. Keeping track of those referred and the outcomes or management plans is a crucial skill. Only when you know for sure that they are in someone else's hands can you really relax.

How might it go better for Dr Willow, Dr Hawthorne, Mrs Silver and Mr Topaz?

Dr Hawthorne ensures that she keeps a close eye on all the incoming mail and is on top of her electronic filing, so that she can check on what happens after referrals. She checks the patient's notes before the consultation so that she is ready with the right attitude and approach, then the best plan can be evolved with the patient.

Dr Willow did call the ward and it turned out that Mr Topaz has been transferred between wards, but that his notes had not caught up with him, so the nurses were unaware of his diabetes. He got his insulin. Dr Willow logged this incident as a Significant Event via his local patient safety system and on the National Patient Safety Agency log. By using these systems, such mishaps can become helpful learning for everyone.

References

1. Marinker M. *Medical Audit and General Practice.* London: Wiley-Blackwell, 1990.
2. Marinker. M. *The End of General Practice.* Bayliss Lecture. London: RCP, 1994.
3. Irvine G, Holden J. The time-efficiency principle: time as the key diagnostic strategy in primary care. *Family Practice* 2013; **30(4)**: 386–9.
4. Buckman R. Breaking bad news: why is it still so difficult? *British Medical Journal (Clinical Research Ed.)* 1984; **288(6430)**: 1597–9.

Resources

Kurtz S, Silverman J. *Skills for Communicating with Patients.* Oxford: Radcliffe Medical Press; 2004.

Chapter 8

The clinical setting, assessment and teaching methods for uncertainty in the Networking Quadrant

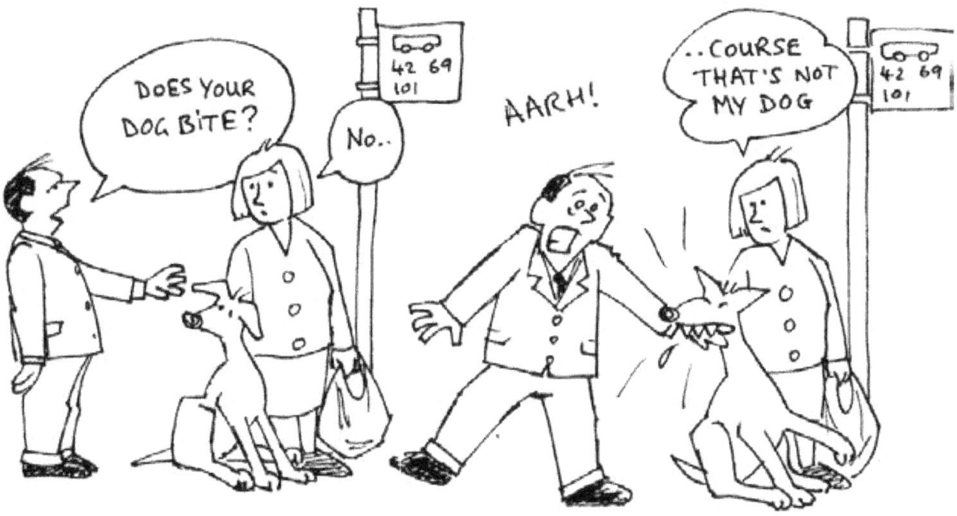

DOES YOUR DOG BITE?
No..
42 69 101
AARGH!
..COURSE THAT'S NOT MY DOG
42 69 101

Effective work in the Networking Quadrant means making sure to ask the right questions of the right people at the right time.

This chapter considers:

- how clinical settings can help the management of uncertainty in the Networking Quadrant
- assessment and teaching methods for uncertainty in the Networking Quadrant.

How clinical settings can help the management of uncertainty in the Networking Quadrant

Doctors now work in a very complex arena. The array of tests, investigations and specialty referral possibilities is huge. Moreover, with the increased fragmentation of the NHS and a multiplicity of providers, it becomes more complex every week. So the settings in which doctors work need to provide accurate and useful information about the network; there is plenty of generic good-quality information available on the internet about referral guidelines, what tests do, and so on. Places where doctors work need to have clear systems for capturing what the network can do locally. Intranets/links to relevant websites covering locally available services should be familiar to all doctors.

Furthermore, in secondary care settings, where referrals back to general practice are commonplace, specialist doctors could recognise that they are really asking the GP concerned for an opinion about the condition in question, rather than directing the referral. If an ENT surgeon says, 'Get a referral to a dermatologist from your GP' she may be expressing her own discomfort with a condition that a GP would be happy to manage without specialist dermatology input. Phrasing such back to GP referrals in terms of 'getting GP advice' allows the GP to use his own expertise and understanding of how the referral network works in primary care.

Organisations and teams can facilitate proper discussion prior to referral; investigation, referral practices, the harms and benefits of referral, and whether referral or investigation are needed at all should all be open to scrutiny. This is especially necessary at induction of juniors and in general practice. The skills required to construct an effective referral or clinic letter should be acknowledged and practised in all settings. Building relationships between referrers and other specialist services can make informal advice more easily available and result in more effective referrals.[1]

Assessment and teaching methods for uncertainty in the Networking Quadrant

Knowledge of the networks available and how to use them effectively can be assessed by asking juniors making referrals to consider alternatives, to establish informal links with providers to get information and advice without referral and by teaching what content is required in referral letters. All doctors should understand how the 'effective use of resources policy' works in their area and be able to explain confidently to patients why commissioners have chosen to allocate funds in particular ways. Money spent on one service is effectively removed from another. All clinicians should be able to see this wider picture and not only fight for their own corner.

Skills can be assessed with audits of referral letters, comparing what is requested with the outcome achieved, ensuring all the relevant information is included. Do letters to other clinicians contain clear statements of the reason for and purposes of referral? The skills needed to write useful clinical letters to GPs are also part of the Networking Quadrant.

All learners should be proficient in identifying the ethical conflicts and constraints in any situation, so that when faced with a novel or difficult situation they have the ethical thinking tools at hand to work through the decision (i.e. replacing a wish for certainty of outcome with certainty of process).

Learners could also debrief situations where referral or investigation has caused harm to the patient (remembering that harm may be physical, psychological or social).

Holding uncertainty and anxiety isn't easy. Some research suggests that the selection of medical students favours those who do not tolerate uncertainty or ambiguity well (see Part III 'Mapping the psychology of uncertainty'). In training settings, leaders can promote and model attitudes that identify, tolerate and even welcome ambiguity and flexibility. Clinicians need to accept the skilled management of anxiety as everyone's business. Thinking ethically and understanding how resource constraints operate is a professional duty. Saying to the patient, 'The CCG won't fund this, which is terrible' may harm the patient.

Box 8.1: Examples of harm caused by network misuse or overuse

Doctors in training could be asked to look out for other such situations they encounter.

A patient in the final stages of lung cancer looks pale and has low blood pressure. The doctor does a blood count, finds that the haemoglobin is 7, and admits the patient for a possible transfusion. The patient then dies in casualty. Holding skills and discussing with relevant colleagues could have enabled the patient to die in her preferred place: at home.

A 35-year-old man with many work worries comes complaining of a funny feeling in his abdomen. Although, clinically, anxiety is the diagnosis, he is referred for an ultrasound that shows a harmless renal cyst. He becomes even more anxious and worries he has really got renal cancer. He insists on a urology referral, increasing the wait for other patients, has a repeat scan (wasting resources) and remains anxious. His work stress is not addressed properly.

References

1. Foot C, Naylor C, Imison C. *The Quality of GP Diagnosis and Referral.* London: King's Fund, 2010, www.kingsfund.org.uk/sites/files/kf/Diagnosis%20and%20referral.pdf accessed [accessed 16 July 2015].

Resources for the Networking Quadrant

Crossley T. *I Don't Know What it is but I Don't Think it's Serious.* London: RCGP, 2008.

Gill P, Wright N, Brew I (eds). *Working with Vulnerable Groups: a clinical handbook for GPs.* London: RCGP, 2014.

Silverman J, Kurtz S, Draper J. *Skills for Communicating with Patients.* (3rd edn). Abingdon: Radcliffe Medical Press, 2013.

The Negotiating Quadrant

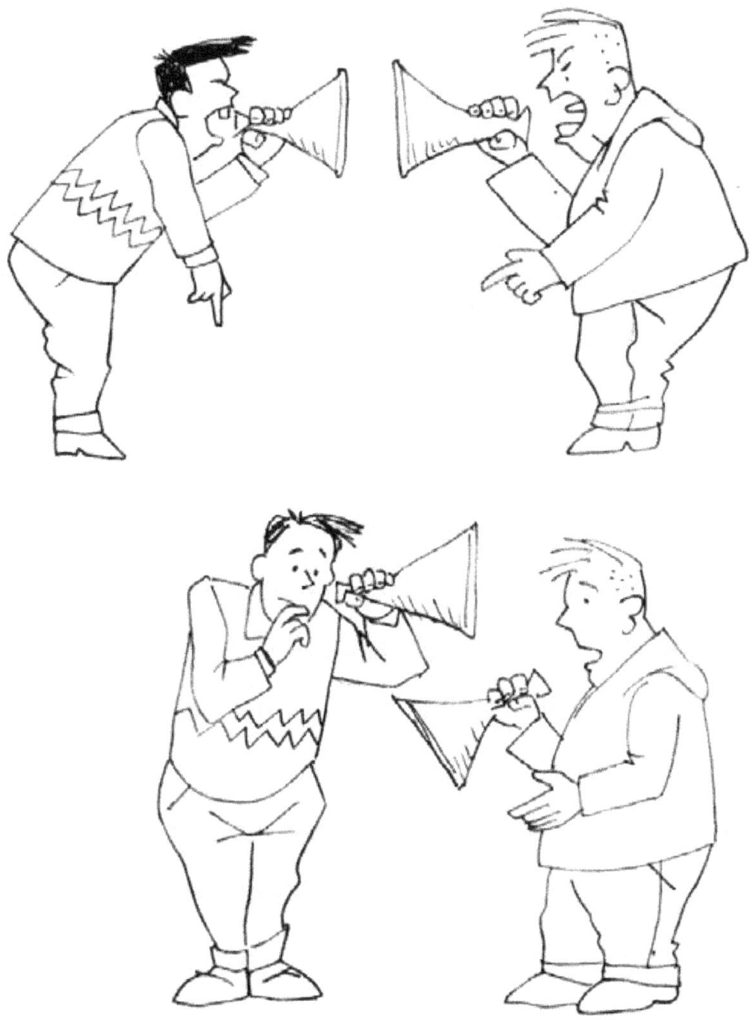

If the Analysing and Networking Quadrants have yielded a complete working diagnosis, or even one that is 'good enough', then most clinicians will concentrate on arranging the right care, assuming that the next steps will be clear. This chapter concentrates on those situations where getting the right treatment into place is not so straightforward.

Chapter 9 is an introduction to uncertainty in the Negotiating Quadrant and also discusses 'dysfunctional ways out'. **Chapter 10** works though examples of common WDYDWYDKWTD situations in the Negotiating Quadrant, explaining 'functional ways through' common problems by identifying the right skills needed for the right situation. **Chapter 11** explores how the clinical setting can help to deal with uncertainty in the Negotiating Quadrant, and suggests assessment and teaching methods.

The key skills in the Negotiating Quadrant are:

- explaining
- negotiating
- talking about risk
- shared decision making
- coping with 'Why don't you … ?' 'Yes, but …'
- motivational interviewing/behaviour change
- engaging with complex problems
- managing 'non-medical' problems
- coping with psychosocial issues in the doctor–patient relationship.

Chapter 9

Introduction to uncertainty in the Negotiating Quadrant

> Seek first to understand and then be understood.
>
> Stephen R. Covey[1]

This chapter focuses on the skills needed to negotiate successful treatment plans with patients. It covers:

- an introduction to uncertainty in the Negotiating Quadrant
- 'dysfunctional ways out' of uncertainty in the Negotiating Quadrant: common pitfalls.

An introduction to uncertainty in the Negotiating Quadrant

This Quadrant concerns the situation where one clinician and one patient are interacting, without referral or team-working being a major feature; the diagnosis is already known but the management gives rise to a feeling of 'I don't know what to do!' This may happen when a management plan preferred by either clinician or patient is impossible to achieve, not available, not acceptable, not understood or not carried out by either party. Perhaps most commonly, a proposed management plan is refused or poorly adhered to by the patient. This situation is frustrating for clinicians and patients alike. Patients may feel that their concerns and needs are poorly understood and clinicians feel that their best efforts are pointless if the patient does not 'cooperate' with the treatment plan. Clearly, all kinds of adverse outcomes can follow if patients do not get the best care for their particular problems. Frustration or conflict can make for unpleasant consultations, which may be followed by complaints, or by either party giving up, or withdrawing from parts of the treatment process. This leaves the patient without follow-up, or with incomplete care.

Sometimes, decisions are not clear cut because of the patient's other health problems. For example, a patient with osteoarthritis may suffer a lot of pain, which is relieved by non-steroidal anti-inflammatory drugs (NSAIDs), such as ibuprofen. However, her doctor may not wish to endorse using this medication if the patient also suffers from high blood pressure, asthma or kidney disease, as all of these conditions can be made significantly worse by NSAIDs. Naturally, the patient wishes to be pain free and explaining the complexities of the prescribing issues can be difficult and lead to an impasse if the doctor and patient cannot agree on what to do next.

If there are two or more relevant diagnoses, particularly where the management of different diagnoses conflict (e.g. prednisolone is good for asthma but bad for diabetes), then the complexity that arises may make it even more likely that the doctor will feel that he 'doesn't know what to do'. Medical complexity requires great stamina from patients and a seeming ability to spin plates from doctors. This can be daunting and sometimes overwhelming (giving rise to the term 'heartsink' in some situations). Doctors will often take refuge in treating only one aspect of the patient's problem in isolation from the rest (perhaps by giving steroids while ignoring the effect on the diabetes). Negotiating uncertainty is often mixed in equal part with feelings of frustration and helplessness. Doctors can feel torn; if they respond with what they perceive as the 'correct' medical approach, conflict with patients and even complaints can follow, even if the doctor is recommending medically sensible treatment. The patient may feel that 'the doctor did nothing for me'. Explaining medical reasoning is not always as easy as it sounds and the patient may not accept the doctor's view. If doctors collude with patients, by concentrating on only what the patient wants, or if they focus on the emotional issues, they feel professionally compromised and fear the censure of their peers for acting in non-standard ways, for example by not following guidelines strictly. Sometimes patients are critical if a treatment that seems straightforward to them is not forthcoming for complex medical reasons, or because it is not funded.

'Dysfunctional ways out' of uncertainty in the Negotiating Quadrant: common pitfalls

Most clinicians will recognise the 'dysfunctional ways out' of these uncomfortable situations.

Deferring the decisions to another time, place and preferably another doctor

Oh yes, we have all been there. After getting stuck, trying and failing to get an effective management plan in place, we say, 'Well let's do some more tests and you can come back next week [when I am on holiday]' or to the 'follow-up clinic in four months', or 'I will refer you to see Dr Clever' (which will get you out of my hair for a bit). Of course the next doctor is unfamiliar with the patient, struggles with the same issue and may take the same (or another) 'dysfunctional way out'. A 'collusion of anonymity' occurs, when the patient may bounce from one specialist to another with nobody taking responsibility for the patient as a person. These kinds of issues are explored in the fascinating books by Enid and Michael Balint.[2,3]

Transferring the responsibility entirely to the patient, also known as 'blaming the patient'

This often happens when doctors' suggestions are not as enthusiastically taken up by patients as we would like. So patients who do not lose weight, or who don't collect their repeat prescriptions, get a label of 'non-compliant'. The doctor may explain the risks and then effectively shrug her shoulders, withdraw and say, 'It is really your decision.'

Blaming the system

If the doctor is not sufficiently aware of how to use his local health resources he may blame others for the difficulty, saying something like 'Well I would prefer to refer you but I am not allowed to because they are trying to save money.' Although this unites the doctor and patient against the system, it also fails the patient who is not being helped to come to terms with reality. The clinician is not facing the gap in his skills either, skills that could perhaps enable him to care for the patient in the same setting, without unnecessary referral.

Conflict and arguments

Sometimes doctors and patients are simply diametrically opposed.

Patient: *I want you to give me some Valium.*
Doctor: *No!*

If the patient leaves with an understanding of the limitations of the situation, all may be well. However, it is more likely that there will be a conflict, stand-off or argument that leaves both parties feeling dissatisfied and upset. When conflict has been ineffectively handled by the clinician, complaints may follow. These are time consuming and demoralising for all concerned.

'Why don't you ... ?' 'Yes, but ...'

Sometimes patients are distressed and asking for help, but seem to turn down every offer. This is the familiar game of 'Why don't you … ?' 'Yes, but …', which some doctors and patients play to the bitter end (and the end usually is bitter).

Trying but failing to share the decision making with the patient

The doctor tries to involve the patient in a complicated or less than clear-cut decision, and the patient retorts by saying, 'You are the doctor, you decide.' If there is equipoise in the decision, or where the decision depends on the patient's own values and attitudes ('Should I have a termination of pregnancy, doctor?'), the doctor may feel overburdened or ill prepared for what can seem a big responsibility.

References

1. Covey S. *The Seven Habits of Highly Effective People*. New York, NY: Simon & Schuster, 2005.
2. Balint M. *The Doctor, His Patient and The Illness*. London: Churchill Livingstone, 2000.
3. Balint E, Norell J. *Six Minutes for the Patient: interactions in general practice consultation*. London: Tavistock, 1976.

Chapter 10

Functional ways through uncertainty in the Negotiating Quadrant

Being able to smoothly negotiate a management plan, which is both medically sensible, and practically feasible for the patient, is no mean feat. Many clinicians spend so much time on the initial information-gathering part of the interview that the second half of the consultation is relatively neglected.[1] When explaining works well, the doctor remains focused on the patient, engages in dialogue rather than instruction and is able to incorporate the patient's thoughts and feelings into the discussion; the plan is then truly shared. Part of the problem is that not all patients want to be involved in decision making to the same degree; people want different amounts of information and may understand it in different ways. We often assume that we have to reach a final plan in a single consultation, especially in secondary care where it may not be possible to see the patient again. This may be too ambitious, yet sometimes the skills needed to manage the decision making in a more timely fashion are lacking. This can work both ways: a woman who has thought hard about her problems, read things up on the internet and talked things over with her GP and her family may be ready to make a decision about having a hysterectomy at her first clinic visit, and may resent being told to 'go away and think it over'. The skills needed to resolve these issues are the subject of this chapter, which covers:

- examples of common WDYDWYDKWTD situations in the Negotiating Quadrant
- clarifying 'functional ways through' common problems by identifying the right skills needed for the right situation.

In summary the skills needed are:

- explaining
- negotiating
- talking about risk
- shared decision making
- 'Why don't you ... ?' 'Yes, but ...'
- motivational interviewing/behaviour change
- engaging with complex problems
- managing 'non-medical' problems
- psychosocial issues in the doctor–patient relationship.

Explaining

Mrs Beryll develops post-coital bleeding and has an abnormal smear. Colposcopy and biopsy show a cancer. She is shocked by this and says that she doesn't want to have any treatment, or see a specialist or go back to the hospital, and she fails to attend several appointments. She comes to Dr Alder saying, 'Please write me a letter for my homeopathy practitioner. She says she has got effective treatment for me.' Dr Alder is pretty sure that the cancer will respond to conventional treatment and is not sure what to do as Mrs Beryll is adamant she will not go to hospital for treatment. They go round in circles.

If you are reaching an impasse in the Negotiating Quadrant, consider first if your explanation is good enough. Successful explanations share the clinical findings with the patient, in a way that enables the doctor and patient to move towards a shared understanding of what needs to happen next. Explanations must be adequate, relevant, understandable and appropriate. All explanations need to begin with knowledge of *where the patient is coming from* to start with. What do they know, fear or anticipate already? What is important to them? Listening for and acting on what the patient is communicating about their 'lifeworld'[2] leads to improved dialogue and more effective planning of care. As Stephen Covey says, 'Seek first to understand, then be understood.'[3]

An *adequate* explanation will cover all the key findings and issues, whereas a *relevant* explanation will ensure that it refers to the patient's own worries and concerns, *even if these are different from the doctor's concerns or views.* Easily understood explanations are free of jargon, technicalities and acronyms, and use short sentences, with pauses for the patient to respond. Language is important; clearly it helps if the clinician and patient speak enough of each other's language to be understood. Using an interpreter can make a huge difference if there is not enough shared language. However, the effective use of language in explanations goes far beyond this. Communicating well will also mean matching the style of the patient's language, the metaphors they use, placing words like 'but' and 'when' to helpful effect. Matching the patient's own language style can be surprisingly effective. There are some examples given in Box 10.1.

Appropriate explanations must refer to the patient's own health beliefs, his own attitudes and values, and what is important to *him*. This means that explaining must necessarily be a dialogue not a lecture and should always include phrases such as:

- 'What is your own response to that?'
- 'How does that fit with the concerns you mentioned earlier on?'
- 'What do you make of what I have been saying?'
- 'What questions have you got at this stage?'
- 'How did you come to be so worried about … ?'
- 'What are your questions now?'

Note that these are all OPEN questions or statements. A closed question – such as 'Did you understand all that?' – will usually receive the answer 'yes', even if the patient is still mystified, as all too often patients don't like to challenge doctors. If this part of the consultation is not going well, it is often because the doctor doesn't really understand the patient's point of view, or does not take it into account fully. Attending carefully to your explanation and linking it clearly to what the patient is thinking about is often enough for things to move on.

To learn more about this subject, see *Skills for Communicating with Patients* by Suzanne Kurtz and Jonathan Silverman.[1] Their chapter on 'Explanation and planning' is full of evidence-based ways to do this better.

Box 10.1: Using language effectively in explanations

- **Ensure rapport**: make eye contact, smile, have an internal attitude of goodwill and desire to help the patient.
- Use effective language in explanations.
- Use '**positive language**' when explaining examination findings or results. Saying 'I can't find anything wrong with your chest' can make the patient think you are too incompetent to find the problem! Instead say, 'Your chest is healthy and the breath sounds are normal.'
- This will be even better if linked to the **patient's own concerns**. 'Your heart and lungs sound healthy, so it is good news that the pneumonia you were concerned about has not occurred.'
- Does the patient want **small chunks or large chunks**? Listen to how the patient answers questions. Does she use a lot of detail or prefer a view of the larger picture? Match the patient's style in your explanation.
- Use '**but**' effectively. Place the thing you want the patient to remember AFTER the 'but'. Compare the following:
  - 'This tablet will give you much less pain from your periods, BUT it can cause nausea, tummy pain and bleeding in a few patients.'
  - 'This tablet can cause tummy pain and bleeding in a few patients BUT it will give you much less pain from your periods.'

  The second example will enhance the effect of the medication more than the first.
- Place '**when**' effectively. Compare the following:
  - 'It is good for your health that you cut down on your cigarettes, and better if you stop altogether.'
  - 'It is good for your health that you have cut down on your cigarettes; when you stop altogether you will feel even better.'

  The positive language in the second example is much more encouraging and subtly nudges the patient into becoming an ex-smoker some time soon.

Note: see David McDonnell's book *How to Communicate Basically Brilliantly*[4] for more ideas about using language effectively.

How might things work out better for Mrs Beryll?

Using explaining skills and starting by understanding what Mrs Beryll already knows about her condition, Dr Alder discovers that she isn't really aware of the fact that cancers have different stages. Mrs Beryll thinks all cancers mean you die within a few months. She watched her mother die from bowel cancer and she would rather not have invasive treatment, which she sees as mutilating. Dr Alder also discovers that she won't go to the oncology service because her sister-in-law works there. 'My ex-husband was furious when I left him because of the violence and I am afraid she will see me at the hospital and tell him I am there and that he will start trying to get to the children.' This gives the doctor a different perspective on Mrs Beryll's thoughts. A plan is negotiated, using the negotiating skills outlined in the next section.

Negotiating

Amber is a 16-year-old girl studying Music, Media Studies and English at a local college. She was discovered to have coeliac disease after a period of diarrhoea and weight loss. Since starting at her new college, she has been increasingly reluctant to see the dietician. Her mother brings her to see Dr Elm and complains that Amber eats takeaway pizza during the day and often refuses to eat the special gluten-free bread her mum gets from the pharmacy. 'It's disgusting!' says Amber. When Dr Elm explains the dangers of eating gluten for her long-term health, Amber grunts and simply spends the time on her mobile phone while her mother gets more angry and frustrated.

If you and the patient agree on what needs to be done, there is no problem. The WDYDWYDYWTD situation arises when the doctor has a plan but the patient is unwilling or unable to follow that plan, or may not agree with the doctor's priorities at all. Sometimes the patient's wishes are unrealistic or not feasible. Being able to negotiate a 'win–win' situation doesn't mean being manipulative, but uses the pragmatic and ethical considerations that you use in all consultations. Begin by understanding what the patient is thinking. Clarify the issues at stake *for the patient*, summarise her position and what you might be able to offer. Identifying common ground ('We are both keen to make sure you enjoy college fully') and looking for shared goals and common interests will build the relationship with the patient and open up areas for discussion. Ensure that you listen carefully to what she says, summarising to show you have listened and understood. Check this explicitly. There may be some small issues on which you can reach agreement (for example, with Mrs

Beryll, 'I can certainly write to your homeopath, as such approaches often work well, alongside more conventional treatments'). This creates a positive framing for the discussion about things where you and the patient might not agree.

Continue to summarise what you have agreed to/achieved so far, remaining positive, respectful and calm. Isolate things that may be difficult and refer back to things you have agreed to already. Be prepared to look for a *less than ideal situation* if it means some progress can be made. Don't stick too rigidly to your own point of view, as you may need to change your direction a bit to help the patient move towards his own reasonable and important goals.

How the negotiation might go with Amber

Dr Elm empathises with Amber and her mother about how difficult coeliac disease can be to manage, and then negotiates that mum waits outside so Amber can be seen alone. Initially tentative, Amber soon warms to her theme when Dr Elm listens in a non-judgemental way. Her mum is always on her case, she hates being different from other people all the time and isn't sure how to tell her new friends at college that she can't eat what they eat. Dr Elm offers to ask the dietician specifically about easy ways to choose safe food from takeaways with her friends. Dr Elm also offers information from the Coeliac UK website (www.coeliac.org.uk) about managing coeliac issues when travelling or with friends. A relationship has been built and Amber agrees to see Dr Elm again to review how she is managing. 'Can I come on my own next time?' she asks. Dr Elm agrees to negotiate this with Amber's mother and a way forwards gradually emerges.

Remember it's good to be creative and flexible; guidelines are not tramlines. It is appropriate and necessary to tailor things to the individual with flexible solutions ('So you don't like taking a lot of tablets. Shall we see which tablets come in suitable combinations?'). If you understand what is important to the individual patient, you can harness her beliefs and attitudes to help negotiate a plan. Try to identify whether you are discussing the past (this is what has always happened before), the present (constraints, priorities) or the future (if I do this, what will happen?). Use the perspective that the patient is most concerned with, exploring assumptions overtly (see Table 10.1).

Table 10.1: What matters to a patient (rather than what is the matter with the patient) – illustrative examples

	Examples of patients' concerns	*Clinicians' responses*
Relating to the past		
Last time this happened I had a bad experience that I am fearful of repeating.	Last time I felt like this I ended up in hospital with pneumonia. The last ward I was on was horrible. I will not go back.	That's a natural worry; let us make a plan to monitor you carefully for any changes in your health. Perhaps a different hospital would suit you better? Or 'I know standards have improved'.
Relating to the present		
There is a lot going on for me at the moment. I cannot do what the doctor is suggesting.	My husband has dementia and gets agitated if I am not there. I have just got a new job and I cannot afford to take time off.	Referral for a carer's assessment could help us identify some suitable sources of help for you. Your job is vital, so let's try to work out how to do this with the least disruption for you.
Relating to the future		
What is going to happen to me? Will the care offered me be suitable?	I hate taking tablets and don't want to end up like my dad on 20 different medicines. If I do not have the knee surgery will I end up crippled?	Let's try and minimise tablets and find some non-drug approaches that could help you. Perhaps a structured decision aid could help you to think this one through?

How the negotiation might go with Mrs Beryll

Understanding her reluctance to attend the local hospital, Dr Alder offers to refer Mrs Beryll to a suitable hospital in a neighbouring town, and explains that at this early stage the cancer discovered will have a much better outlook than if left untreated. This will offer her a much longer life than her mother could have expected with a late diagnosis. Mrs Beryll's own children won't have to experience what she herself went through, watching her mother suffer. Mrs Beryll agrees to see a different specialist and gets her treatment. The doctor does also write a letter for the homeopath as Mrs Beryll finds that treatment comforting and supportive.

If you find negotiating difficult, seek out more detailed information from the sources cited at the end of this chapter.

Shared decision making

What matters *to* the patient is as important as what is the matter *with* the patient. This section considers how we can incorporate this insight into caring for the patient in situations where, initially, there may seem to be a WDYDWYDKWTD situation. Failure to understand patients' preferences as well as their illnesses has been termed the 'silent misdiagnosis'.[5]

Mrs Limestone has rheumatoid arthritis for which she has been put on NSAIDs and a course of steroids. She also has hypertension and mild chronic kidney disease. She smokes heavily and gets indigestion. The NSAIDs put her blood pressure up and affect kidney function, but Mrs Limestone says they are the only things that help her to sleep. They also allow her to keep moving in her busy job as a manager of a shop. Her rheumatologist wants to stop the prednisolone and put her on methotrexate. Mrs Limestone has read about chemotherapy on the internet and feels it will be too toxic. Can't she just have some more of the steroids that seem to help so much? Mrs Limestone and Dr Pine go round in circles, Dr Pine warning of the dangers of her current treatment, Mrs Limestone wanting to continue, because she feels the current approach is the only way to keep her job.

In many situations, agreeing a way forward with a particular individual is straightforward. In other situations this does not happen. This may be because:

- the patient does not accept the usual approach because he has different ideas
- there are several options of roughly equivalent predicted effects
- the effects of interventions are uncertain
- the situation is complex and the interaction of different factors (multiple drugs, multiple comorbidities) cannot be readily predicted.

How do doctors then share the decision effectively with the patient, without simply shrugging and passing off the responsibility? Here is a useful description of a good 'shared' decision: 'the quality of a clinical decision, or its patient-centeredness, is the extent to which it reflects the considered needs, values, and expressed preferences of a well-informed patient'.[6] It is not the doctor's values, needs or preferences that take priority, and yet the decision is shared, not simply passed over to the patient. Better outcomes follow when patients are involved in decisions.[7,8] The decisions that most need to be shared are those where there is an element of equipoise (i.e. the decision has significant and balanced pros and cons),[9] where the treatment may significantly interfere with elements of her life that the patient values, or where the usual approach (for example, major abdominal surgery for bowel cancer) is not acceptable to the patient. It follows that, to achieve effective shared decisions, we need to complete the following tasks.

Identify clearly the decision to be made

Clarify *how much* the patient wants to be involved. Identify the patient's *own priorities and preferences*, as well as what information she has already. Find out *what other information* she would like and what form it should take. Possibilities include a diagram, a decision tool or a Cates plot[10] that sets out the expected probability of various alternatives. Cochrane reviews are now including Summary of Findings tables, which compare the risks of an event in patients who receive treatment with the outcomes for those who do not receive treatment. These tables are not visual like Cates plots. It is helpful to have such resources easily available wherever decisions are being made with patients about their treatment.

Bringing the clinician and patient together to make a plan that is acceptable and feasible needs three phases. These have been termed 'team talk', 'option talk' and 'decision talk'.[9]

Team talk

This conveys the idea of the clinician and patient working together to get to the best answer for that individual. Ideally, the clinician and patient have developed a relationship in earlier consultations, or the earlier part of a consultation where a decision is being made. The 'team talk' should recognise the existence of alternative actions or options, including the patient's preferred ideas; the clinician seeks the patient's point of view actively, using open questions as in the explaining section.

Option talk

This refers to the clinician and patient working out together the possible benefits and harms that may result. Identify advantages/disadvantages from the *patient's* point of view. A jargon-free way to talk about this is to say, 'What would be your reasons to say "yes" to this option?' 'What would be your reasons to say "no" to this?' The clinician can explain her own reasons for her recommendation and clarify the patient's understanding of the clinician's reasoning. Benefits and harms may not simply be matters of physical health: impact on relationships, work, self-image and other health conditions or constraints may all come into the picture.

Decision talk

Finally, the patient's preferences are articulated and integrated into the final decision. The clinician does not stand back and say, 'You decide', but has a part to play in weighing things up. The clinician does have extra knowledge and understanding of what the benefits and harms may be and brings this to the discussion. The clinician has a responsibility to help the patient recognise what impact the benefits and harms could be for him. Simply giving patients information and asking them to make an 'informed choice' risks abandoning them to indecision or poor decisions, if factors are not weighed up appropriately.

Shared-decision discussions are easier if accurate information, including absolute risks, is readily to hand. Be prepared. In health, making 'no decision' is still a decision with consequences, as it effectively means taking the option of 'not doing anything'. If a decision is deferred, for example, to allow for a discussion with family members to take place, a specific time frame should be specified to ensure that the decision is actually made. Ensure that a relevant way of conveying the decision is in place; this may mean seeing the patient, speaking to her on the phone or the patient talking to your secretary. Make sure you have a failsafe system for chasing up decisions and recording them, with reasons, in the notes.

Remember that making decisions about care is not just about *effectiveness*, although doctors often focus on that. We also have to think about *preferences*, when plans have inherent risks and benefits, which for patients will always include *trade-offs* between different possibilities. For example, one patient may happily trade off having to go to the gym and do intensive physiotherapy against the need to take unpaid time off work. However, another individual may not wish to take time off work, preferring to trade off a better income against slightly more pain or a longer recovery time from an injury. Patients may value trade-offs very differently from doctors. Explicitly recognising and discussing the effects of a patient's preferences may be enough to create a way forward.

How might this decision go better with Mrs Limestone?
Dr Pine invites Mrs Limestone to identify some key goals. For her, being pain free, enough to work, is crucial. When Dr Pine talks about the rising blood pressure, it emerges that Mrs Limestone's mother was disabled for years after a stroke, and she wishes to avoid that risk as much as possible. The reasons for and against her various treatment options are discussed, in the light of these two core goals, and Mrs Limestone's priorities for care are examined. She decides to trade a temporary increase in pain, while the steroids are reduced, against a lower risk of stroke. Prednisolone is gradually reduced and replaced with methotrexate, and NSAIDs replaced with alternative analgesia. Mrs Limestone manages to stay at work, and takes her various treatments regularly.

Talking about risk

Mr Slate is 72 years old and has ischaemic heart disease, peripheral vascular disease and recurrent mild rectal bleeding from his piles (which have been treated but with mixed success). He has a mild, but chronic, thrombocytopenia, which the haematologists say needs no special treatment. He develops atrial fibrillation. Should he be anticoagulated to try to prevent a stroke? What if the treatment just causes him to bleed? His situation is less than clear cut because of the risk of bleeding from his low platelet count.

Modern medicine often seems to be more about risk management than the treatment of actual diseases. Making decisions about whether to anticoagulate a patient like Mr Slate, or at what level of blood pressure to treat hypertension, or cholesterol levels, is all about calculating the 'risk' and trying to explain that to patients. Decisions about chemotherapy and many other treatments are often couched in terms of relative risk, so we say things like 'with this treatment you are 30% less likely to have a heart attack'. Or, 'This treatment will halve your chances of recurrent breast cancer.' The newspapers are full of these relative risk reduction statistics because they look dramatic,

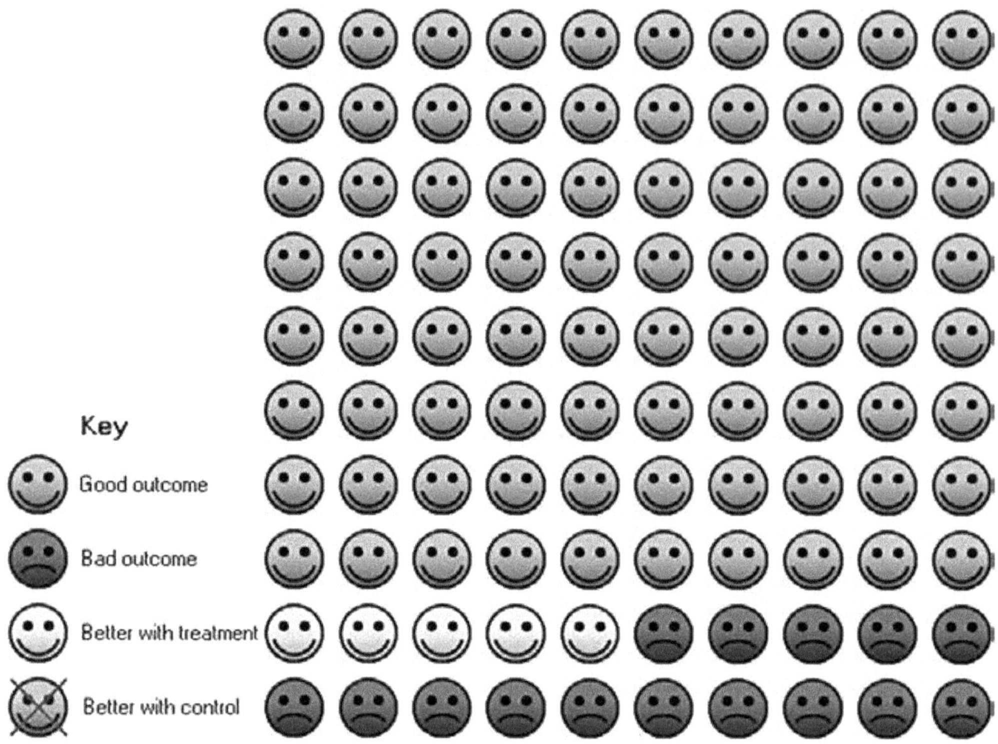

Figure 10.1: Cates plot

and seem easy to understand. However, when working with patients we should instead talk about *absolute risks* using natural frequencies. So, instead of talking about a 30% reduction in risk, this becomes:

> *Of 100 patients like you, 20 will have a heart attack or stroke in the next ten years. With treatment we can reduce that by a third so that means only 14 will have a stroke or a heart attack. Of course that means that 86 of the patients taking this drug will get no benefit and moreover 14 of those who take the drug for ten years will still have a heart attack.*

Patients faced with this sort of accurate information are better informed about the implications of the decision to take tablets or not. Cates plots[10] are one way to show this to patients but even simple decision trees are very helpful as long as risk is explained in ABSOLUTE not relative terms. Figure 10.1 is an example of a Cates plot.

How might this work out better for Mr Slate and Dr Sycamore?
Mr Slate and Dr Sycamore look at the Cates plots referring to anticoagulation with warfarin and look at the absolute risks for him. Using his CHA2DS2-VASc score it seems that the risk of anticoagulation is probably

less than the risk of bleeding. Warfarin will be easier to reverse if his low platelets trigger bleeding from some other precipitating cause (e.g. an injury) than the newer anticoagulants like dabigatran. In spite of this knowledge, Mr Slate reveals that he would prefer not to be anticoagulated until he comes back from a long anticipated trip to Ireland, to see his brother. 'I don't want to have to go to clinics there, doctor. It will mess up my visit.' Dr Sycamore agrees to arrange anticoagulation on his return, even though it is not his preferred outcome, but does take into account Mr Slate's thoughts and preferences.

Being confident with absolute risk and explaining it to patients is a key skill for doctors in all specialties. The books by Gigerenzer or Paling (see resources at the end of this section) make fascinating reading and will help to improve your confidence in explaining things.

'Why don't you … ?' 'Yes, but …'

Mr Crystal, aged 55, is overweight, smokes heavily and has been in hospital several times with chest pains of musculoskeletal origin. The practice nurse asks Dr Oak to see him because his HbA1c is borderline and he is at risk of developing diabetes. He won't change his diet or do any exercise. He wants a 'sick note to sign me off so I can go back to work next week'. He says he does not want to give up smoking, 'my only pleasure', and does not believe he is overweight. 'I do not eat that much', he comments. He did not take the diet advice leaflet the nurse got ready for him. Dr Oak gets a bit frustrated reiterating the same information as the nurse talked about, the consultation does not go well and as he leaves Mr Crystal is heard to say, 'Well that was a big waste of time.' The next HbA1c is in the diabetic range.

Impasse can occur in the negotiating part of the consultation when the doctor makes suggestions about management and the patient responds with, 'Yes, but', going on to explain why he can't do what the doctor asks.

Ever had this conversation?

Patient: *I want some help losing weight.*
Doctor: *We have an excellent weight management clinic here.*

Patient: *Yes, but I can't get time off work during the day except when I have holidays.*
Doctor: *Well we have locally sponsored cheap rates for evening weight loss support groups.*
Patient: *Yes, but I don't like going out at night.*
Doctor: *Well, I can recommend some good diet books.*
Patient: *Yes, but I can't afford to buy them.*

And it goes on until the doctor gives up, which allows the patient to take the view that her problem is really too difficult and she can't be expected to solve it. This is dysfunctional, although, in an odd way, satisfying for the patient who is able to let go of responsibility for dealing with her problem. If you want to understand the process more read *Games People Play* by Eric Berne.[11] In the consultation watch out for the 'Yes, but' line from the patient. After one round *stop making suggestions.* Instead, enquire what kind of approaches the patient had in mind, how was he proposing to proceed? This is the antidote but needs to be applied calmly, kindly and without trying to get one over on the patient.

How might this work out better for Mr Crystal and Dr Oak?
Dr Oak refrains from continuing the 'Why don't you ... ?' 'Yes, but ...' conversation with Mr Crystal. Instead he asks, 'How are you seeing your health at the moment?' Mr Crystal explains his relief at being able to go back to work. He has few friends and work gives him social contact. He often goes to the pub after work, which he really enjoys. The doctor empathises with this and builds some 'team talk' about wanting to help Mr Crystal remain well enough to be at work, and uses motivational interviewing skills to see what behaviour changes might be feasible for Mr Crystal.

Motivational interviewing/behaviour change

This issue commonly causes frustration or bad feeling between clinicians and patients, and often gives rise to the WDYDWYDKWTD question for clinicians. Clinicians identify changes that would benefit health in their patients, who find it hard or impossible to make those changes. When those important changes don't happen, clinicians can feel they 'don't know what to do'. This may be about common issues like weight loss or smoking that adversely affect many disease processes, and may lead to premature death or disability. Watching a patient you know well, drinking himself to death yet still consulting about his abnormal liver function tests, can be disturbing for clinicians. 'You must stop drinking!' the clinician feels like yelling, as the patient drags himself in, still smelling of beer, for another sick note.

Effective work here means changing the clinician's stance from that of director ('Your symptoms are caused by thyroid deficiency, and the effective treatment is …') to that of a well-informed guide, with the destination being chosen by the patient, not the clinician. This means a shift from 'telling' to listening, understanding where the patient is coming from and listening for, and using, the patient's own motivations to change. Encouraging 'change talk' from patients means working in collaboration, emphasising the patient's autonomy and building on her motivations for change. The skills needed are often referred to as motivational interviewing.

Motivational interviewing has been defined as 'A collaborative, person centred form of guiding, to elicit and strengthen the motivation for change.'[12]

This involves the clinician recognising that being in two minds (ambivalence) is an intrinsic part of the process of change. Helping the patient to identify her ambivalence, examine it and perhaps evolve it in a positive way builds the doctor–patient relationship. It moves towards mutual understanding and lets the doctor off the hook of having to 'always be right' and 'always be responsible'. The use of open questions, drawing out rather than imposing solutions, allows the doctor to come alongside the patient from her own point of view. Lasting change comes when patients discover their own reasons and motivation to do things differently.

Setting the agenda for change is the first step. Often there may be several changes to consider (should the patient try to lose weight, or stop smoking, or work to stick to the drug regime recommended by a specialist?). Clearly working on what is most important to the patient is likely to succeed better than working on something the individual sees as of little current significance.

Finding a patient-centred way to start talking about these issues is important. Start in a neutral way, for example with 'Where are you in your thoughts about your weight/drinking/smoking?'

The doctor will need to listen carefully to what the patient says to elicit evidence that change is something the patient is prepared to discuss. Then using the mnemonic OARS (see below) the doctor can start to elicit the patient's own motivations, and support these with suitable information and strategies.[13]

O = Open questions

The aim of open question in this situation is to understand the patient's position, listening for evidence of ambivalence or motivation through asking evocative questions and working sensitively with the answers. Expressing empathetic identification is key, builds the relationship and enables the doctor to pick up on cues about where the patient is in his thinking and planning. Help the patient to explore decisional balance by identifying benefits and downsides in the status quo: 'What do you like about smoking?' 'What are the benefits of drinking for you?' Affirming and recognising the gains will help doctor and patient to start to identify other ways to get the same benefits. Then explore any downsides again using positive language, 'Are there any downsides you can see?'.

A = Affirmation

Affirming, rather than opposing, the patient's point of view helps to keep the doctor alongside the patient, rather than in opposition. Accepting and understanding the patient's current position is, paradoxically, the best way to initiate change and overcome resistance. A comment like the following can help a patient feel supported rather than lectured: 'So, stopping smoking feels like it would be overwhelmingly difficult just now. That makes sense.'

Explore the patient's ability to change using decision scales:

- 'On a scale of 1–10 how **important** is it to you right now to (stop smoking)? How did you choose that position? What would make it a zero? … What would make it one or two grades more important than where you are at present?'
- 'On a scale of 1–10 explore how **confident** you are that change could happen. What would make you more confident?'

This helps to clarify motivation and blocks to change. If the motivation is low, how does she see the future if nothing changes? What could happen that would make this change more important in the future?

R = Reflection/rolling with resistance

This also known as 'resisting the righting reflex'. All clinicians tell people to stop smoking. However, only a few patients comply. Often they explain why they can't or won't make a change; clinicians carry on telling them what to do anyway. RESIST the reflex to tell the patient he has the wrong plan, roll along with it and stay alongside … agree with him. 'Yes, I can see that smoking offers you regular breaks from your difficult boss at work.' Encourage the patient to elaborate his thoughts and concerns, and use empathy to show that you really understand his position.

'For you it's more important to see your friend in the pub than it is to have better liver test results, so maybe this just isn't so important to you right now.' Then, you can use the 'What would make this a bit more important?' question to open up the discussion further.

S = Summarise

Summarising is an opportunity to build the relationship by showing the patient that you have really understood her position. You can also summarise any commitments she has made to changes, any agreements made about follow-up appointments and so on.

At all points in this dialogue eliciting the patient's point of view can lead to an opportunity to offer (rather than impose) information. For example: 'You are saying that you aren't confident that you could give up smoking even if you wanted to. Would you like some information about things that have helped other patients in your situation to become non-smokers?'.

Having shared relevant information, elicit the patient's reactions to and thoughts about that information: 'Where does that leave you now?'.

Being explicit about recognising the difficulties for a patient, and that maybe now is not the best time to change, can paradoxically help patients to change. This happens when patients feel accepted and understood, rather than in conflict with their clinician. This may seem troubling to doctors and nurses who are not used to handing over a measure of control to their patients. However, the improved relationship going forwards will often show that the patient is influenced by the clinician, even if that is further down the line.

The clinician will need to listen carefully, retain a strong input over the direction of the consultation and have the right information to share; however, the responsibility for change remains with the patient. Open-ended questions work better and a genuine curiosity to understand how it is for him will go a long way to build a relationship supportive enough to move things forwards.

Box 10.2: Some useful opening questions to help the conversation focus on behaviour change and the patient's motivation

- What changes would you most like to talk about?
- How important is it for you to change? How confident do you feel about changing?
- What benefits are you aware of? How do you see the downsides?
- What would make the most sense to you/work best for you?
- How might things be different if you … ? In what way … ?
- Where does this leave you now? It will be up to you to decide when and how to do it (emphasising the patient's freedom of choice) but I am wondering how do you see yourself succeeding with this?

Having this conversation with Mr Crystal is not going to be a one-off event. Building a supportive and positive relationship may require some time and doctors should try to construct continuity in their care so that the relationship can develop. Having information about services such as smoking clinics to hand can be helpful if there is a moment when the patient recognises that he would like more information.

How might things go better with Mr Crystal?

Dr Oak increases his understanding of Mr Crystal's social isolation and the pleasure he gets from being at the pub and at work. Dr Oak is affirming of this and Mr Crystal relaxes, recognising that he is not just going to be told off again.

Dr Oak asks if he is allowed to smoke at work, and Mr Crystal acknowledges that he doesn't smoke at work, which may offer a way to reducing his smoking. They discuss the reasons for and against stopping smoking, and Mr Crystal says he has tried before to stop but has always failed. His confidence is very low. Dr Oak empathises and says that if Mr Crystal finally decides to stop smoking he has some good information about techniques that have worked for other men of his age. Dr Oak explains how stopping is usually an iterative process that may take several attempts before success is achieved. Mr Crystal takes a leaflet about the smoking cessation clinic and how to access it. One step along the road to giving up smoking has been taken.

Engaging with complex problems

> Mr Granite is a 48-year-old man who is new to the practice. At his first appointment with Dr Juniper he produces a list of problems on his mobile phone. These include worries about occasional incontinence of urine and his urine 'looks funny at the weekends'. He has an eye condition that means he needs an urgent referral to the Eye Hospital for special contact lenses, has constant headaches, needs some more inhalers for his asthma, wonders why he is sneezing all the time, has aches in his arms and shoulders that mean he can't carry shopping, worries he may have got HIV from a 'sexual indiscretion' last week, has Type 2 diabetes and is grossly obese, which 'all came on from the shock of my sister dying in a car accident two years ago'. When Dr Juniper tries to say something, Mr Granite interrupts to say he especially wanted to mention that his friend, who is a top cardiac doctor, has recommended he takes propranolol to help his fear of flying, and he is going on holiday to Tunisia on a stag do next week, and does he need some vaccinations for that? When Mr Granite has been talking for ten minutes without stopping Dr Juniper feels overwhelmed and doesn't know what to do next.

Some conditions are complicated: arranging the treatment of end-stage kidney disease means organising dialysis, diets, financial benefits, the investigations for the transplant list, etc. However, there will be a protocol to help and a tick list to complete. Care gets much more difficult when things are *complex*, that is, where there are several morbidities, psychological issues and social problems with competing requirements. Managing such situations is sometimes easier for specialists who can say, 'I will just deal with my bit.' The GP faced with the list in Box 10.2 could be forgiven for feeling overwhelmed; the patient is probably feeling that way too. Finding a way to share this thought, creating a structure that helps to deal with the problem bit by bit, can help things. One helpful initial step is to make a mind map of the patient's issues with the patient contributing.

Draw a circle in the middle of a piece of paper with the patient's name in the centre. Draw lines out to circles representing the patient's problems, trying to put linked problems adjacent to each other. If the patient is taking a lot of drugs, then try to link each to the problem for which they are being taken. Use this information to generate a priority for today. Remain calm but firm in explaining that all the problems cannot be dealt with at once, even though they are all important.

When Mr Granite's problems are mapped out, some new connections may suggest themselves (are his STI worries and observations about his urine connected?), some connections that could have been overlooked are identified (his sister's death, obesity, Type 2 diabetes and anxieties), and some hazards highlighted (propranolol would be dangerous in a patient with asthma). In the initial confusing consultation these could easily have been missed; mapping them also provides a way to structure the discussions and may help both clinician and patient to feel less overwhelmed.

Such mapping also offers a way to use future consultations effectively: going through the problems one by one or in groups. Continuity is crucial here, to build a sound doctor–patient relationship and create the basis for effective decision making. Getting to know each other well will facilitate trust and understanding for both parties.

The clinical course of patients with complex comorbidities is rarely straightforward and will not be predictable in a linearly understandable way; many different issues will interact to produce the outcome. At times this will result in outcomes that feel more like chaos, as uncertainty increases and the degree of agreement between people about what should be done decreases. Acknowledging (perhaps even enjoying) the uncertainty that such non-linearity brings can help make such consultations more understandable, and sometimes release some creativity in the interaction.[14]

Mr Granite's mind map might look like Figure 10.2.

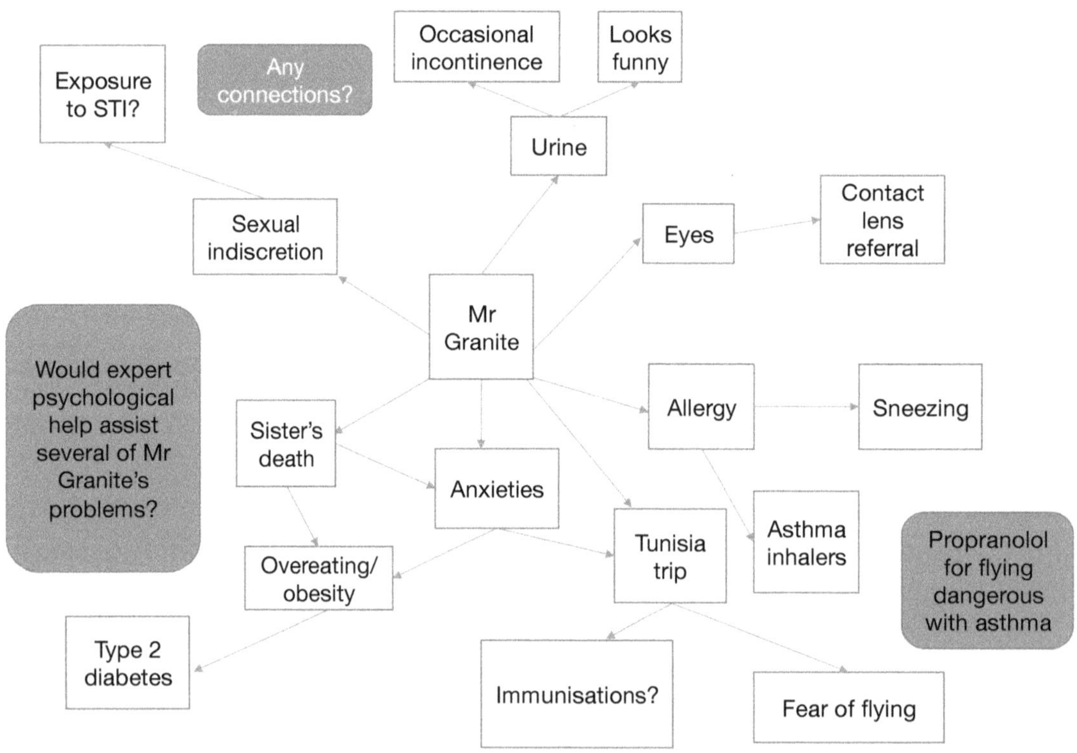

Figure 10.2: Mind map

Dealing with non-medical problems

Ms Opal is a 32-year-old woman with borderline personality disorder, who has previously self-harmed quite a lot. She is on antidepressant therapy and a small dose of zopiclone at night as required, recommended by her previous psychiatrist. She has completed several courses of psychotherapy and cognitive–behavioural therapy (CBT) and has recently been discharged from another CBT course. The psychiatry team has also discharged her. Ms Opal comes yet again complaining of feeling anxious, upset by a mix-up over her contract at her new job, and is in conflict with a neighbour about a noisy dog. 'I need some help!' she wails. Dr Hornbeam is now at a loss, having exhausted all the obvious avenues for helping Ms Opal.

BATHE the patient in empathy

Sometimes the WDYDWYDKWTD question arises when patients bring non-medical problems to clinicians and seem to want clinicians to help them manage the problem better. The patient in the above scenario has a defined mental health condition; however, this label will not help her deal with life's common problems. Another patient, usually managing her life easily, may come complaining that her children's school is too far away from her new house, that the stress of getting the children to school is too much, that the bus fares are too expensive now they have sold the car, etc. Realistically the doctor can do nothing about these issues even if completely empathetic about the upset it is causing the patient. A tool that is helpful here is called the BATHE technique, as developed by a family doctor in America. It is fully described in the useful book *The Fifteen Minute Hour*.[15] Think of this as 'BATHEing the patient in empathy'. It goes like this.

B = Background

Use open-ended and evocative questions to understand what the background to the problem is. Use empathic and specific comments to show the patient that you understand his predicament and empathise with it.

A = Affecting the patient

How is the patient feeling about the situation? What impact is this situation having on them/on others around them? Again use empathy to help the patients feel understood and supported.

T = What aspect is Troubling you the most?

This is a very helpful way to focus the conversation on something specific; as it is also the most troubling thing, this will focus on what is most important to the patient. It is quite common for patients struggling with many issues to say something like: 'There is no one thing. What is troubling me is that there are so many problems coming all at once!' An empathic comment, that it seems as if 'being overwhelmed is the most troubling thing', can often deepen rapport. This leads into:

H = Handling

This is as in, 'How are you handling this?' Or, 'How are you tackling this/ dealing with this/approaching this problem?' This helps the clinician to mobilise the patient's own resources and to endorse or support actions that she is taking. In the above example, when overwhelmed, strategies like making a list and doing one thing at a time seem simple and yet are valid ways to help the patient move forwards.

E = Empathy

The clinician needs to respond not only to the cognitive and decision-making parts, but also to the emotional experiences, feelings and relationship-building elements of the conversation.

Sometimes seeing a patient for long-term follow-up for intractable chronic disease may mean the clinician feels helpless and 'doesn't know what to do' or why the patient keeps coming back. Here a technique called the 'positive BATHE' can be useful to direct the conversation, emphasising positive experiences.[16] There is good evidence that focusing on positive emotions is beneficial for wellbeing. The 'positive BATHE' goes something like this:

- **B** = What is the **Best** thing that has happened this week/since we met?
- **A = Affect.** How did that feel? How can you account for that? How did it happen?
- **T = Thankfulness**. What are you most grateful for at the moment?
- **H = Happen**. How could you make those things happen more often/ more regularly?
- **E = Empathise/empowerment**. Give positive regard to what has been achieved. 'It is great you have managed to stay at work in spite of the difficulties', or 'I think the plan you have mentioned sounds really good and I am sure you will find a way to do it.'

Which is more appropriate, the BATHE or the positive BATHE?

With a relatively new patient or problem, BATHE will work best. If you are following up a patient or seeing him often with a chronic problem use the positive BATHE to promote empowerment and energy. Positive psychology research clearly shows that positive feelings and experiences release endorphins and are stimulating. Negative thoughts increase adrenaline, which affects bodily function adversely.

How this could go better for Ms Opal?

Ms Opal, who is 'post therapy', is likely to seek support from Dr Hornbeam for some time. Initially, using the BATHE technique Dr Hornbeam starts to build a supportive relationship and help Ms Opal find a way through. At follow-up appointments asking Ms Opal to notice anything good that happens and then doing the positive BATHE technique will help Dr Hornbeam to give a framework to the consultations. Dr Hornbeam feels less helpless in the continuing relationship.

Psychosocial issues in the doctor–patient relationship

Dr Hazel has recently coped with serious illness in a close family member, without taking any time off work. Things are better now. Mr Glass comes in insisting on a sick note because 'my mother-in-law's sister is unwell and I am too anxious to go to work'. Unconsciously the doctor may resent this suggestion; after all, Dr Hazel herself coped without time off work, didn't she? Dr Hazel says 'no' to a sick note, rather than fully exploring what the patient is experiencing. Mr Glass gets angry, storms out and immediately books an appointment with a more sympathetic colleague.

Remember we used that dreaded word 'metacognition' in the preface? Applying 'metacognitions' to the psychological issues between clinician and patient can help to identify how things are going awry. Unconscious psychological processes may interfere with the smooth progress of a consultation. Being self-aware can help. First, take note if something the patient says strikes a personal chord and seems irritating, unreasonable or gets a disproportionate emotional reaction. This may mean that there is something going on for the doctor, other than the surface meaning of the consultation.

The processes to be aware of include:

- transference: when the patient behaves towards you as she behaves elsewhere (someone who bullies her spouse may try to bully the doctor)
- counter-transference: when the doctor behaves towards the patient as if he was someone else (the doctor who was bullied at school either rolls over to bullying patients or over-reacts and is unnecessarily rigid)
- projection: when uncomfortable parts of the self are projected into others (Mr Granite may not acknowledge his own helplessness, but project that onto the doctor).

Some things that patients are experiencing are too painful to articulate. If being overweight makes you feel embarrassed and ashamed, you may just switch off when it is mentioned. Doctors and patients may both find certain subjects hard to talk about, such as domestic conflict or abuse, and tacitly avoid the clues and cues that show its presence. Often discussion with seniors, or a Balint group/Schwartz round-style discussion, is the best place to learn about these issues. Being able to recognise the gut feeling that all is not well will tell you some metacognition is needed. This is a key skill for doctors to develop. Knowing that you have to start a different thinking process creates more options and room for manoeuvre and may reduce doctors' stress.

How it could go better with Mr Glass
Dr Hazel makes a conscious effort to put her own experience aside and to try to understand Mr Glass. It transpires that his family members are not well off and the sick lady has no children. He is the only one with a car and feels that he should help out by taking his mother-in-law to see her sister in hospital. Although sympathetic, the doctor asks about the possible impact such absences will have on his employer/work. Mr Glass confesses that he is on a second warning for taking unpredictable time off. The doctor explains about financial help for bus fares to hospital, which the patient didn't know about, and offers a short sick note while things get organised.

References

1. Silverman J, Kurtz S, Draper J. *Skills for Communicating with Patients.* (3rd edn). Abingdon: Radcliffe Medical Press, 2013.

2. Barry CA, Stevenson FA, Britten N, *et al.* Giving voice to the lifeworld. More humane, more effective care? A qualitative study of doctor–patient communication in general practice. *Social Science and Medicine* 2001; **53(4)**: 487–505.
3. Covey S. *The Seven Habits of Highly Effective People.* New York, NY: Simon & Schuster, 2005.
4. McDonnell D. *How to Communicate Basically Brilliantly.* Lancaster: NLP Healthcare, 2013.
5. Mulley AG, Trimble C, Elwyn G. Stop the silent misdiagnosis: patients' preferences matter. *British Medical Journal* 2012; **345**: e6572.
6. Sepucha KR, Fowler JF Jr, Mulley AG Jr. Policy support for patient-centered care: the need for measurable improvements in decision quality. *Health Affairs* (Millwood) 2004; Suppl Variation: VAR54–62.
7. Levit LA, Balogh EP, Nass SJ, Ganz PA. *Delivering High-Quality Cancer Care: charting a new course for a system in crisis.* Washington, DC: National Academies Press, 2013.
8. Elwyn G, Frosch D, Thomson R, *et al.* Shared decision making: a model for clinical practice. *Journal of General Internal Medicine* 2012; **27(10)**: 1361–7.
9. Elwyn G, Edwards A, Kinnersley P, Grol R. Shared decision making and the concept of equipoise: the competences of involving patients in healthcare choices. *British Journal of General Practice* 2000; **50(460)**: 892–9.
10. Dr Chris Cates' EBM website. Cates plot. www.nntonline.net/visualrx/cates_plot/ [accessed 27 July 2015].
11. Berne E. *Games People Play.* Harmondsworth: Penguin, 1987.
12. The Motivational Interviewing Page. www.motivationalinterview.net.
13. Miller W, Moyers T. Eight stages in learning Motivational Interviewing. *Journal of Teaching in the Addictions* 2006; **5(1)**: 3–17.
14. Innes AD, Campion PD, Griffiths FE. Complex consultations and the 'edge of chaos'. *British Journal of General Practice* 2005; **55(510)**: 47–52.
15. Stuart M, Lieberman J. *The Fifteen Minute Hour: therapeutic talk in primary care.* Abingdon: Radcliffe Publishing, 2008.
16. Stuart MR. Accenting the positive: putting an affirmative spin on the BATHE technique. www.marianstuart.com/Accenting-the-Positive-Affirmative-BATHE.pdf [accessed 27 July 2015].

Resources

Gigerenzer G. *Reckoning with Risk: learning to live with uncertainty.* London: Penguin Books, 2003.

Paling J. *Helping Patients Understand Risk.* Gainsville, FL: The Risk Communication Institute, 2006, www.riskcomm.com.

Chapter 11

The clinical setting, assessment and teaching methods for uncertainty in the Negotiating Quadrant

Effective work in the Negotiating Quadrant can be supported by the clinical setting clinicians work in. When this Quadrant goes well complaints are less likely, which reduces stress on clinicians, and keeps their seniors or organisations happy. Win–win as they say!

This chapter considers:

- how clinical settings can help the management of uncertainty in the Negotiating Quadrant
- assessment and teaching methods for uncertainty in the Negotiating Quadrant.

How clinical settings can help the management of uncertainty in the Negotiating Quadrant

Many of the situations and difficulties described here are predictable and occur quite often. Shared decision making is essential to involve patients in their care[1] and support for this using decision aids is available through the NHS Shared Decision Making programme.[2] The educational or workplace setting can have a big effect on how well doctors deal with uncertain situations involving negotiating with patients. We need opportunities to *share* experiences of these types of uncertainties and to discuss how others cope. Teams should create such opportunities for discussion and peer review in calm, supportive encounters. As individuals, we can develop our skills by making the most of opportunities for discussion and feedback. This may mean video analysis, shared consulting with difficult patients, and discussions in Balint or Problem-Based Learning groups. Even a specific time set aside to have coffee and talk can help, and team meetings should have time set aside to discuss these kinds of difficulties.

Tools such as Cates plots should be available to doctors where they consult, perhaps on computers or folders relevant to the job. If you want to go through a shared decision-making conversation about starting warfarin, it is better not to waste time struggling to find the Cates plot during the consultation.

Seniors in teams often say, 'Well, this is the right thing to do…'. However, they can also lead the way in incorporating the patient's viewpoint and demonstrating how to do this. Managing patients flexibly, recognising that guidelines are not tramlines, can model patient-centred care for junior staff to emulate.

Assessment and teaching methods for uncertainty in the Negotiating Quadrant

Reading something about the theory of negotiating or motivational interviewing does make it easier to put into practice. The resources at the end of this chapter are a good start and the bibliography covers more extensive resources. Stress levels tend to decrease as you learn to work alongside patients instead of against them. Some of the resources are online, but reading a book is still a good way to go.

To develop a skill, try to see it done well by a senior colleague or online. Practise explaining things in absolute terms with your peers/senior colleagues, rather than using relative risks when discussing patients. This will help improve familiarity with this method. Practise the skills in real consultations and also in skills rehearsals or role plays, and GET FEEDBACK from a senior, peer or, better still, a patient. Learning how to use explanatory diagrams like Cates plots will pay dividends.

Video assessment is a good way to see how things are going. GPs are very familiar with this and anyone can do it these days. Digital cameras are widely available and cheap. Even your mobile smartphone can do a video that is good enough. Make sure to get permission from the patients using a standard form.[3] Getting specific feedback from patients about shared decisions can also be helpful. Patients who consult with others or check their treatment plans with other clinic staff may be revealing problems with explanations or shared decisions.

It is helpful for senior clinicians to model shared decision making with patients, and for juniors to have the opportunity to talk through how to approach complex or difficult decisions before meeting the individual patient concerned. Using resources such as Health Talk Online (http://healthtalk.org) to help understand the patient's point of view and see the effects of health care from a totally different perspective can help to change attitudes to shared decision making. This is covered in more detail in Part V 'Exploring uncertainty from the patient's perspective'. Understanding what it is like for patients to experience illness and the difficult decisions they have to make can be a humbling experience. This can help doctors build the empathy and engagement that is needed for effective negotiating.

References

1. Coulter A, Collins A. *Making Shared Decision-Making a Reality: no decision about me, without me.* London: King's Fund, 2011.
2. NHS. Shared decision making. http://sdm.rightcare.nhs.uk/ [accessed 28 July 2015].
3. RCGP. Patient consent form for video/digital recording for training purposes. www.rcgp.org.uk/gp-training-and-exams/mrcgp-workplace-based-assessment-wpba/~/media/Files/GP-training-and-exams/WPBA/Patient-Consent-Form-for-Video-Digital-Recording.ashx [accessed 28 July 2015].

Resources for the Negotiating Quadrant

Crossley T. *I Don't Know What it is but I Don't Think it's Serious.* London: RCGP, 2008.

McDonnell D. *How to Communicate Basically Brilliantly.* Lancaster: NLP Healthcare, 2013.

The Motivational Interviewing Page, www.motivationalinterview.net.

Platt FW, Gordon GH. *Field Guide to the Difficult Patient Interview.* (2nd edn). Philadelphia, PA: Lippincott Williams & Wilkins, 2004.

Silverman J, Kurtz S, Draper J. *Skills for Communicating with Patients.* (3rd edn). Abingdon: Radcliffe Medical Press, 2013.

Stuart M, Lieberman J. *The Fifteen Minute Hour: therapeutic talk in primary care.* Abingdon: Radcliffe Publishing, 2008.

THE TEAM-WORKING QUADRANT

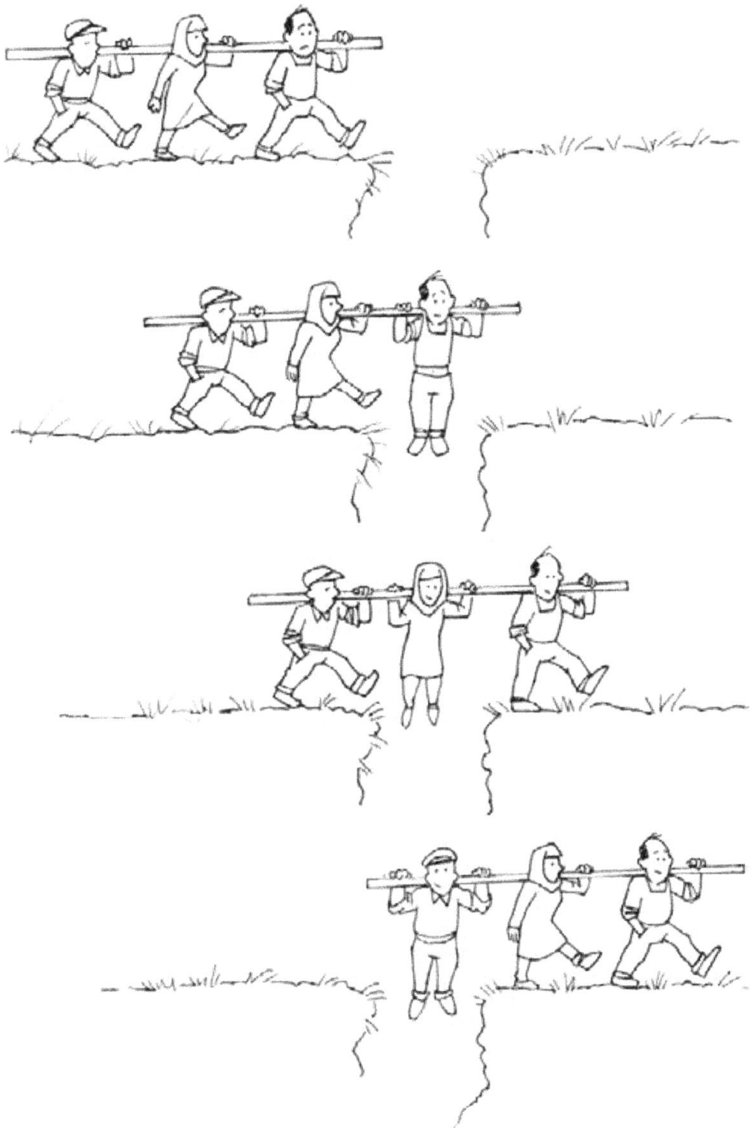

Although effective team-working is essential for almost all aspects of caring for patients, all professionals have experienced problems when working with others and uncertainty about how best to proceed.

Chapter 12 is an introduction to uncertainty in the Team-working Quadrant and also discusses 'dysfunctional ways out'. **Chapter 13** works though examples of common WDYDWYDKWTD situations in the Team-working Quadrant, explaining 'functional ways through' common problems, identifying the right skills needed for the right situation. **Chapter 14** explores how the clinical setting can help to deal with uncertainty in the Team-working Quadrant, and suggests assessment and teaching methods.

The key skills for uncertainty in the Team-working Quadrant are:

- creating a good team
- making meetings work, including skills in chairing meetings
- managing boundaries
- being good enough
- managing difficult situations.

Chapter 12

Introduction to uncertainty in the Team-working Quadrant

> If you wish to travel quickly, travel alone; if you wish to travel far, travel with other people.
>
> N'gambai proverb

So, you have analysed your patient's problem, used your diagnostic network skilfully and precisely, and reached a working diagnosis (or maybe even diagnoses). The management plan is clear because you and the patient have shared some important and useful decision-making discussions, and you even have a multidisciplinary team of professionals to work together on behalf of the patient. Everything should be plain sailing now, surely?

All clinicians get WDYDWYDKWTD moments connected with team-working issues. This chapter covers:

- an introduction to uncertainty in the Team-working Quadrant.
- 'dysfunctional ways out' of uncertainty in the Team-working Quadrant; common pitfalls.

An introduction to uncertainty in the Team-working Quadrant

When teams work well together the results can be joyous for patients and professionals alike. Patients are well cared for, supported and reassured that they are in good hands; good outcomes follow. Team members feel the same: cared for, supported and aware that they are performing as well as possible. Good camaraderie leads to high morale, a sense that improvement is continuous and that professional development and job satisfaction are good.

Having different disciplines and different personalities in a team gives the advantage of multiple perspectives, a greater amount of information relevant to the patient can be considered and tasks can be divided and achieved by the most suitable personnel.

Yet, every healthcare professional is able to think of times when the care of patients was not good enough because the teamwork didn't happen properly, because teams turned away, messed up, bullied each other or their patients, or where teamwork existed in name only but didn't happen in day-to-day practice. If 'teamwork' is not working well, it can be hard to fix and may produce grim outcomes for all concerned. This may lead to WDYDWYDKWTD moments that can seem especially puzzling for inexperienced members, while remaining challenging for senior practitioners.

Teams of well-intentioned people, individually trying hard but overall failing to work effectively together, can still end up with undesirable outcomes. Truly awful team failure is not usually the result of individual incompetence, although that may play a significant part. It has been remarked that 'Accidents happen; disasters require organisation'. Teams that are not working well can slide into dysfunction and, at worst, disaster. Moreover, teams need to maintain high levels of function to work in ways that are kindly towards patients. Where this doesn't happen we see consequences such as the abuses at the Mid Staffordshire Hospital as described in the Francis Report.[1]

To resolve a WDYDWYDKWTD question in relation to teams, familiarity with the principles and skills of effective teamwork and knowledge of alternative approaches are needed. Teams are more than the sum of the individuals in them and effective teams have structures and ways of working that require specific skills, attitudes and values. Such skills can be learned; the need for such skills must first be recognised and access to appropriate learning made available.

Ideally, a team whose members have different skills and perspectives will mean that issues are less likely to be overlooked, or aspects of care omitted. Ensuring that tasks are delegated to the right people can promote efficiency, enable resources to be used effectively and get the right care happening in the right place at the right time. However, individuals working in established teams can feel that trying to influence a team is like shifting the trajectory of a super tanker: languid and frustrating. Not knowing what to do, or how to do it in the Team-working Quadrant, can lead to the slow development of incomplete, chaotic, uncoordinated care, with unethical, incompetent or difficult behaviour remaining unchallenged. Frustrations in teamwork are common in community settings where teams may meet at weekly or monthly, rather than daily, intervals. Such teams may be of fluid membership, have members with unclear roles and team boundaries complicated by the effects of hierarchy and incompatibility between different organisations. Such difficulties may not be explicitly discussed or worked through.

In effective teams, leadership is, at least partly, devolved; this means that all team members have to step up and support the leadership functions. If this happens, teams cannot be hijacked by the loudest, strongest or most vocal, to the detriment of the contribution of less powerful members. Effective teams need to promote attachment and affiliation, encouraging staff to feel part of things by attention to joining and leaving processes. Health care is emotionally difficult work and teams need to contain emotion, providing a culture of safety that is both emotional (staff feel supported) and addressed to the safety of patients in the work carried out. Effective teams communicate well, and are open so that difficulties or conflicts can be reflected upon and resolved appropriately. A sense of involvement, such that members feel their work is acknowledged and valued, is crucial. When these aspects are in place a culture of empowerment can develop, in which all members of the team participate in its running and decision making to a relevant and appropriate degree. Clearly understood relationships between teams will also make for more effective work. Turf wars, demarcation disputes and the uses and misuses of 'inclusion criteria' (which are really 'exclusion criteria') can create fertile grounds for disagreement, disillusionment and failure.

The work of teams is often made more complex by the hidden and unacknowledged roles of patients and their families, friends and carers, who have important contributions to offer. These may be overlooked, especially if people are not able, or do not wish, to fulfil traditional expectations. Behaviour complicated by multiple diagnoses, or by drug or alcohol misuse, may make it harder for professionals to fulfil their own responsibilities. Conversely, the devoted, unpaid, highly skilled caring done by family members or other carers enables the overall care of the patient, in partnership with professionals, to reach the highest standards.

This chapter will explore how effective teamwork skills can unlock some WDYDWYDKWTD situations. The formation, leadership, maintenance and training of teams is a complex subject that cannot be treated fully here. However, in discussing some common issues, this chapter highlights the importance of mastering the knowledge and skills that help teams along, and emphasises the need for everyone on a team to be able to develop helpful attitudes towards each other, and to value the skills needed to maintain effective teamwork.

'Dysfunctional ways out' of uncertainty in the Team-working Quadrant: common pitfalls

Without becoming frankly dysfunctional, or abusive, there are many ways in which teamwork problems can give rise to 'dysfunctional ways out'.

Ask 'X' to do it

To work well, teams need to know the roles and capacities of their members and use those effectively. Team members also need to feel confident to undertake their specific roles. Sometimes within teams, the statement 'Ask "X" to do it' is an indirect way of really saying, 'I am too busy/lazy/stressed/resentful/overloaded/unskilled/scared … to do what is being asked of me.'

Left unaddressed, this kind of failure can have a demoralising effect. If the task is always passed on, no one takes responsibility for it and it may end up not being done. Bullying leadership or hectoring, with imposed targets or frameworks, are sometimes attempts to deal with this issue. Addressing the underlying issues – lack of time, skills, morale or leadership – needs a different team development approach.

The converse 'dysfunctional way out' is to 'do everything yourself and do not rely on others'. At first sight this may seem like admirable conscientiousness. However, teams are there to share skills as well as workload and responsibility, and patients may miss out if too much is taken on by a single person working alone.

Deferring decisions (and hence actions too)

Sometimes one team member involved in a complex process (for example palliative care, repeat prescribing, surgical theatres, childbirth) identifies a problem, which may even be discussed, but no decisions are made and no actions follow to correct the problem. This tends to be when there is a lack of clear team structure or accountability. The problem will tend to recur or escalate.

Passing the buck

A social worker once described this process to me as 'passing on a bundle of anxiety to someone else'. Under the guise of a 'referral' or 'protocol' a little package of anxiety and uncertainty is passed from one practitioner to another. Clinicians may groan when they receive this message at 6 p.m. on a Friday evening: 'The District Nurse left a message to say she is going off duty but just wanted to let you know that Mr Smith seems a bit poorly. She told his wife she would let you know.'

We know when 'passing the buck' has happened because the effect is different from the usual process of referral. In a straightforward handover or referral the action needed (even if it is extra work) is clear, within our remit and we tend to buckle down and get on with it. When a buck is being passed we get a feeling that 'we don't know what to do', a sinking feeling of anxiety and uncertainty. That is probably the uncertainty and anxiety of the person who has passed the buck to us, and who in turn has got *her* feeling of uncertainty or unease from the patient or relative, and pressures from their own management structure or even their fear of the media.

Retreat because it is too difficult

Sometimes problems seem too difficult to deal with. Instead of proactively trying to solve difficulties, teams retreat, give up or simply fire-fight a tricky situation without getting to the bottom of things. Team-work difficulties are complex because they involve the patient, the team and the individuals working in the situation, and it is hard to know where to start. It can be tempting to offer the routine, the restricted or the 'obvious' solution and then withdraw if this is unacceptable or not feasible for the individual patient. Sometimes, an individual team member retreats, or reacts badly, because the situation really is too difficult for him. A clinician who has recently suffered a painful bereavement may need to avoid caring for dying patients for a while. The human, psychological needs of the team deserve as much attention as those of the patients; if we do not care for each other, it becomes hard to care for patients.

Blaming others

Perennially popular! When things are uncertain or difficult a common 'way out' is for the team to retrench, pull together and pass the blame for difficulties on to someone else. This is sometimes another team ('That department never do things properly'), or perhaps blame is attached to the patient ('She won't cooperate with what we need to do, well that's her choice'), or sometimes a particular team member ('Things always go wrong when "X" is in charge').

Burnout, depersonalisation, unkindness

Health care means working in situations that can be emotionally very demanding and fraught for everyone; it isn't easy to contemplate suffering and pain all the time, especially if it can't be relieved easily. The emotions of patients and staff can run high because of fear and anxiety. If difficult feelings can't be processed within a team, then dysfunctional behaviours, failure of compassion or bullying can follow. The pressures of trying to do high-quality work, sometimes with insufficient resources of time, personnel or money, can create intolerable stress in health workers at times, especially if they are unsupported in their efforts by their management structure or institution. This may make them detached and accepting of low standards, as a survival mechanism.

Conversely, aiming to be perfect (a strategy doomed to failure) can lead to chronic anxiety. Feeling guilty or helpless when things can't be perfect may lead to an exaggerated fear of making mistakes, an inability to 'let go' and a desire to try to control everything, often through exhaustive checking or what seem to others to be excessively high standards. This can lead initially to depersonalisation and a sense of detachment from the patient (inimical to truly compassionate care) and later to burnout, chronic anxiety or depression.

Reference

1. Francis R. *Report of the Mid Staffordshire NHS Foundation Trust Public Inquiry* (3 vols). London: TSO, 2013, www.midstaffspublicinquiry.com [accessed 29 July 2015].

Chapter 13

Functional ways through uncertainty in the Team-working Quadrant

When working successfully, good teamwork skills can be inconspicuous. The need for teamwork skills often becomes really obvious only when they are missing. This section aims to make the skills explicit, so that they can be identified and learned. Practising such skills and honing them to a high level takes a long time, and much experience. Senior practitioners who have these skills are usually seen as wise and desirable team members! This chapter covers:

- examples of common WDYDWYDKWTD situations in the Team-working Quadrant
- clarifying 'functional ways through' common problems by identifying the right skills needed for the right situation.

In summary the skills needed are:

- creating a good team
- making meetings work, including skills in chairing meetings
- handover skills: SBAR
- managing boundaries
- being good enough
- managing difficult situations.

Creating a good team

Drs Firtree and Cone have been delegated to run a practice that has been taken over by their own larger practice, when a single-handed doctor retired. Several staff retired with the doctor, so new administrative staff have been recruited, and their inexperience shows. The clinics are busy, with far more appointments needed than expected, and many extra patients are booked in by receptionists, who often interrupt doctors mid-consultation, asking what seem to be trivial questions. Administrative staff often say, 'Please get "X" to do that' when the doctors ask them to do things, and Dr Firtree often rushes out to visits, looking over her shoulder saying, 'I think Dr Cone can sort that one out.' There never seems to be any time to sort things out properly. Eventually Dr Firtree loses her temper and yells at Rose, an administrative colleague, who goes home in tears and then makes a complaint. 'I don't know what to do', groans Dr Firtree when she discusses this with the senior partner.

All medical care, especially general practice, requires teamwork to be effective. Drs Firtree and Cone have perhaps assumed that medical care happens in the consulting room and have concentrated on that. Meanwhile, all around them, problems are building up and not being solved. Effective teamwork begins with creating a good team. What skills could help Drs Firtree and Cone here?

Knowing that teamwork is crucial means taking decisive action to create, build and develop the team. Team members need to get to know each other as people and to understand their professional roles and capacities. Using small-group skills will help teams to get to know each other, decide how they will work together, and establish a team's overall purpose and methods. Being open to identifying problems to work on initially brings conflicts out into the open. However, this can also lead to resolution if all parties have developed some trust in each other.

This team framework can be remembered as:

- *forming* (everyone getting to know each other and the team's purpose)
- *norming* (agreeing how the team will work, who will lead it, what the team is for)
- *storming* (identifying and dealing with conflicts and difficulties)
- *performing* (what the team needs to be doing to fulfil its particular purpose).

These steps are not single, one-off processes in a team's life. They are iterative processes that have to happen at different times and in varying forms over and over again to maintain team functioning.[1]

Drs Firtree and Cone discuss the problems together and with Ms Sage, the manager from the main organisation. They reflect on what the new team needs, and introduce an experienced worker from the main surgery to introduce consistent ways of doing things, and to support and train the inexperienced staff. They arrange for the whole clinic team to meet every week for an hour to discuss issues arising and plan how they will work effectively together. The initial sessions centre round everyone getting to know each other, building trust with some straightforward team exercises and gaining an understanding of what everyone's job entails. This helps the administrative staff to understand why interrupted consultations can be stressful and even counterproductive, and helps the medical staff to realise how difficult it is for the administrative team to negotiate with angry patients.

Once a month they have a longer meeting that includes problem-solving training and team-building processes. It takes time and sensitive handling of the meetings, and the administrative team flourish when their issues are given the attention they need. Everyone feels that their work is more recognised and valued by others, which leads to better performance.

After a few months they all go on an outing and enjoy each other's company. The time and effort gradually pay off, the work is managed more smoothly, interruptions are reduced, and no one goes home in tears.

Managing meetings, including skills in chairing meetings

Organisational issues

It is Monday afternoon and the doctors are having their usually weekly meeting. It is supposed to start at 2 p.m. but by 2.15 p.m. only half the doctors are there. Dr Apple rushes in late clutching a sandwich and immediately starts talking about a difficult patient. She makes colleagues laugh as she describes a funny incident. Dr Pear is reading his mail. Finally, everyone is there. Many issues are discussed without decisions being made, although the meeting is cordial, kindly and respectful. There are no minutes so some issues from last time are discussed again. Just before the end Dr Orange mentions an important issue that he would like to discuss, which he hasn't mentioned before. The meeting finishes late, patients are kept waiting and yet no decisions were really made. Dr Juniper sees this happening nearly every week and is getting very frustrated. He cautiously mentions this and Dr Pear says, 'No problem, you chair the meeting next time.' Dr Juniper sighs. Now he doesn't know what to do; he has never chaired a meeting in his life.

Almost all professional and business life involves meetings. They can be time consuming, ineffective, boring and slow. And yet other meetings can be productive, enjoyable and fly by. So what skills will Dr Juniper need to work more effectively with the team of doctors at the next meeting?

There are specific skills for running meetings that can be learned. Dr Juniper can read about these and develop his skills by getting some feedback from his partners on how he is doing. In summary, in meetings he needs to *unite* the group, then *focus* the group, and then *mobilise* the group into action.

Uniting

Uniting the group means what used to be known as 'calling the meeting to order'. Some committees still do this and have a nice big gavel to bang on the desk and attract everyone's attention. This works best if the time and day of the meeting are conducive to everyone being there … and it is key to start on time. This may need to be negotiated outside the meeting by the new chairperson. In the meeting the chairperson needs to ensure that everyone knows who the participants are, and that they all have the agenda. This needs to be prepared in advance, usually with some draft timings to stop everyone spending 50 minutes on the colour of the new toilet signs, and five minutes on the action to be taken about a massive complaint. Uniting the group needs some discipline from participants (to turn up on time for example), and from the chairperson, to stick to the agenda and the timings. Dr Juniper would be wise to mention these ideas before he starts and perhaps to tighten up on the meeting gradually.

Focusing

Focusing the group means bringing the group's attention to the task or agenda item in hand, in a timely and precise way. The chairperson needs to encourage relevant contributions, tactfully get some people to stop talking, encourage the contributions of others and make sure the digressions do not waste time. The purpose of the agenda item should be clarified. Is it to inform people about something? To clarify what decisions need to be made? To make the decisions? Is this an operational meeting? ('Who is going to see Mrs Smith?') A strategy meeting? ('How will we meet the new targets we have been set?') A policy meeting? ('What are our most important priorities?') Does all the work need to be done in the meeting? Can the group delegate someone to get information, make a proposal and come back with a recommendation?

Mobilising

Mobilising the group means getting to a decision and clarifying who is going to act and when she is going to complete her actions. This can be reviewed at the next meeting (with the minutes of course). It also means keeping moving through the agenda to finish at the agreed time.

So how might it go better for Dr Juniper?

Before the next meeting, Dr Juniper speaks to everyone individually. He gets the agenda items together, asks everyone to be on time and soon realises that Monday lunchtime isn't the best time for a meeting as there are so many competing claims on people's time and attention. Some agenda items don't need to be discussed at the meeting; the manager has the skills to make certain decisions and needs only to inform the group of how things are going. So Dr Juniper focuses the group next time on two questions:

- What is this meeting for? Information? Chat? Policy? Strategy? Day-to-day organisation?
- And when should the meeting happen?

It turns out that the doctors use the meeting for several purposes: exchanging support and information about clinical care, making day-to-day decisions about practical matters like holidays and more important questions like plans for the future and staffing.

After discussion Dr Juniper mobilises the group to decide how they will meet. They decide to do the chat and support stuff over coffee while they read the clinic letters and laboratory results. It won't matter if people come and go or are late. They decide to have a separate meeting for day-to-day issues every two weeks before clinic, so they will have a good incentive to finish and get on with their work. Once every six weeks they will have a longer meeting to discuss weighty issues, with all doctors bringing reports and information about a specific topic they have responsibility for.

This meeting finishes on time, and Dr Juniper looks forwards to chairing the next one.

The same skills are useful in clinical settings as well as organisational ones. Teams often meet to discuss the care of patients and try to ensure that everything works smoothly. Sometimes healthcare staff come away from team meetings frustrated and none the wiser about how everyone will work together for the patient.

Clinical issues

The primary healthcare team meeting starts late because some of the doctors are on visits. Rosemary is a new district nurse attending her first meeting. She gets lost on the way and arrives feeling a bit flustered. A new system for continence aids is being introduced and discussing this takes up a lot of time. Near the end Rosemary hesitantly mentions Mrs Amethyst, who has been having dressings to an infected wound after a hip replacement. The wound is nearly healed, but Mrs Amethyst doesn't want the nurses to stop coming and keeps ringing them up, asking them to re-dress the wound even though it has already been done. Will it be OK for them to pull out when the wound is healed?

This seems reasonable. No one has any better suggestions and the team move on to other matters, without getting much detail. Two weeks later the doctors find that the patient is requesting frequent visits from *them*; now everyone feels a bit stuck.

When teams meet they sometimes make helpful decisions, delegate the work and things move on. However, as in this example, sometimes an individual member's feeling of WDYDWYDKWTD is echoed by the whole team not seeming to 'know what to do'. Nothing is decided, care drifts and the uncertainty is somehow glossed over.

Part of the effectiveness of a team lies in adherence to effective running of meetings. In the meeting described, no introductions were made, the agenda seems unclear, and no commitments to decisions were made. To 'make meetings work' attention needs to be paid to all those issues. Having someone chairing the meeting who will manage the relationships, the timing and the actions will make the meeting work smoothly. However friendly and informal the relationships between team members are, a meeting will work better if these formal principles are followed. In this primary care meeting no one took overall responsibility for the chairing of the meeting, not enough detail was elicited from the rather hesitant new member and an opportunity to plan care effectively was missed.

Ideally, teams can also help to maintain continuity of care for patients, who benefit from and greatly value seeing the same people. Could the chairperson identify the doctor most involved and encourage care from him after the nurses finish their own care?

How could it go better for Mrs Amethyst and Rosemary?

At the start of the meeting the person chairing is clearly identified, and gets everyone to introduce themselves and their role, and agrees a list of patients and issues to be discussed with clear timings. The meeting starts with the agenda and introductions rather than drifting to a start when everyone arrives.

Rosemary feels more welcome and able to discuss the problems with Mrs Amethyst a bit more fully. From the discussion it emerges that Mrs Amethyst seems to forget that her wound has been dressed and may have some cognitive decline. Her current state could also be triggered by a postoperative depression. It is agreed that Dr Blackberry, who knows her best, will visit to assess this, that the administrative team will arrange her medication to be delivered in blister packs and that Rosemary will continue to attend until the outcome of all this is known. By the next week it has become clear that Mrs Amethyst is actually suffering from an agitated depression; she responds well to treatment and starts attending the practice again so the nurses can reduce their input appropriately. This reduces their stress too.

Handover skills: 'SBAR'

Mr Moonstone is an 80-year-old patient with Type 2 diabetes. He is on twice-daily insulin. His wife died six months ago. Her care had masked his vascular dementia. He became unable to cope at home and has gone to live with his daughter, Iris, who lives at the edge of the practice area. She refuses to give Mr Moonstone his insulin as she is 'too busy'. Rosemary and the other district nurses are finding it hard to get there twice a day and in the primary healthcare team meeting emphasise how difficult it is to get there in time for Mr Moonstone's breakfast insulin. His evening insulin is given late because they are so short staffed.

The GPs in the meeting pick up on Iris's difficulty in coping with her father and wonder whether she is getting too stressed, whether residential care should be considered and whether it would be feasible for them to find a nursing team closer by. The meeting ends with no definite conclusions about what is to be done and Rosemary feels unsupported and frustrated.

This a good example of decisions being discussed, but no real conclusions reached, with actions deferred to some unspecified later date. Could there be a better way? Perhaps improving the handover structure could help here.

Why are 'handing over' skills so important? The most risky time for patients is when their care is handed over between individual nurses, doctors or teams, or when they are transferred from one part of the service to another different service, or when one part of the team seeks advice and guidance from another. The loss of continuity and tacit knowledge about the patient risks the loss of significant information when handover occurs. Some handovers give rise to the feeling of a buck being passed. Yet this can be largely and effectively mitigated by attention to the skills needed in handover.

Handover can be a time of difficulty for the professional and great anxiety for the patient. For someone who suspects that she has cancer to have to wait two weeks to see a consultant can feel like torture. Waiting for an appointment with a physiotherapist or being told 'a nurse will come and visit' without knowing when it will happen creates unease. For the doctor or nurse, referring to someone else can be a relief ('Someone else will sort this, take responsibility, make a decision') or trepidation ('What will they think of me so far?').

Sometimes handovers and referrals are more about 'hoping and hinting', rather than explicit requests: 'hinting' about the real issues or difficulties and 'hoping' that the receiver will pick up the hint and act in a helpful way. This is almost like hoping the recipient will read your mind and do what is needed without you telling him very much; this is not a reliable strategy.

So what method can we use for effective handover? A useful tool is called 'SBAR', which stands for: **S**ituation **B**ackground **A**ssessment **R**ecommendation. This is a handover tool originally developed for handovers in the US Navy and adopted as a useful patient safety strategy.[2] It uses a standard structure to overcome barriers to effective communication, when there may be differences of hierarchy, communication styles, jargon or team culture. Gender, ethnic background and institutional loyalties can further impede effective communication. A standard structure reduces vagueness, hints or reticence and ensures that misunderstandings or assumptions are avoided, especially if there is what has been called an 'authority gradient', for example when someone is talking to someone else who she sees as more senior or more authoritative. Having a memory prompt encourages proper preparation for handover or referral and reduces the time needed for the handover.

S = Situation

They key to effective handover is to attract the *focused* attention of the receiver, and to orientate him immediately to what is likely to be required of him.

Ensure the right demographic information is stated clearly, at the start, including your name and role if on the telephone. Then immediately explain what the main problem is, clearly stating the reason you are referring or handing over the patient. It helps if there is a clear question or statement. Saying, 'Please review this man with ENT problems' is vague and doesn't sum up the situation or question. Saying, 'Would this man with chronic rhinitis benefit from a surgical procedure to his polyps?' prepares the receiver for the information that is coming and helps her make best use of it. Ideally, the opening of a handover should be summed up in a single sentence or question.

B = Background

Next, explain the background to the situation that you are handing over. This might include the present problem and the previous medical history. This should be concise, relevant and brief. Prepare by noting down the key points as an *aide-mémoire.*

A = Assessment

How did you interpret the information summarised in 'Background'? What further assessment have you made? This section should include relevant physical findings, laboratory results, responses to treatment so far, and other relevant information. In the example with the nurses it could include an assessment of the risks or problems with the current approach or information about what is happening in the patient's home environment.

R = Recommendation

Explain what *you* think needs to happen now. If you need your colleague to do something, being specific and clear about your request and specifying your time frame will help him act appropriately. Don't just 'hint and hope'!

How could things go better for Mr Moonstone, Rosemary, the other nurses and Iris?

Instead of hinting and hoping that a change of insulin will make things easier, Rosemary, assisted by the chair of the meeting, decides to try out an SBAR approach. She says, 'Could we consider changing Mr Moonstone to once-daily insulin now?' (S).

The (B) background is that we can't get there on time in the morning because we are short-staffed and he is far away at the edge of our area. His daughter can't get back from work on time to do his evening insulin. Our (A) assessment is that once-daily insulin could be safe and suitable for him, and Iris would agree to give it in the morning with his breakfast and we would only go when needed. We would like to (R) recommend a once-daily insulin regime now.

With the issue clearly stated, the discussion does not digress down a dead end. A suitable regime is agreed and Mr Moonstone's care is streamlined. Iris is relieved, Mr Moonstone remains at home for longer and the nurses get more time for other patients.

SBAR can be used to structure communication at any stage of handover, perhaps between colleagues, when writing referral letters or when communicating discharge information back to the GP. The initial statement about the situation should ensure that the reason for communication is explicit, and underpins the assessment and recommendations.

SBAR is also a good tool for juniors asking for advice from seniors within a team, and makes for more effective teamwork. Consider the following scenario:

Dr Guelder is working in general practice as an ST1 trainee. She asks her trainer, Dr Elm, for advice and gives the following information: 'I need your advice about Mrs Marble, a 26-year-old who is married to a civil engineer. She has been on the oral contraceptive pill for four years and is stable on it. Her BP is 118/78, she doesn't smoke (has never smoked actually because her dad died of lung cancer, which put her off) and she is up to date with her smears. She doesn't want to be pregnant because she and her husband are going to Costa Rica, she is doing a Spanish course there, and then they have six months off to go travelling as he has finished a series of international placements with the posting to South America and then he can take a career break until his post in London starts in a year's time. She has never had problems with the pill, her periods come regularly, she has no inter-menstrual bleeding and her weight is stable, BMI 22, she is very adherent with treatment and never misses pills and gets no side effects since she started taking the pill in the evening instead of first thing in the morning which used to make her faintly nauseated…'. Dr Guelder continues in this vein for a while hoping Dr Elm will pick up on her hints about the problem and tell her what to do.

In this scenario it's Dr Elm who doesn't know what to do. Can he interrupt this fluent history and find out what on earth is the problem? Will that put Dr Guelder off? After all, there is a good history here and the point must be coming soon.

Preparing handovers or requests for help means that you are more likely to get the support needed; thinking it through beforehand will help your own decision making and assessment processes to develop. SBAR makes for active rather than passive handover, and has been shown to be more time efficient too. This particularly helps those who are inexperienced or who are communicating to someone higher up a hierarchy. Using SBAR avoids the 'hinting and hoping' that means the right information might be overlooked or not acted upon. If Dr Guelder used SBAR the discussion might go like this:

How might things go better for Dr Guelder and Dr Elm?

Dr Guelder says, 'Is it OK for me to give Mrs Marble a prescription for 12 months of the oral contraceptive pill? She has been stable on it for three years, all examination findings and a recent smear are normal and she is going abroad for a year with her husband, travelling lots of the time, with less access to medical care. She doesn't want to change her contraception in that time so I think it will be OK … but am I allowed to do that?'

Dr Elm replies, 'Yes, it's a good idea and acceptable practice.'

This gets the job done quickly, more effectively and has helped the learner to develop because she had to get her thoughts in order first.

Managing boundaries

Professional issues

Amber is now 17 years old and has developed a helpful relationship with Heather, the practice nurse. Heather is in her twenties and also has coeliac disease. This has stabilised Amber and all seems well. One evening, a member of the administrative team is waiting outside a local music venue to collect her daughter after a concert by a famous rock band. She is surprised to see Amber emerge arm in arm with Heather, both smoking, and then they disappear into a night-club next door. Not knowing what to do, she reports this to Dr Guelder, a GP trainee, the next day. Dr Guelder in turn, having been quite friendly with Heather, doesn't want to 'get anyone into trouble' and isn't sure what to do either. After all, Amber is over 16 now isn't she?

In teamwork there are two kinds of boundaries that need to be understood and managed: first, the boundary between the personal and the professional life and, second, the boundary between what 'our team can and will do' and what 'belongs' elsewhere. The situation with Amber described here illustrates the first of these boundary issues.

Patients need comfort and closeness as well as technical care. In a time of fear and anxiety because of illness, being 'accompanied' by someone who has been there before, and who can navigate the unfamiliar territory of disease and illness, is crucial. This is why patients with serious or complex illnesses like to get to know the professionals looking after them and want to feel that they are 'known and understood' as individuals. However, healthcare professionals also need care and closeness; looking after patients well can make us feel good about ourselves and satisfied with what we do, overcoming our own sense of isolation or anxiety.[3] This mutual dependence may mean that either party can start to see in the other a means to meet personal needs, rather than the professional needs of a working relationship. The risk here is that the boundary between professional and personal roles becomes blurred. Amber is 17, her professional relationship with Heather the nurse started before that age, and it is professionally inappropriate to have a relationship outside work with a patient. Moreover, if the dependence increases on either side, the other party may start to resent the vulnerability perceived in himself or in the other, and that can spill over into resentment, anger or hostility.

What is needed is an emotionally safe place to discuss the feelings that patients arouse in us as healthcare workers. Team meetings may be set up to do this, especially if taking the format of a Balint group or similar discussion, with explicit methods used to manage the emotional content. Sometimes a one-to-one discussion is more suitable. Helping others to recognise and maintain suitable personal/professional boundaries is not 'getting them into trouble', but rather a means to 'keep them out of trouble' in the longer term. One of the higher-order skills needed to work in teams is the ability to recognise emotional issues, reflect on them and discuss them, while maintaining a safe emotional climate.[3] The leaders of such teams need to develop opportunities to discuss the boundaries between personal and professional needs and behaviours. Any difficulties that arise can then be discussed in a way that promotes self-awareness and learning from mistakes, and which provides emotional support in situations of difficulty. This work comes more easily to some teams than others.

How could things go better for Amber, Heather and Dr Guelder?

Dr Guelder discusses the issue in a private conversation with Dr Elm, the GP trainer, who discusses it with Ms Lupin the practice manager too. They decide to discuss the matter discreetly with Heather.

It transpires that Heather herself has been feeling that the relationship with Amber has been becoming difficult. Amber met her at the concert unexpectedly and 'I just sort of got sucked in'. Tactful ways to re-establish professional boundaries were considered and carried through. Amber's appointments are made with Poppy, the other practice nurse, while Heather is 'away'. Poppy develops skills in coeliac disease, guided by Heather. At a subsequent team training day, general issues about professional boundaries were discussed and everyone shared some of the difficulties they themselves had experienced.

Professional issues II

Dr Oak is doing some paperwork when Lily, a member of the nursing staff, comes in and asks, 'Can I have a quick word?' She sits down and says how exhausted she is feeling. She has not been sleeping very well. Would it be OK for her to take next week off to rest? Does Dr Oak think she should ask her GP for some sleeping tablets too?

She says the sleepless nights are caused by worry and stress in her working role; she feels that the office manager, Ms Swan, is bullying her by insisting she see extra patients, by criticising her methods of ordering vaccines ('I always like to have plenty in. I don't know why she makes such a fuss about the money. We only have to discard a few out-of-date ones!') and by not being very flexible about her having time off at short notice ('I want to take next week off because I can get a cheap deal. Don't you think that's reasonable, doctor, as I have not had any holidays for three months?'). Some sleeping tablets for a good night's sleep would help her get all this in perspective....

Dr Oak may well feel that this is a WDYDWYDKWTD moment. There are several types of boundaries being broached here, which makes it confusing.

First, this staff member does deserve to be listened to and supported in any work difficulties. In a hospital setting this is part of good teamwork, and in a GP setting the doctor is likely to be the nurse's employer. Knowing about these stresses may help to resolve some difficult issues. However, advising a staff member about treatment is crossing a professional boundary. It is the nurse's own GP who should be making decisions about prescribing matters.

There are other boundary issues here too. Who is the line manager for this nurse? Probably not Dr Oak directly. Managing sickness absence, holidays, budgets and so on is usually the responsibility of a relevant manager. Lily may be trying to outflank her own manager by appealing to Dr Oak, who may not be aware of what the issues really are and what the manager is doing to put things on a better footing. Dr Oak has sympathy for both parties involved. After all, he doesn't like having lots of extra patients either! Dr Oak is being asked to act, at least partly, as a clinician but also as employer, confidante, colleague and possibly even referee between the manager and the nurse. Given the confusions about his role he risks losing focus on the clinical issues and making an incomplete or erroneous assessment, and also risks affecting the way the team as a whole functions.

How might it go better for Dr Oak?

Dr Oak listens carefully, without saying much and without committing himself to answering the questions about sleeping tablets. He expresses empathy for the nurse who seems to be struggling with her present situation. He then explains his thought processes about crossing boundaries explicitly. Not being her GP, he really cannot advise about whether sleeping tablets are a good idea or not. The oversight of clinic times, holidays and vaccine expenditure is the responsibility of the office manager and it is not really appropriate for him to intervene at this stage in those matters. He suggests Lily asks for a discussion with Ms Swan, in the first case.

Talking with Ms Swan afterwards, it emerges that Lily tends to book her holidays at very short notice, which makes it hard to organise the clinics. Dr Oak is relieved to hand this problem back to Ms Swan, the office manager, who says they have it in hand with the appropriate staff processes.

If things feel tricky, always consider what boundaries are relevant, and whether they are being transgressed appropriately or not.

Team and turf issues

Mrs Beryll's cancer has spread widely and she wants to stay at home. She has patched things up with her husband now. The Macmillan and district nursing teams withdraw because her husband gets drunk and won't let them in. They are worried about their personal safety because he is threatening and angry. The pharmacist, trying to be helpful, responds to pressure and phone calls from Mrs Beryll's daughters and delivers drugs before getting the prescription. Mrs Beryll takes more drugs than she needs and ends up in casualty, drowsy and confused. Her two daughters constantly ring the Macmillan and general practice teams with opposing demands, one daughter insisting that she stays at home and the other constantly asking that her mother be admitted to the local hospice for care. When Dr Alder tried to visit he was also turned away by the husband; speaking with Mrs Beryll on the phone, it seemed that she had quite mixed feelings and 'just wanted to have no pain and for everyone to get along'.

It can be helpful to remember that 'only simple problems have simple solutions' and that difficult issues require patient, repeated and multiple interventions. End-of-life care can be complex and challenging even when the team is welcomed, focused and skilled. In the case of Mrs Beryll it seems that the team is withdrawing in the face of the family's distress and their dysfunctional ways of expressing it. If nothing is done, a messy, painful and protracted phase of end-of-life care may well result in painful memories for the family and complaints or even litigation for the care team.

So given that it seems that no one quite knows what to do here, what skills could help?

First, this kind of messy, difficult problem is hard and this must be acknowledged by the team. There are no easy answers and no magic bullets. This alone is sometimes enough to put professionals off, knowing that all they have ahead is a long, thankless set of tasks that may go wrong in spite of their best efforts. If members of the team know Mrs Beryll well they may also be grieving over her suffering and imminent death (albeit in an unconscious and unexpressed way). For health professionals involved in palliative care it can seem that all care ends in failure: we postpone death but cannot prevent it. If the emotional meaning of this is not open for discussion the team may withdraw from difficult situations 'blaming the patient', or in this case blaming the husband. Furthermore, there are many problems in parallel here, which can seem overwhelming; managing Mrs Beryll's symptoms, her grief at facing her own death, her husband's emotional outbursts and problem drinking, and the confusing and contradictory demands of her daughters, who are also understandably distressed.

In order for a team to work effectively here, it must become a functioning team again and that will start with meetings. First, the professionals involved will need to meet each other to discuss the situation. Then, they will need to meet with the whole family. This could be with all of the primary care team, or perhaps just with Dr Alder and the district nurses. The team itself will have to be clear about the identity and roles of various members, how they are going to communicate (frequently in this case, maybe with an email group, a daily telephone call, a weekly meeting?) and how decisions are to be shared and plans adhered to.

When this preliminary work is done, a meeting with the family can begin to allow their fears, concerns and needs to be understood. Using Covey's maxim 'seek first to understand',[4] the priorities of family members can be identified. Perhaps one member can become the representative for the family so that the care teams get and give a consistent message to the family? Perhaps an alcohol treatment worker could help to deal with some of the problems that the medical team are struggling with?

Team members will need to agree ground rules and boundaries with the family, and, crucially, with each other. Who will have overall charge of the prescribing? How will the regime be reviewed and updated? Having the pharmacist involved in the discussions could help to smooth the path. Administrative team members will also need to be involved so that they can have support for the difficult phone calls they receive and so they can give consistent messages to the family.

How might things go better for Mrs Beryll?

Dr Alder and Ms Drake the Macmillan nurse talk about the situation and agree to work together to try to resolve things, explaining the situation at a meeting of all primary healthcare team members to clarify what may need to be done. Dr Alder and Ms Drake then arrange to meet the whole family at Mrs Beryll's house and hear all points of view. This is time consuming and needs skilled handling, which Ms Drake does well, having experienced something similar before. Afterwards, there is much better agreement and cooperation about what needs to be done. Mr Beryll expressed his regrets and agreed to see the alcohol worker who will arrange counselling, support and detoxification. Their daughters accepted how difficult it is if they both ring up and eventually agreed that the older one will be the spokesperson. Mrs Beryll expressed her wishes; although she wants to be at home (which she told her younger daughter), she doesn't really want to die there and had been hoping that if her symptoms were bad she could be referred to the hospice (which is what she told her older daughter). She is admitted to the hospice, initially as a day care patient; the care and counselling the family receive enable them to accept finally her peaceful death in the hospice some weeks later. Working relationships within the primary healthcare team were further reinforced when they hold a 'debrief' after Mrs Beryll's death, celebrating the effective work they had done and drawing out lessons for the care of patients in the future.

Delegating skills

As usual, Dr Guelder is pretty much the last to leave the building. As she is getting her coat on the practice manager says, 'Are you always this late leaving? I decided to stay late tonight and finish off because I am going to my little girl's nativity play in the morning, but why are you here so late?' Dr Guelder replies, 'There is so much to do. I can't get through it all, and I have to check things after the clinics. I like to type all my own letters and there are so many phone calls to make, results to chase up and so on ... to make sure I haven't missed anything. It's really all my responsibility isn't it? My husband is getting very fed up with it but I don't really know what else to do about it.'

Is Dr Guelder right when she says 'it is all my responsibility'?

Health professionals rightly expect high standards of themselves and others. However, expecting perfection will ultimately be soul destroying. Trying to do everything yourself is the antithesis to 'ask X to do it', and rarely feasible in a complex health setting. Knowing the skills and roles of other team members and learning to delegate appropriately is a key teamwork skill. This is not the same as 'dumping' a task on someone who is unprepared, unqualified, unsupervised or in some other way inappropriate. That should be avoided.

At induction, and then subsequently as she gets used to the job, Dr Guelder needs to learn the roles, skills and limitations of other members of the team, and to learn from others about what is appropriate to delegate. Remembering that delegation does not mean passing the buck, and does not transfer final responsibility for the task, may help Dr Guelder to feel sufficiently in control to 'let go' of parts of the job.

Effective delegation includes the following steps, which can be followed when designing pathways for work in teams:

- *define the task* that might be delegated
- select the right team member
- *ensure* they have the skills
- *explain the task* and the required results, and what the *limits of responsibility* are
- agree deadlines
- remain *available for feedback*, support and advice.

Within Dr Guelder's clinic team, the administrative staff are probably qualified and experienced in chasing up results, typing letters, preparing referrals, communicating with patients and many other tasks. Having opportunities for peer review, and talking with senior colleagues or managers about what can be delegated, will help her to pass on specific tasks that others can do and free up her time. Dr Guelder's repeated checking over of work she has already completed needs to be sympathetically examined with her. Is she lacking in confidence? If so, is that justified or not? Is she feeling that everything not perfect is a 'failure'? There need to be limits and boundaries around what a doctor can be expected to do; Dr Guelder may need to learn about concepts such as being a 'good enough' rather than a 'perfect' doctor. It is sometimes said that the 'excellent drives out the good' by creating impossibly high standards.

How might it go better with Dr Guelder?
A training session with the manager is arranged. They go through all her tasks for the day and the manager is able to explain how many can be performed by the administrative team. Methods of supervising and checking are discussed. Dr Guelder still spends time checking her own work rather too much, to the detriment of her time management and personal wellbeing. The manager refers her on to a senior trainer for advice and coaching as to how to manage things better. Dr Guelder also takes a time management course and an assertiveness course, learning how to ask effectively for things she needs, and also how to say no effectively. She gets home to dinner with her husband rather more often. ...

Managing stressful situations (a.k.a. s**t happens)

Dr Firtree arrives at work feeling stressed; her car got a flat tyre half a mile away and she had to jog the last bit into work. Her daughter's nursery have called to say they are closing for a week because of an outbreak of norovirus and her husband has had to take the morning off his work to care for their child. He is hoping she will take over at lunchtime. At work it turns out that two doctor colleagues have gone off sick with influenza, the computer system has crashed and the operations manager has discovered that twice the usual number of patients has been booked in to the clinic as is usually feasible. Dr Firtree finds herself the most senior doctor around, just when she was feeling more stressed than usual. She doesn't know what to do.

Some teams feel as though they function like this almost every day or every week. Other teams seem to rise above such crises or at least keep them hidden from view. Being able to cope with teamwork crises is part of professional development. Surviving and coping will mean that important skills are honed, and resilience (the ability to thrive in spite of potential adverse circumstances) will increase. In the short term, what skills could help?

Clearly a plan of action is needed and here are some ideas to get the ball rolling. The exact details of the solution will depend on the team and department and these processes will help that solution along.

Start by thinking *helpful thoughts*. Initially, the thoughts in everyone's head are likely to be something like:

Oh no, this is too bad!!! We are all going to have the worst day imaginable! What else is going to go wrong? There will be loads of complaints from the patients!

Consciously replace those thoughts with helpful ones like these:

Well, even this will pass and when I get off duty I am going to treat myself to....

In this situation anything we can do will be better than nothing. I am sure we can all come up with a plan.

Then identify *helpful actions*. Sitting around moaning won't help; neither will it help if Dr Firtree rushes in and starts trying to see double the number of patients, without attending to the whole picture. Helpful actions will include identifying priorities, making a plan, identifying who is around to help and what they can do best.

The third essential is to identify *helpful people* who are in the situation too. It helps if good teamwork relationships have been established in the 'forming and norming' stages, but, if not, here is an opportunity to build some camaraderie and mutual help. Dr Firtree could set up a brief crisis meeting with the relevant people (operations manager, administrative team leader, the remaining clinician) and use the time to make a reasonable plan. Although this will expend time, it will save time overall, as the day will be better planned.

How might it go better for Dr Firtree?
Dr Firtree reminds herself that 'this too will pass' and that at the end of this busy week she is going to enjoy a peaceful family weekend. There had been similar crises in the Accident and Emergency department and they got through all right. Checking who is around, she meets with all her colleagues; a short meeting results in a viable plan for the day. Mr Byrd, the manager, is delighted to have a group to discuss things with because he had been feeling stressed too. Priorities and a sequence of actions are organised, and tasks are clearly allocated (finding staff to help, cancelling non-urgent patients, apologising to those who are delayed and so on). Dr Firtree asks Mr Byrd to call a local sandwich bar to deliver some lunch and everyone takes a 15-minute break at that point to eat, regroup and review the situation. Dr Firtree takes five minutes out to call her motoring

organisation; their man takes the car keys, fixes the tyre and brings her car back to the car park. Her husband calls to say Grandma will step into the breach.

On the whole the patients understand. The organising group praise and thank their team-mates and patients for their forbearance and hard work. The team pull together and 6 p.m. comes. Dr Byrd has a plan for the next few days and Dr Firtree goes home tired, but also feeling that she has made the best of the opportunity to deal with a tricky situation. She will be less fazed in future and her professional resilience has increased.

References

1. Tuckman B. Developmental sequence in small groups. *Psychological Bulletin* 1965; **63(6)**: 384–99.
2. NHS Institute for Innovation and Improvement. SBAR: situation – background – assessment – recommendation. 2008, www.institute.nhs.uk/quality_and_service_improvement_tools/quality_and_service_improvement_tools/sbar_-_situation_-_background_-_assessment_-_recommendation.html [accessed 30 July 2015].
3. Ballatt J, Campling P. *Intelligent Kindness: reforming the culture of healthcare.* London: RCPsych Publications, 2011.
4. Covey S. *The Seven Habits of Highly Effective People.* New York, NY: Simon & Schuster, 2005.

Chapter 14

The clinical setting, assessment and teaching methods for uncertainty in the Team-working Quadrant

How clinical settings can help the management of uncertainty in the Team-working Quadrant

Managing the setting in which teamwork problems arise is crucial if they are to be solved; it is hard to separate a team from its context. In healthcare settings professionals are often expected to work in a 'team' in which no time, effort or respect is offered towards such issues as induction, introductions, understanding and setting up 'group rules' or terms of interaction. Many teams are under so much pressure to 'perform' that the prerequisite 'forming, norming and storming' phases of a team are routinely neglected. Trainers and clinical teachers teaching teamwork skills can make opportunities to demonstrate these in practice and explain them to learners. Inductions are crucial elements of this: new team members need to be introduced, welcomed and their roles clarified and reinforced. Active participation by all members in the team discussion can be encouraged by the chairperson of any meeting. Ensuring that members of teams talk to each other informally, as well as formally, and have opportunities to work alongside each other can help to build trust and cooperative working. This may happen fairly naturally in some ward or Accident and Emergency department settings. Outpatient and general practice clinics can give rise to feelings of isolation if these issues are not addressed by having arrangements to share coffee and informal discussion, having social events for the whole team or regular debriefing opportunities.

Making decisions in teams can be difficult, and yet good decision-making skills result in safer and more effective approaches to the patients' problems. Trainers and teachers can model good decision making that incorporates the expertise of other team members. When discussions are difficult it may be helpful to use formal tools such as DODAR, which is used in aviation to help decision making.[1] This refers to:

- DIAGNOSE (What is the problem? What exactly is the decision to be made?)
- OPTIONS (What possibilities do we have, including doing nothing?)
- DECIDE (What is the action to be taken?)
- ASSIGN (Who is going to take responsibility for the action? When will that happen?)
- REVIEW (What happened and was action effective? Are further actions needed? Does further diagnosis need to happen and start the cycle again?).

Sometimes an extra R for RISK is added, to help teams reflect on what the risks and time frames are connected with the decision to be made.

At best, teams combine the expertise of their members to solve the problems at hand. Sometimes, this can give way to 'group think', where a particular view becomes the normal and cannot be challenged. Sometimes a drift in the wrong direction can be noted by a team member, who nonetheless feels herself powerless to change things. Members and leaders of teams can explicitly allow for what has been called the 'two challenge rule', to allow the team to remain open to dissenting voices, especially on matters of patient safety. Like many developments in safety systems, this came from the aviation industry, where senior pilots are encouraged to listen to feedback and requests for explanations of reasoning from junior pilots.[2]

In health care, this means expecting team members to advocate for the patient even if a particular viewpoint is unpopular or in opposition to the prevailing view or authority. Team members having differing points of view should be encouraged to voice concerns and to provide evidence or data to support their point of view. If a particular view is stated twice, by the same or different team members, the team should be encouraged to ensure that the concern is heard, understood and acknowledged. The 'two challenge rule' suggests that, if that does not happen, the team member is justified in taking a stronger course of action or enlisting the help of a senior. This overcomes our natural tendency to believe that the team is always right. Clinical errors and malpractice claims sometimes follow situations where team members have not been able to advocate assertively for their patients. Teachers and trainers can model this kind of behaviour towards other team members.

The setting in which the team is working can also improve the learning of teamwork skills by allocating appropriate time and structure to 'debriefing' processes. This can be both for times when the team worked well, or for times when there was a problem. Informal debriefing ('Phew! We got through that difficult situation' or 'That was the hardest death I have ever had to deal with') should be encouraged.

Sometimes a formal debrief needs to be instituted by the team leader. This can be structured to ensure that the following questions are addressed, in an atmosphere of trust, where errors are seen as learning opportunities for all. What went well? What should change? What do we need to improve? All teamwork settings should develop the expertise to do Significant Event Analysis, or Root Cause Analysis, although a detailed description of this cannot be given here. Discussions of this nature can help teams to develop shared understandings of how to use handover tools such as SBAR (see p. 151) and how to maximise the contribution of all members (e.g. having a 'two challenge rule' or by having formal decision-making processes).

Other elements of the setting that promote effective teamwork include an emphasis on supporting continuity of care, and, where that is not possible, having explicit and structured handover, so that problems are not 'left hanging' with no one accepting responsibility. The organisation of work within a service can encourage follow-up by identified individuals who know the patient. When proposing changes to the organisation of care (perhaps considering telephone follow-up rather than face to face), continuity should be supported.

Members of clinical teams need to support each other. This begins with knowing each other as people, perhaps having some social time together ('work hard, play hard'). Members of teams need to model praise and warmth, encouraging empathic listening to the stress and difficulties experienced, at times, by everyone who works in health care. If the clinical setting denies, ignores or belittles the difficulties of healthcare work, team members are more likely to become stressed, burnt out and, consequently, less effective.

Assessment and teaching methods for uncertainty in the Team-working Quadrant

Some learners may not appreciate that teamwork skills are like any other skills: they have to be learned. Asking learners to observe teams at work and identify the skills used can be a good way to start. Then learners can identify which skills they may need themselves, and their trainers can give them opportunities to practise those skills. Initially this may be straightforward: make sure new members in a team get to know who everyone is, make friends with them, and understand and respect their unique roles and skills. It is surprising how often these simple steps are omitted, and they should form crucial parts of any induction programme. Educators can do exercises, producing a series of tasks and asking juniors to prioritise them. Identifying the person to whom parts of the task can be delegated can lead on to learning about delegation skills. Supervisors or trainers could teach the SBAR method explicitly for handing over or asking advice; educators can model this themselves to ensure it becomes embedded in the way of doing things. Educators need to model respect for others' opinions and roles in team meetings.

Learners can then go on to learn higher-order teamwork skills, perhaps chairing a meeting after learning about what the chair does and using formal feedback tools (see resources) to get feedback on how effective they were. Multisource feedback assessments can assist in focusing learners' attention on the teamwork issues; colleagues may need to be encouraged to write free-text comments to illustrate their thoughts.

Teams are often involved in complex tasks; operating theatre teams or palliative care teams in the community are two such examples. To work well, all team members need to be clinically confident in their tasks. Where such tasks are demanding or unfamiliar (e.g. developing an Advance Care Plan for a patient with dementia dying in the community from cancer), educators need to help identify learning needs and put learning opportunities in place, with increased supervision and support until skills are embedded.

Attitudes are important. Supervisors and trainers need to set attitudinal goals as well as knowledge- and skill-related goals. For example, ask the learner to find ways to demonstrate that she has the attitude of 'valuing the input and opinions of team members from other disciplines'. How would a learner show that she respects the input of another team member? How would someone observing her deduce that her attitude respected others' skills or input?

Team members need to value and respect others, and to see that, however skilled and senior they are, no effective health care takes place in isolation. We all have a responsibility to participate in, build and develop our teamwork. Reflecting on teamwork cultures, 'how do we do things around here', may be quite challenging for learners and teachers; juniors see things with fresh eyes and teachers must remain open to comments and even criticisms.

Comments like 'It is pretty stressful. I don't feel supported' need to be seen as teamwork and training issues, not opportunities to blame the learner for incompetence or frailty.

References

1. Aviation Knowledge. DODAR, http://aviationknowledge.wikidot.com/aviation:dodar [accessed 31 July 2015].
2. Pian-Smith MC, Simon R, Minehart RD, *et al.* Teaching residents the two-challenge rule: a simulation-based approach to improve education and patient safety. *Simulation in Healthcare* 2009; **4(2)**: 84–91.

Resources for team-working

Ballatt J, Campling P. *Intelligent Kindness: reforming the culture of healthcare.* London: RCPsych Publications, 2011.

Covey S. *The Seven Habits of Highly Effective People.* New York: Simon & Schuster, 2005.

NHS Health Education North West. Medical leadership development tool: chairing a meeting, www.nwpgmd.nhs.uk/sites/default/files/Chairing%20a%20Meeting%20MLDT.pdf [accessed 31 July 2015].

Part III

Mapping the psychology of uncertainty

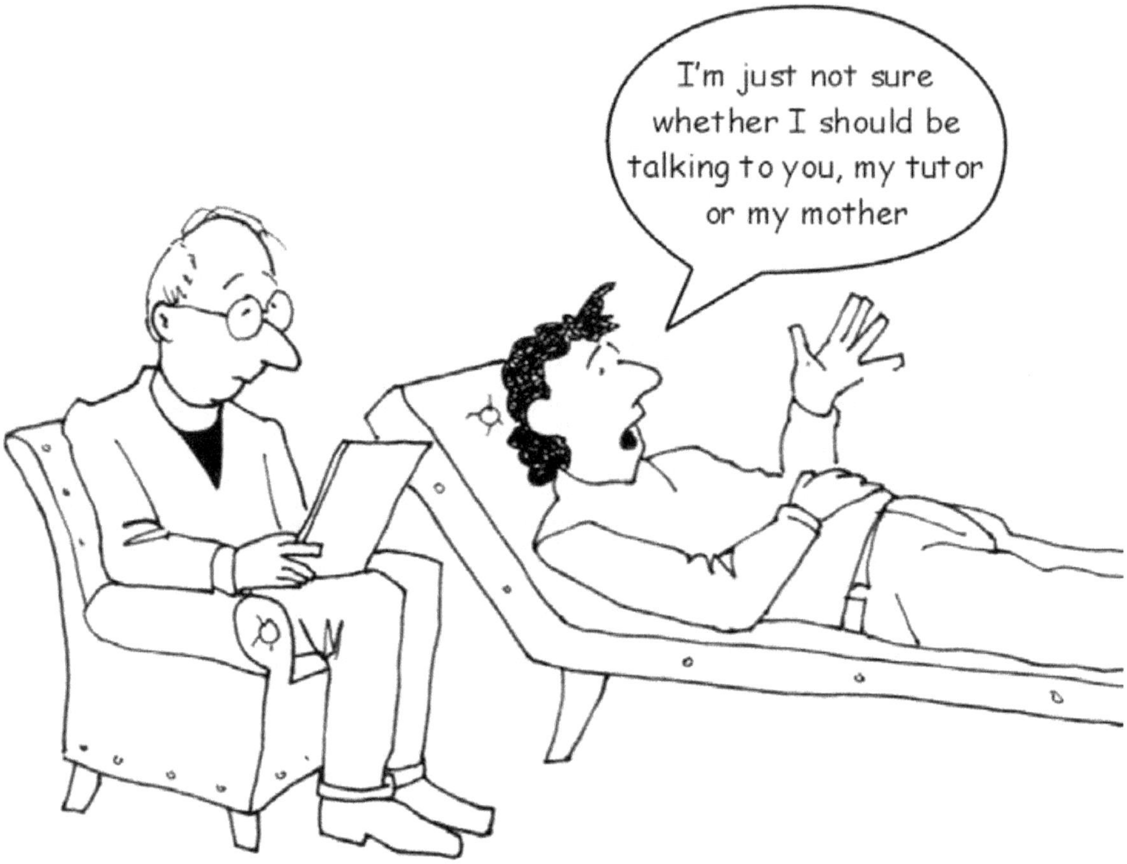
I'm just not sure whether I should be talking to you, my tutor or my mother

Uncertainty is complicated from a psychological point of view and involves thinking (cognitive) and emotional (feeling) aspects; furthermore, psychological insights illuminate how uncertainty affects relationships and behaviours within organisations. This part of the book examines these issues in more detail.

Chapter 15 discusses some of the broader psychological issues that influence clinicians in situations of uncertainty. **Chapter 16** examines how psychological aspects of uncertainty are manifested in the different types of uncertainty that were identified and explored in Part II.

Chapter 15

The psychological themes that underpin clinicians' responses to uncertainty

> In theory, a person should make decisions about life and death matters analytically, on the basis of the facts. But the facts were shot through with holes and uncertainties.... No clear predictions could be made. Making choices required somehow filling the gaps, and what my father filled them with was fear.
>
> Atul Gawande[1]

Uncertainty is experienced in all branches of medicine and by practitioners of all levels of seniority, and also by patients. Many clinicians are disturbed by uncertainty, even though it is a common experience, and try to avoid it as much as possible, sometimes by employing the 'dysfunctional ways out' described in the Quadrant chapters. Action rather than inaction, referring or deferring to someone else, are all methods used to relieve the discomfort of uncertainty. How do uncertainties in the different Quadrants affect clinicians?

This chapter addresses some of the psychological components of uncertainty. Some responses to uncertainty are unconscious; understanding these responses more explicitly gives rise to the possibility of adopting better ways of tolerating and managing uncertainty in medical practice. This chapter is divided into:

- definitions and some psychological elements of uncertainty
- how clinicians think about uncertainty
- two key underlying themes: error and 'existential' issues
- strategies for maintaining resilience to uncertainty.

Definitions and some psychological elements of uncertainty

Can we define 'uncertainty' psychologically speaking? If we do, will it help us understand how our minds work when faced with uncertainty, and even offer some better strategies? Uncertainty is found in all fields of endeavour: economics, sport, mathematics, philosophy, theology and computer science[2] as well as social work, nursing and management. It is hard to imagine an area of life where uncertainty does not play a significant part. Ambiguity, signifying 'inexactness or double meaning', is a crucial part of uncertainty, also thought of as a 'fact or condition that lacks firm predictability'.[3] To be uncertain about something, there also has to be a consciousness, an awareness, that not all the required information, knowledge or skill is available. This is a 'metacognition', an awareness of the process of thinking. This concept leads Han *et al.* to define uncertainty as 'the subjective perception of ignorance'. In contrast, Han refers to 'meta-ignorance', when the unknown remains unconscious. In that situation the ambiguity or uncertainty remains unrecognised.[4]

Time can also be incorporated into a definition of uncertainty:[5]

> *Uncertainty is a present orientated state that is influenced by perceptions of the past and future reflected in precognitive sensations (feeling in your gut that it is right) or cognitive processing (consciously choosing a path to meet a desired outcome).*[6]

This definition elaborates the subjective experience of uncertainty into an *emotional*, feeling, part, and a *cognitive*, thinking, part. The subjective nature of uncertainty is crucial; an ambiguity, or lack of complete knowledge tolerated by one person, may be perceived with great anxiety by another. The cognitive elements of uncertainty relate to knowledge, analysis and decision making. This is familiar territory to clinicians, who often feel more comfortable talking about decisions than they do talking about the emotions affecting those decisions, whether these are their own emotions or those of their patients.

In clinical practice, uncertainty is made more complex because it inevitably involves other people. In other words, uncertainty in clinical practice always involves personal *relationships*: with patients, relatives, colleagues and managers.

Uncertainty also has *organisational* components. Clinical settings, and organisational and regulatory structures, may exacerbate or contain uncertainty. Clinicians' awareness of others in related departments or institutions also has an impact on their own subjective perceptions of uncertainty.

In Chapter 16 the impact of these four components of uncertainty (feeling, thinking, relationships and organisational aspects) will be mapped against the Quadrants of Analysing, Networking, Negotiating and Team-working. This will cast some light on how these psychological elements affect clinicians during their work.

Although clinical work has its own specific kinds of uncertainty, clinicians are also affected by responses to uncertainty that are basic to all human behaviour. Our brains are organised to recognise uncertainty, which indicates that there is a decision to be made. We then weigh up the possible outcomes and choose a course of action or inaction. Our neurological systems are continually monitoring our environment and modifying our responses to that incoming information. Learning to cope with uncertainty is evolutionally advantageous, and essential to survival, wellbeing and productivity.[7] Fast, intuitive Type 1 thinking in response to uncertainty, described in Chapter 3, is probably helpful from an *evolutionary* point of view. It is safer to assume that speckled shadow could be a leopard and take evasive action quickly, than to waste time wondering if, perhaps, it is just a pattern from overhead leaves. Otherwise, a leopard, if present, will soon be enjoying a bit of your leg for lunch. Type 1 thinking is still very useful in non-clinical life: when driving, Type 1 thinking will take over and result in rapid braking when something moves out from behind a parked car. We don't wait for Type 2 thinking to analyse whether it is a child, a dog or a harmless plastic bag blowing in the wind.

Anxiety is another response to uncertainty; noradrenaline release in uncertain situations heightens the subjective experience of anxiety, with raised heart rate, tremor and hyperventilation, the typical 'flight or fight' response. Fear is likely to be elicited by threatening situations with clear strategies for avoiding the threat. If there is no clear strategy for evading the threat then anxiety is the more likely response.[8]

Uncertainty arises in situations where a choice of action, or interpretation, has to be made; anxiety actually increases with the simple fact of increased choice. When faced with an increased choice of products, consumers become more anxious despite the minimal consequences of choosing one product over another. Some anxiety in response to uncertainty is simply the result of having to choose between options, rather than concern about choosing wrongly.[9]

However, total certainty is not necessarily preferable. When everything is known and predictable, life can seem boring, lacking in excitement or unrewarding. Clinicians, in particular, enjoy problem solving and puzzling things out; getting the 'right answer' when things initially seem confusing is psychologically rewarding.

How clinicians think about uncertainty

Uncertainty in clinical practice has been explored by many writers. As long ago as 1957 Fox discussed the different impacts of uncertainty like this:

> *The first results from incomplete or imperfect mastery of available knowledge. No one can have at his command all skills and all knowledge of the core of medicine. The second depends upon limitations in current medical knowledge. There are innumerable questions to which no physician, however well trained, can as yet provide answers. A third source of uncertainty derives from the first two. This consists of difficulty in distinguishing between personal ignorance or ineptitude and the limitations of present medical knowledge.*[10]

Although this is helpful in understanding how clinicians may encounter uncertainty, we also have to consider what professional responses to uncertainty actually are. Do clinicians accept and acknowledge uncertainty, or do they take refuge in defensive dissociation or denial responses that disavow the uncertainty?

One physician cannot possibly have all the relevant and current medical knowledge to hand at any given time. For many clinicians, the difficulty in 'distinguishing between personal ignorance' and 'the limitations of present medical knowledge' can provoke anxiety. In practice, clusters of symptoms may take time to become apparent, or delays in investigations will mean that most physicians will face a period of uncertainty during the care of an individual patient. This may or may not be shared with the patient or with others. Outcomes are often uncertain; there are so many factors that impinge on individuals, meaning that the effects of treatment can be unpredictable. Research helps a bit here, but medical research rarely provides all the answers. Clinicians know that the validity and generalisability of most medical research is itself uncertain. Applying research findings to the individual patient can be difficult, as patients often differ in important respects from those who have been researched. Even robust research does not completely change practice immediately; many findings from research need to be consistently replicated before doctors feel happy deviating from usual behaviours.

A more nuanced approach to uncertainty in clinical practice recognises technical, personal and conceptual uncertainties.[11]

Technical uncertainty includes physicians' lack of knowledge and the unknowns of medical knowledge. To some extent, these may be reduced by advances in technical knowledge, the outcomes of further research and by the physician gaining more information or experience.

Personal uncertainty arises from the doctor–patient relationship and includes uncertainties that arise because of inadequate data gathering or not understanding the patient's wishes.

Conceptual uncertainty includes having limited resources, the inherent uncertainty of the effects of treatment on individuals, and unexpected or unpredictable outcomes. Bias from past experience may affect current decisions.

Personal and conceptual sources of uncertainty have been described as 'meta uncertainty' because the amount of uncertainty present cannot be easily defined or measured; there is 'uncertainty about how uncertain one is'.[12] The uncomfortable and complex uncertainty encountered in primary care has been evocatively described as:

> *The confusion, conflict, stuckness, unease, and/or discomfort an individual primary care clinician experiences when confronting a predicament in an individual patient who presents a diagnostic, therapeutic, general management, clinician-patient relationship, prognostic, ethical dilemma, or some combination of these dimensions.*[13]

Multiple themes beyond the individual patient create uncertainty; these include patient–physician relationships, physician–colleague relationships, professional norms, self-esteem as a physician, bad outcomes, missed diagnoses, malpractice worries, patient referrals and investigation requests. Clinicians show a variety of reactions to uncertainty, and doctors' self-reporting methods are inconsistent. For example, many doctors feel uncertainty should be shared with the patient, but few actually admit to doing this.[14/15] The personality traits of individual clinicians also affect their behaviour in uncertain situations. For example, clinicians scoring highly for agreeableness, conscientiousness and openness to experience were significantly positively associated with communicating uncertainty.[16]

When dealing with uncertainty, clinicians need to possess more than clinical knowledge and experience. They have to develop the cognitive processes involved in decision making, understand the limitations of their knowledge and recognise the impact of emotion and of relationships on how they respond to uncertainty. That makes things complicated enough, but the complexity is increased when we start to consider some deeper, perhaps fundamental, issues.

Key underlying themes: error and 'existential' issues

There are two overarching themes that provide a powerful background for clinicians responding to uncertain situations. First, there is the undefined relationship between uncertainty and error. Second, and unique to healthcare work, is the fact that uncertainty for clinicians exists within a wider uncertainty of illness, disability and death itself.

Much of the literature about how doctors think is primarily concerned with how doctors come to make errors. In situations of uncertainty, where there are several possible options for decisions, doctors are aware that they may make a 'wrong decision'. Unless paralysed by the anxiety of choice (which can happen), a clinician will usually make a decision, articulating implicitly or explicitly what their reasoning process has been. The consequences of a 'wrong decision' may then be seen as following from faulty reasoning or decision making. This is sometimes only apparent with hindsight, which all doctors, but fewer patients, know is a wonderful thing. However, many decisions regretted in hindsight were reasonable at the time at which they were made. Inherently unpredictable events may overtake the clinical situation, however appropriate the initial decision making. As emphasised in the very first chapter of this book, much uncertainty in medicine is irreducible.

Reasonable decisions, which are later deemed 'wrong' decisions, can sometimes occur when the clinician is not overtly uncertain. Many errors occur when clinicians feel perfectly comfortable with their decision making or actions. This may be because they have succumbed to bias in their thinking (as outlined in Chapter 3), or because they have resorted to a 'dysfunctional way out'. Both of these cognitive strategies have the effect of reducing or even eliminating uncertainty for the clinician. The uncertainty is met with denial in the clinician ('this is the answer'), or deflected to somewhere else ('let's just get a scan'). Thus, error is just as likely to be associated with apparent certainty, as with apparent uncertainty.

Most clinicians live in fear of error, especially perhaps diagnostic errors, but also errors of judgement or practice. They fear causing harm to patients (with all the attendant guilt) or the scorn of peers or regulators (with the attendant shame). So strong is doctors' aversion to being thought in error that errors may not be acknowledged or discussed. Investigation by the General Medical Council (GMC) into *potential* wrongdoing may be enough to trigger suicide, even before the outcome of the investigation is known,[17] clearly showing how threatening the possibility of being in the wrong can be. This fear of error underpins some doctors' distinct intolerance to uncertainty. Doctors need to feel that they are 'doing the right thing'. Maintaining a state of ambiguity or ambivalence, which precludes decisive action, simply renders doctors so uncomfortable that they jump to an action or decision. This can mean making premature decisions, which is, paradoxically, a key cause of error.

Furthermore, clinicians may not distinguish situations in which they really were at fault from those where there was an unpredictable deterioration in a patient. Most doctors will be able to describe 'lucky escapes' where performance was poor or a mistake was made but there were no bad outcomes. Both of these situations seem to provoke intense guilt, which is again linked to anxiety as doctors ask themselves disturbing 'what if' questions. Danielle Ofri is a physician who has written frankly about the intense emotions that doctors feel in relation to the pressures of their work. The narrative that follows describes her response to what she saw as her own incompetence.[18]

When she discovered that a patient who had self-harmed had left the hospital without a formal psychiatric opinion, Danielle Ofri vividly described feeling 'scared witless', 'negligent' and 'stupid', although basic assessment revealed he was not suicidal.

Yet, the patient had been transferred by ambulance to a private psychiatric hospital, with the full involvement of his family and had said, 'it's not like I want to die or anything'. In spite of the fact that *no harm came to him at all*, she felt that she should apologise and that she had 'endangered his life'. This surprising reaction came about because she had relied on a basic risk assessment by her team (who established that he was not trying to kill himself and was not actively suicidal) and had authorised transferring him to the care of his own psychiatrist without seeing a psychiatrist in her own hospital first. She felt that only a psychiatrist could take the responsibility of establishing that the patient was safe to travel to another hospital.

Taking responsibility for a potential outcome to such a degree (when nothing adverse actually happened to the patient), and for the doctor to feel such guilt, seems to absolve the patient of any responsibility or agency, and seems only partly driven by worries about litigation. Doctors can use a kind of 'defensive omnipotence' in the face of uncertainty, by trying to be in control of all eventualities. This is a way of avoiding uncertainty by planning ahead. With this thinking approach, the intrinsic uncertainty of illness may seem to be tamed. Even if the doctor made an error, she nonetheless controlled the outcome.[19] However, if this strategy is used, clinicians may feel unreasonably responsible for unpredictable or uncertain outcomes. Letting go of the sense of total responsibility means accepting a disturbing degree of uncertainty.

Such uncertainty may be particularly difficult for clinicians, because error and any harm that results directly affects the person they are supposed to be caring for and the clinician–patient relationship is one of profound trust in the clinician doing the 'right thing'. This is why failure, or the causing of deliberate harm (such as happened with Harold Shipman), is so deeply disturbing. Errors in other fields of work may also cause harm up to and including death. However, such harms are usually accidental. If, say, an engineer designs a faulty bridge, this might unintentionally lead to injury or death if the bridge fails, but the engineer does not have to look the victims in the eye first. Moreover, a team is much more likely to be involved in an engineering project, so that errors will be picked up by other people before the final decisions are made. In health work, clinicians face the risk of causing someone harm or death by their intentional actions, applied directly to the person being cared for, without so many opportunities to check our actions with other people. Any breach of trust through error, and the possibility of real harm or death, is painful for all participants to contemplate. It links fear of error to the second overarching theme of uncertainty, which is the threat posed to us by illness and death. This 'existential' issue is one of the basic problems that being human poses. Our fear of death takes its place alongside our fear of being alone, our need for meaning in life and our difficulties with making choices and decisions, as one of the key 'existential' issues everyone faces.[20]

Clinical work brings us frighteningly close to suffering and death. This makes our own vulnerability as humans painfully apparent; clinicians are just as scared of death and pain as anyone else. The psychological defences of denial ('It will not happen to me'), disconnection ('I will not allow this patient's suffering to impinge on me'), displacement ('Let's really concentrate on getting all these drug dosages correct') or distraction ('I have an important meeting to attend') will probably be recognised by most clinicians, although often not articulated.

Daily contact with disease and death is inevitably stressing and distressing, and using up reserves of energy, kindness, intellectual capacity and physical stamina makes all healthcare work particularly demanding. All front-line health staff have to deal with the 'overwhelmingness' of disease up to and including death. Coping with the attendant uncertainty is tricky. Too much denial of uncertainty can lead to premature decision making and errors; too little denial of uncertainty can result in paralysing anxiety.

Strategies to maintain resilience in the face of uncertainty

Although uncertainty is uncomfortable, clinicians find ways to cope! Many writers have recorded the black humour of clinicians, sometimes even called 'gallows humour', and even non-clinicians enjoy television programmes such as *House*, which explores clinical work through the eyes of a team led by a misanthropic, yet clever, physician. Humour also helps us diffuse feelings of aggression, frustration or anxiety in the face of clinical problems that seem too ambiguous, too difficult or too demanding. All clinicians have their favourite funny stories that cast a light on situations of uncertainty, death or failure.

Clinicians have cognitive strategies for coping with uncertainty too. We have already described many of them. Perhaps the least acceptable is to unconsciously maintain a state of 'meta-ignorance', a state of not knowing that you are ignorant. This is a strong method of keeping uncertainty at bay. Doctors who are comfortable with practical, cognitive decision making may, in effect, decide that they 'know enough' and adhere to comfortable routines. Others may deny that there is any relevant knowledge in the fields of psychology, theories of effective teamwork or the social science of medicine. Such knowledge may be airily dismissed as being 'touchy feely' and thus not needing to be taken seriously. Meta-ignorance is more comfortable for the clinician than it is for his colleagues or patients. Experience may lead to a greater 'equanimity' as William Osler had it,[21] but the risk is that emotional blunting or unhealthy interpersonal distancing will occur. This can be ameliorated through healthy discussions with others.

Relationships can help clinicians be more resilient to uncertainty. Creating opportunities to talk about uncertainty, whether informally over coffee, or more formally in meetings or supervision sessions, helps clinicians to articulate their thought processes, to acknowledge the emotional effects of uncertainty and to learn that others also have similar experiences. This can help protect doctors against the idea that they should be 'perfect', 'know everything' and be the doctor who 'never makes mistakes'. Trying to avoid the stresses of uncertainty by 'being perfect' can become extremely stressful; burnout and its associated problems of depression, substance abuse and poor family relationships may follow. Organisations can take steps to foster such discussions, to build time into teamwork to allow healthy relationships to develop; this can increase opportunities for learning effective ways to deal with uncertainty.

Things can become more serious if clinicians start to believe their own publicity about being certain. If a doctor cannot tolerate or accept a degree of uncertainty or ambiguity in her clinical practice she may start to see things in a rather black and white way, either taking refuge in 'being perfect' or seeing the alternative as 'being a failure'. This may even encourage some doctors to take refuge in a narcissistic view of their practice; in effect they may deny uncertainty and say 'I am doing the right thing' and therefore 'What I am doing must be right'. Needless to say, the latter view is neither healthy for the individual clinician nor safe for the patient. Discussing problems with peers allows triangulation and a sense of what is 'reasonable' or 'good enough' to be established.

There are pressures on clinicians to be certain. The earlier part of this chapter reflects on how internal psychological factors can mean doctors place themselves under pressure to be certain. Patients may also prefer certainty, which can influence clinicians to act as if they are more certain than they really feel. Patients' reactions to uncertainty are considered in more detail in Part V. The organisations in which clinicians work also prefer certainty; they want their clinicians to make decisions and get on with doing the job of caring for the patient appropriately. 'Sitting' with uncertainty, reflection and discussion take precious time that may simply not be available when resources are tight, clinics are full and organisations are under pressure to keep waiting to a minimum. Clinicians occupy a position among all these competing pressures, and learning to deal with attendant uncertainty is one of the requirements of professional life. This aspect of uncertainty is considered more deeply in Part IV.

References

1. Gawande A. *Being Mortal*. London: Metropolitan Books, 2014.
2. Halpern J. *Reasoning About Uncertainty*. Cambridge, MA, and London: MIT Press, 2005.
3. Luther V, Crandall S. Ambiguity and uncertainty: neglected elements of medical education curricula? *Academic Medicine* 2011; **86(7)**: 799–800.
4. Han P, Klein W, Arora N. Varieties of uncertainty in health care: a conceptual taxonomy. *Medical Decision Making* 2011; **31(6)**: 828–38.
5. Penrod J. Refinement of the concept of uncertainty. *Journal of Advanced Nursing* 2001; **34(2)**: 238–45.

6. Penrod J. Living with uncertainty: concept advancement. *Journal of Advanced Nursing* 2007; **57(6)**: 658–67.
7. Friston, K. The free-energy principle: a rough guide to the brain? *Trends in Cognitive Sciences* 2009; **13(7)**: 293–301.
8. Hirsh J, Peterson J, Mar R. Psychological entropy: a framework for understanding uncertainty-related anxiety. *Psychological Review* 2012; **119(2)**: 304–20.
9. Iyengar S, Lepper M. When choice is demotivating: can one desire too much of a good thing? *Journal of Personality and Social Psychology* 2000; **79(6)**: 995–1006.
10. Fox RC. Training for Uncertainty. In: RK Merton, G Reader, PL Kendall (eds). *The Student-Physician: introductory studies in the sociology of medical education.* Cambridge, MA: Harvard University Press, 1957.
11. Beresford EB. Uncertainty and the shaping of medical decisions. *Hasting Centre Report* 1991; **21(4)**: 6–1.
12. Hall K. Reviewing intuitive decision-making and uncertainty: the implications for medical education. *Medical Education* 2002; **36(3)**: 216–24.
13. Sommers LS. Introduction. In: LS Sommers, J Launer (eds). *Clinical Uncertainty in Primary Care: the challenge of collaborative engagement.* New York, NY: Springer, 2013, pp. 3–18.
14. Gerrity M, Earp JA, DeVellis RF. Uncertainty and professional work: perceptions of physicians in clinical practice. *American Journal of Sociology* 1992; **97(4)**: 1022–51.
15. Gerrity M, De Vellis RF, Earp JA. Physicians' reactions to uncertainty in patient care. A new measure and new insights. *Medical Care* 1990; **28(8)**: 724–36.
16. Schneider A, Löwe B, Barie S, *et al.* How do primary care doctors deal with uncertainty in making decisions. *Journal of Evaluation in Clinical Practice* 2010; **16(3)**: 431–7.
17. Horsfall S. *Doctors who Commit Suicide while under GMC Fitness to Practise Investigation.* London: GMC, 2014, www.gmc-uk.org/Internal_review_into_suicide_in_FTP_processes.pdf_59088696.pdf [accessed 1 August 2015].
18. Ofri D. *What Doctors Feel: how emotions affect the practice of medicine.* Boston, MA: Beacon Press, 2013.
19. Collins ME, Block SD, Arnold RM, Christakis NA. On the prospects for a blame-free medical culture. *Social Science and Medicine* 2009; **69(9)**: 1287–90.
20. Yalom ID. *Existential Psychotherapy.* New York, NY: Basic Books, 1980.
21. Osler W. *Aequanimitas,* www.medicalarchives.jhmi.edu/osler/aequessay.htm [accessed 17 December 2015].

Chapter 16

Mapping the psychology of uncertainty against the Analysing, Networking, Negotiating and Team-working Quadrants

This chapter looks in more detail at how the emotional, cognitive, relationship and organisational components of uncertainty are involved in the different types of uncertainty, mapped against the four Quadrants that were explored in Part II. The chapter covers psychological components of uncertainty in the:

- Analysing Quadrant
- Networking Quadrant
- Negotiating Quadrant
- Team-working Quadrant.

Psychological components of uncertainty in the Analysing Quadrant

- Emotional reactions: anxiety, guilt.
- Cognitive strategies: bias, premature closure.
- Relationship issues: trust in the clinician–patient relationship.
- Organisational components: time, access to information.

Emotional reactions to uncertainty in the Analysing Quadrant have two components. First, uncertainty is closely tied up with concerns about making mistakes for clinicians and this colours their emotional stance when making diagnoses. Second, emotions affect the cognitive (thinking) processes that clinicians bring to the diagnostic process.

The main emotional reactions in the Analysing Quadrant relate to anxiety and guilt. Diagnosing skilfully is a crucial part of any examination or assessment process for clinicians. Clinicians' self-esteem is bound up with the ability to make the right diagnosis, or at least a plausible differential diagnosis. Uncertainty in this area is therefore closely tied up with notions of 'error', or 'getting it wrong'. Uncertainty about diagnosis drives a fear that the diagnosis will be missed or wrong; all doctors have lain awake at night, suffering from anxiety that they may have 'missed something', or made an incorrect diagnosis. Guilt can follow.

Guilt is a powerful feeling of internal conflict that arises when someone does something he thinks he should not have done (on moral or legal grounds), or when he considers himself to have failed to do something that he was legitimately expected or even required to do (e.g. make the correct diagnosis). Guilt can occur owing to internal conflict alone, or as a result of actual harm to others. Doctors often feel guilty, and blame themselves, even if no actual harm comes to a patient, or if others think that the harm could not have been avoided. Anxiety and continual worry about 'missing things' can be seen as a way to forestall the unpleasant guilty feelings that would be experienced if something 'went wrong'.

Feelings of guilt and anxiety can be also be forestalled if the clinician responds to uncertainty by premature closure; this strategy may be favoured more frequently by clinicians who are less tolerant of ambiguity. Action is favoured over inaction, driven by Type 1 thinking; difficult feelings associated with uncertainty are avoided because the uncertainty itself is denied or rapidly avoided. This process drives some of the 'dysfunctional ways out' discussed in the Analysing Quadrant (see Chapter 3, p. 27).

Clinicians' emotions related to uncertain diagnosis also influence *cognitive* (thinking) processes. Negative emotions tend to drive the reduction of uncertainty by anchoring bias, that is, latching on to particular information early on and ignoring other information that does not 'fit'. This process has already been described in Chapter 3. In contrast, positive emotions may lead to attribution bias, when the problem is blamed on some aspect of the individual patient (perhaps the fact of her alcohol misuse) rather than on the situation (her confusion may be due to delirium in the presence of an infection, rather than due to alcohol). Positive emotions favour a view of the bigger picture ('the forest'), whereas negative emotions tend to favour the smaller details ('the trees').[1] In uncertain situations the general emotional 'tone' of the clinician may affect which bias she tends towards. Sometimes clinicians can simply rationalise away difficult feelings about uncertainty if important things, at least, are ruled out. As one clinician remarked: 'The emotional response to uncertainty is a function of the consequence of being wrong. I may feel uncertain about the cause of chest pain but comfortable in my uncertainty if important causes are excluded.'[2]

Emotion influences analysis in other ways too. Information transmitted by emotions is part of the 'data that should be considered' in consultations.[3] Emotional intelligence is important both for accurate diagnosis (emotional or mental health are always among the diagnostic possibilities) and for building an effective doctor–patient relationship, which is an intrinsic part of effective care.

Much research on the *cognitive processes* in the Analysing Quadrant has focused on how errors in thinking occur. Individuals tend, possibly unconsciously, to choose an approach to diagnosis that requires least cognitive effort, which tends to favour fast, intuitive Type 1 thinking.[4] Avoiding uncertainty through intuition or heuristics ('rules of thumb') is a kind of 'cognitive "short circuiting" where a decision is reached even though the reasons for the decision cannot easily be described'.[5]

Intuition or heuristics tend to make complex tasks more simple, or decision making faster, and so can mean that uncertainty (and its associated feelings) can be avoided. Although intuitive thinking can lead to error, unless 'checked' by subsequent analytical thinking, intuition remains a crucial part of clinical reasoning.[6] Pattern recognition strategies (another type of heuristic or 'rule of thumb') often lead to assessments that are just as accurate as those achieved analytically (and with less effort). Intuitive Type 1 thinking and analytical Type 2 thinking work in interacting and complementary ways.[3]

Following strict guidelines for practice (there are very many available to follow) is one way to reduce the cognitive effort of clinical practice. One important limitation of guidelines is that they do not always apply to the individual patient concerned, because of age, comorbidity or other complex factors. In this situation 'rules of thumb' may result in experienced clinicians making rapid, apparently intuitive, decisions that do not conform to guidelines. Although this may be rational and effective, over-reliance on rapid decisions using 'heuristics' can mean that prejudice ('this patient is too old to benefit') or lack of skill ('I do not know how to get the patient involved in this decision') over-ride appropriate reasoning.

Decision making is also affected by the clinician's own level of acceptance of ambiguity, for example where symptoms are complicated or vague, a common situation in clinical practice. People who are less tolerant of uncertainty prefer to avoid such complex or contradictory situations, whereas people who are more tolerant of ambiguity enjoy problem solving and are more at ease making complex decisions.[7]

Relationship issues are important for uncertainty in the Analysing Quadrant. The patient's question 'Can I trust this doctor to see me as an individual?' or 'Will the doctor listen carefully to what I have to say and take me seriously?' reflect a need to trust the clinician. Conversely, the doctor needs to feel that the patient trusts and respects her, as that allows the doctor to have enough self-confidence to navigate any uncertainty in diagnosis. Malpractice claims, which occur when that trust has disappeared, can damage a doctor's ability to work well, *even if exonerated of any wrongdoing.*[1] Doctors who have been sued for wrong diagnosis make changes in their behaviour to become 'more defensive'; an ability to manage a reasonable degree of uncertainty is replaced by over-reliance on tests or referrals, checking and rumination, which may actually become counterproductive.

The *organisational* setting in which diagnosis is occurring also has a strong influence on how uncertainty is perceived and acted upon. The amount of information available to clinicians (such as test results, patient notes, reference literature, access to online information) and the kind of training that is supported by the institution (are trainees allowed access to study, are seniors given time to supervise, teach or reflect on difficult situations?) will influence how much uncertainty is expressible. For example, if the institution 'implies or permits' only a short response time before a diagnosis is to be made, perhaps expecting a doctor to see 20 patients in three hours, 'intuition is the mode that the institution expects'.[8] If time and information are in short supply the only way to manage uncertainty will tend to be 'premature closure'.

Psychological components of uncertainty in the Networking Quadrant

- Emotional reaction: shame, contempt for others.
- Cognitive issues: over-diagnosis.
- Relationship issues: subjective experiences of uncertainty.
- Organisational: lack of continuity, unfamiliarity.

Emotional reactions to uncertainty in the Networking Quadrant are related to the fact that there is a wider audience; guilt develops into shame, an even more toxic emotion. The dividing lines between guilt, shame and embarrassment are not clear cut in medical practice. Even in the privacy of a consultation, the doctor may be working to anticipate and avoid errors that could lead to potentially shaming experiences with the GMC or a courtroom. However, as generally understood, shame is a social experience; it occurs when other people are (or we imagine them to be) critical, disapproving, dismissive or contemptuous of our actions. Guilt implies regret and responsibility for *actions* that violate norms. Shame is applied to the person himself, rather than the event or action. Shame can be anticipatory ('I would be ashamed to do that'), or inward, as it is possible to feel ashamed of thoughts or even actions that no one else knows about, if discovery is feared. Shame is an acutely self-conscious state in which we imagine ourselves under scrutiny, and found to be inadequate, wrong or unacceptable.

Studies of doctors' reactions to uncertainty have emphasised the 'fear of personal inadequacy and failure'.[9–12] Thus, doctors may not disclose uncertainty to colleagues because of the shame involved in being seen as inadequate. 'Education by humiliation' still occurs in medical practice and can result in a deep-seated fear of being shamed for 'not knowing'. When referring within a network, doctors face a complex emotional situation: if they are uncertain in diagnosis, referral to another clinician may be a 'functional way out' if the referral is generally deemed appropriate. However, clinicians also risk shame if, on referring, they expose unacceptable ignorance or inadequacy.

The *cognitive element* in the Networking Quadrant is about decision making, choosing a plan for investigations and enacting that with the patient. Thus, the psychological effects of choice return. In the previous section, it was apparent that choice can, of itself, create anxiety. Knowing that a wide array of tests, investigations and specialists are available will add to the uncertainty experienced by many doctors, especially if they are unfamiliar with 'using time as a diagnostic tool' or if they lack the confidence to 'hold' uncertainty for a time. Confusing their own uncertainty ('Am I sure I have the right diagnosis?') with the intrinsic uncertainty of medical practice ('Is this child's sore throat the first sign of leukaemia, or just a sore throat?') compounds this anxiety. Experience may mitigate this anxiety to a point; however, while learning, trainees may:

> *find it difficult to exercise restraint in their investigations and to tolerate ambiguities in the undifferentiated, minor and self limited problems of family medicine and may feel inadequate and professionally unfulfilled if they are unable to establish an exact diagnosis.*[12]

Of course, investigations do not always ease uncertainty; they can also add to it. False positives, false negatives or inconclusive results need to be explained to the patient (a difficult task); more detailed, costly and risky investigations may follow with a real risk of harm to the patient. As medical practice becomes more regulated and more complex, referring for tests and investigations is also becoming more regulated. Doctors defend themselves against any shame attached to over-referral by blaming the system ('they won't fund this type of referral') or, in the USA, getting into conflicts with insurance companies over what they will fund. Blame and contempt for the other party involved can also be seen as defence mechanisms that protect clinicians from feeling shame if their 'unsuitable' referrals are exposed and criticised.

Resolving uncertainty by investigation or referral can also be a way for clinicians to bolster their sense that they are doing everything possible for their patients, which may provide another avenue for disguising any sense of inadequacy. However, denying uncertainty in this Quadrant, together with an attitude that requires doctors to seem to be 'in control', can also be seen as part of a very big problem in modern medical practice, as it tends to result in over-investigation. This can be a strategy for avoiding uncertainty and yet can lead to harm through over-treatment, with the attendant risks of iatrogenic harm.

> *Denial of uncertainty, defences against criticism and management of patients to maintain dominance, if they are common products of training have important consequences for medical practice. They may be predisposing factors behind overtreatment and iatrogenesis.*[14]

How do *relationships* affect uncertainty in the Networking Quadrant? Uncertainty is not necessarily a result of inadequate knowledge, rather of how a particular individual (or partnership if shared with a patient) *feels* about their state of knowledge, and whether or how uncertainty is talked about. Being uncertain is a subjective state; nobody can deny another's feeling of uncertainty. One person may have all the required knowledge to make a decision but still feel uncertain, whereas another individual may have much less knowledge but be more decisive.[14] Such variations in the perception of uncertainty exist for patients too. This can influence the pressure on doctors to refer onwards, if they and the patient have a different perception of uncertainty. Referral is a frequent cognitive 'way out' of uncertainty; the difficulty is transferred to someone else.

Organisational factors play a part in how wider networks are used in times of uncertainty. How the practice or clinic was set up (for example the criteria for referral, the expertise available), the funding (which may preclude certain activities), the investigations available (promoting or restricting some 'dysfunctional ways out') and the appointment schedule all affect the handling of uncertainty. If a clinic is full, referral may be seen as a short cut to keeping to time. Being able to 'hold' situations over time requires continuity of care; many organisational structures do not facilitate this, with doctors rotating frequently or having their work split over several sites. There may simply be no 'culture of continuity', which implies a personal commitment to an individual patient's care. Limiting commitment to an individual clinician–patient relationship may be one of the ways in which clinicians avoid the emotional or relationship effects of uncertainty, by effectively deferring care to the next clinician.

If multiple clinicians are involved in the care of a patient, the quality of the note keeping is also under scrutiny by other clinicians all the time. In effect colleagues are constantly making judgements about each other.[15] The effect on decision making is likely to lead to increased referrals to ensure 'nothing is missed' and the clinician will thus avoid painful guilt or shame. The loss of the personal clinician–patient relationship is not recorded and risks not being valued.

Clinicians in training may also feel heightened stress from uncertainty while trying to familiarise themselves with the organisational factors involved in the patient network, such as how to order investigations and what services are available. This adds further complexity to a consultation and often requires advice from colleagues. Juniors may be uncertain about how to resolve such uncertainties, or worry about being a burden on their supervisor. A complex mixture of guilt ('I can't interrupt my supervisor yet again') and shame ('I probably ought to know this') can ensue. This may mean that, although some trainees appear over-anxious, others, fearing shame or guilt, may simply deny their uncertainty and act over-confidently. Organisational factors in training can mitigate the psychological stresses of uncertainty to some degree, if wise supervision is readily available.

Psychological components of uncertainty in the Negotiating Quadrant

- Emotional reactions: guilt.
- Cognitive strategies: anxiety of choice.
- Relationship issues: blaming the patient.
- Organisational components: uncertainty avoidance.

The *emotional* experiences of doctors in the Negotiating Quadrant are again dominated by the obligations that clinicians feel towards patients, trying to avoid 'doing something wrong' and failing the patient. Thus, again, guilt is a predominant emotion in the background. When interviewed about caring for dying patients who had unexpected outcomes, physicians most often blamed themselves, often disproportionately to their involvement in the patient's care.

> *When physicians use the pronoun 'we' while discussing mistakes, this suggests a willingness to include themselves in the sometimes faulty decisions and actions of others … an effort to assume control over bad outcomes by conceptualizing them as related to a mistake, rather than the randomness and inherent risk that pervade medicine.*[16]

In contrast, junior doctors, whose uncertainty or lack of experience led them to make errors, may use a variety of strategies to ameliorate the guilt and self-blame that they feel. Errors may be approached with denial, or with discounting or distancing remarks. In particular, as part of a distancing approach to error, blame was placed on patients, either because they presented in an unusual way or because they failed to provide adequate information or gave an incoherent history.[17] Patients may also be 'blamed' for not adhering to treatment plans, or not changing unhealthy behaviours.

Cognitive issues in the Negotiating Quadrant centre on uncertainty about how the patient's treatment or care is to be organised. This Quadrant is dominated by issues of choice (of treatment or plan). Modern medicine produces an unprecedented array of choices,[i] with multiple guidelines, protocols and pathways available, and choice creates anxiety of itself. If shoppers get anxious choosing washing powders (when failure to get the right one has no serious consequences), it is no wonder that clinicians feel anxious choosing between or within guidelines, many of which run to hundreds of pages. For clinicians, unlike consumers in supermarkets, the consequences of getting it wrong are serious: from inconvenience up to and including disability or death for the patient, and professional failure and expulsion for the clinician (professional 'death'). This difficulty is exacerbated when patients have complex comorbidities, which mean that guidelines may contradict each other, be too onerous to enact in full, or simply not be applicable to the specific patient. Anxiety may be a way of forestalling guilt about making the right choice.

Uncertainty may also be dealt with, in effect, by the clinician reducing the choices or simplifying the decisions that have to be made. This may be by rigid adherence to guidelines, to pre-empt criticism and reduce the number of alternatives; this may result in difficult negotiations with patients who may not always accept 'the guideline'. Resorting to 'meta-ignorance' (acting as if the complexity or uncertainty does not exist) or defaulting to apparently intuitive choices, using heuristics or 'rules of thumb', are cognitive strategies that clinicians sometimes use when uncertainty seems too much.

Relationship issues are of particular importance in the Negotiating Quadrant. Clinician uncertainty has, in the past, resulted in patients being kept in the dark with regards to investigations, likelihood of diagnosis and success of treatment. Doctors perceive that sharing uncertainties with patients causes unnecessary anxiety and loss of trust.[18] Sharing uncertainty means having actually to recognise its existence, rather than being in denial about it. Clinicians often feel that they should be in control (thus if things go wrong the clinician can be blamed and should feel guilty and ashamed).

---

i One example: a Google search on chronic kidney disease produced 15,550,000 results on 22 October 2014 with guidelines from at least five different authoritative sources (the National Institute for Health and Care Excellence, the Scottish Intercollegiate Guidelines Network, the Renal Association, the National Kidney Foundation and the International Society of Nephrology). Even choosing which guideline to follow may not be easy. Applying such information to individuals is not straightforward, as many patients differ in important ways from those researched in the evidence from which the guidance is derived.

Feelings of frustration among clinicians when patients do not agree with the clinician's plans are mirrored by patients' frustrations at being ignored. This can lead to difficulties in arranging optimum care, as patients may not cooperate if their concerns are not recognised and acted upon. Some writers have commented on how it can be reassuring for patients to have a clinician who seems to be in control:

> *The dominant relationship reassures many patients. They do not want to hear all the complexities and ambiguities. Reassurance, a simplified explanation and a prescription (even where none is needed) are gifts cherished by many patients.*[19]

However, this attitude can seem old fashioned and patronising, and does not recognise the contribution of patients who prefer to be involved in decisions about their care. This will mean sharing some uncertainty with patients, which we assume to be a good thing. However, patients have been found to be more satisfied if the doctor seems certain. In particular, verbal expressions of uncertainty such as 'I don't know' or 'It's not clear' made patients less confident; actions such as looking things up were seen as neutral (at worst) or inspiring confidence (at best).[20] It is likely that the exact nuances of phrase and expression make a difference here too. Can strengthened relationships enable uncertainty to be discussed more readily? In general practice, doctors have the advantage of building up trust via long-term relationships with their patients, which may allow disclosure of uncertainty to seem less threatening. The patient's perspective on uncertainty is discussed more fully in Part V.

Organisational factors also influence how uncertainty in arranging care is handled. Clinicians have to respond to uncertainty in a complex context, comprising individual clinician–patient relationships, institutional and regulatory concerns, with variations in the availability of resources and uncertainties about the limits of medical knowledge. If uncertainty is not accepted or discussed then adherences to guidelines, structures or rules will be promoted. This minimises uncertain situations and avoids risk-taking behaviour.[21] Avoiding ambiguity by rigid adherence to guidelines tends to deflect responsibility for actions away from the individual clinician and on to others (the patient, the institution, 'the system'). This may allow the individual clinician to avoid any unpleasant feelings about their own actions being judged as inadequate. They were after all 'following the guidelines', which may be seen as a way to pre-empt or deflect any censure, whether from themselves or others.

Insistence on rigid protocols or guidelines by regulators or institutions is likely to increase the stress that uncertainty causes for clinicians. If they cannot reconcile what is expected of them with what seems appropriate for the individual patient, then they will resort to 'dysfunctional ways out'. This may lead to 'blaming the patient' or neglecting the patient in favour of pleasing the institution or regulator (spending more time assessing suicidal risk and less time listening to the patient's concerns, or discharging patients too rapidly to keep 'length of stay short', would be obvious examples). Intolerance or lack of understanding of ambiguity and complexity on behalf of institutions tends to lead to an over-emphasis on goals that are clear cut, measurable or endorsed by authority, rather than those which support patients and clinicians struggling with uncertain or complex situations. This can lead to spectacular organisational failures like the problems described in the Francis Report.[22] A previous Care Quality Commission inspection of the Mid Staffordshire Hospital focused on clear-cut, measurable goals, but failed to notice serious shortcomings in the actual care that patients were receiving.

Psychological components of uncertainty in the Team-working Quadrant

- Emotional reactions: shame and embarrassment.
- Cognitive strategies: group 'norms'.
- Relationship issues: boundaries, team style.
- Organisational components: projection, conflict.

From an *emotional* perspective, uncertainty in the Team-working Quadrant relates to the social consequences of exposing uncertainty. Shame and embarrassment can be the feared outcomes for individuals discussing their own uncertainty or inadequacy. Trainees seem less likely to acknowledge and discuss uncertainty, whereas qualified doctors may recognise a stress response from uncertainty, but still be reluctant to share this with colleagues.[23] However, teamwork also creates the potential for powerful bonding between team members, providing emotional support and a 'group' approach to problems that can mitigate individual feelings of uncertainty. Affiliation and social connectedness are crucial for good mental health and when teams have a strong emotional connection this can be protective to its members facing the difficulties of clinical work.

In *cognitive* terms, uncertainty in the Team-working Quadrant is dealt with by the group or team developing defined boundaries to their area of work (e.g. clear inclusion or exclusion criteria for accepting patients) and by developing team protocols and norms about how work is to proceed. These may be explicit, but implicit norms about 'the way we do things around here' can also be powerful drivers of behaviour. This will include the extent to which uncertainty is acknowledged or discussed. If the team encounters an issue that is ambiguous or potentially outside its remit, the cognitive approach can be to refer the problem to someone else, for example another team or department. Having firm boundaries about what the team can do seems 'rational' or 'logical' while also having the effect of limiting exposure to painful ambiguities or uncertainties.

Collective decision making and accepted 'norms' ameliorate uncertainty and provide a stable supportive environment for staff to work in. This is important in medicine when there are so many ways to provide care and treatment to patients, and where many patients do not fit into 'the guidelines'. In the past, the 'Bolam test' has been applied to potential medical negligence cases in the UK; practice was legally judged to be adequate, if what was done would be considered reasonable by other medical professionals, working in the same field. This still applies to diagnosis and treatment options. However, the shelter of a 'group norm' was removed by the case of Montgomery when the Supreme Court ruled that information given to a patient should be determined by what a reasonable person would want to know.[ii] The law for consent to treatment is now that a doctor should follow the GMC guidance on consent, and that information must be given to patients in line with what they themselves require (the onus is on the doctor to find this out) and not what other doctors would usually disclose about the risks and benefits of treatment. This creates new opportunities for uncertainty in the Negotiating Quadrant, and will require that all doctors develop the skills of accurate information sharing and shared decision making.

The danger of collective 'norms' is that they may not be evidence based, and do not take into account the psychological processes within teams. The

ii The Supreme Court judged that the doctor should have informed the patient, who was a pregnant Type 1 diabetic of small stature carrying a large baby, that there were risks of shoulder dystocia, and also of brain and other injury to the mother and the unborn child if shoulder dystocia occurred, these being risks that the patient wished to know about, and that any reasonable person would wish to know about. See www.scottishlegal.com/2015/03/12/montgomery-in-the-supreme-court-a-new-legal-test-for-consent-to-medical-treatment/ [accessed 4 April 2015].

reports into health scandals over the past 20 years have made similar observations: appalling care was being given and, furthermore, many professionals allowed poor care to continue without acting to change it. This is the downside of group thinking. There will always be individual rogue members of any profession, but the real danger is when a group follows blindly, rather than constantly questioning and adapting to changing circumstances, changing evidence or changing outcomes. How do teams move from uncertainty to develop such potentially damaging acceptance of poor practice?

'Groupthink' is the evocative term that describes the thinking that occurs when people are so deeply involved in a cohesive group striving for unanimity that this 'overrides their motivation to realistically appraise alternative courses of action'.[24]

This does not fully explain why groups make risky decisions or perform badly, especially in healthcare contexts. Other factors also influence decision making in team settings. Groups are known to tend to select the option supported by the majority at the outset ('social decision schemes'). Furthermore, if individual members of the group are generally oriented towards risk at the outset, 'it is reliable that the decision of the group will be even riskier than that of the average group member'.[25]

If there is a strong pressure towards uniformity, members of the team or group try to avoid raising controversial issues and don't question weak arguments. These group phenomena can be observed in healthcare teams: senior, dominant members tend to take the lead and as a result of experience or authority may be more willing to 'hold' risk. At times this is appropriate. However, other members of the team may be unwilling or unable to question weaker arguments, for example because they are juniors 'trying to fit in' or because they are hierarchically less powerful (for example practitioners other than doctors may find themselves in this position). Doctors are driven by a powerful *personal* sense of responsibility and expectations of decision making, which may mean that they need specific training to accept the expertise of others, and work effectively in teams.

The *relationship* issues connected with teams are complicated: there are the relationships within teams to consider, relationships between different teams and relationships between teams and the organisational structures within they operate, as well as the relationships with the patients under the care of the team. Team-working relationships can both generate or suppress uncertainties and teams may help to ameliorate or exacerbate responses to uncertainty. The nature of discussions about uncertainty will vary between teams and institutions; there will be different group 'cultures' around this theme.

Relationships within teams could be thought to echo the four different doctor–patient relationships proposed by Emanuel and Emanuel (which are discussed in more detail in Part V 'Exploring uncertainty from the patient's perspective').[26] These are referred to as paternalistic, informing, interpretive and deliberative relationships, and they exemplify different approaches to uncertainty. These concepts can be applied to teams also.

In *paternalistic* teams, a strong hierarchy and clear, even rigid, roles may inhibit expressions of uncertainty, or at best defer decisions to more 'senior' members of the team. Uncertainty (and the possibility of error) is not well tolerated in such teams and thus such teams tend to prefer to follow guidelines, structures or rules. Trainees or teams members often face uncertainty when starting a new placement; they have to work out the implicit rules of the team quickly, and conform to these:

> *Trainees try to 'act professional', learning the language and mannerisms of their mentors. Ironically through this process of impression management, trainees get taken in by their own act until the self-conscious process of role simulation becomes the real thing.*[19]

This dissimulation is partly driven by the potential shame or embarrassment of seeming 'not to know what to do'. Confidence (short of arrogance of course!) is seen as a worthy trait in healthcare professionals, especially in teams having a paternalistic style.

Paternalistic teams

Dr Strongbow has been a GP in a small town for many years and has gradually built up a strong practice team of salaried GPs, with the practice nurse and practice manager all having worked with him for many years. They are tight knit and supportive to each other, but everyone knows that Dr Strongbow is the dominant figure and 'boss' of the practice. All major decisions go through him and the rest of the team do not have to handle much uncertainty as they get 'told what to do'.

Mr Arrow is the senior surgeon in the ENT department. He has loyal secretaries and clinic nurses who work closely with him. His junior staff follow his instructions to the letter. Although he can be very strict he also backs up his team if they have followed his procedures and will defend them vigorously against any complaints or attempts to change practice from outside.

In these teams uncertainty is largely managed through denial that it exists, or by sticking to rigid protocols that do not admit of ambiguity, or by deferring to the authority of a senior figure.

In *informing* teams the predominant interactions are around information and decision making. Multidisciplinary teams may overtly encourage contributions of information from all members, with decision making deferred to the relevant clinician. When large groups make decisions they may become more than the sum of their parts and make more risky decisions than individuals or smaller groups. Such teams can view medical care in transactional, rather than relationship, terms. What is the diagnosis? What needs to be done? Who will do it? The emotional needs of team members or the priorities of individual patients may not be seen as relevant. Overt uncertainty may be buried under adherence to guidelines and protocols. Psychologically this reduces the anxiety associated with uncertainty, which does not have to be 'held' by the team but can be devolved to the patient, or to other teams. Shame and embarrassment will be minimised.

The informing team

The multidisciplinary team of a cancer unit is meeting to decide what to do about Mrs Salix's cancer of the bowel. They decide she would be best treated with some chemotherapy, followed by a surgical removal of the cancer. A doctor who knows her from the ward says, 'She is not keen on having any surgery at all and wants to go home today.'

The team make a decision to explain the options and risks, and then let her make her own choice.

Uncertainty is managed by effectively giving it back to the patient. Difficult emotional or holistic care issues are kept in the background.

In *interpretative* teams, a more holistic view can be incorporated, taking into account the emotional needs of the team members and a wider view of the wishes and priorities of the patient. Such teams may be able to discuss uncertainty more overtly; the emotional aspects of the patient's care and even the emotional aspects of the professional responses are open to discussion. Decision making may become being more difficult as all points of view are valued.

The interpretative team

The primary healthcare team consisting of GPs, district nurses, Macmillan nurse, practice nurse and active case manager are discussing the care of Mrs Salix, who came home after being diagnosed with cancer, having refused all treatment in hospital. The hospital consultant telephoned the GP feeling frustrated and upset that Mrs Salix would not accept treatment that he regarded as being 'probably curative'.

The GP has discussed things with Mrs Salix, who is aware of what will happen. Her over-riding priority is to stay at home, near the garden she has spent 50 years tending. She is not afraid of dying – 'We all have to go, doctor' – and just wants to be comfortable. The nurses and doctors discuss practical plans, and also how it feels to be caring for someone who refuses treatment. It is agreed that one doctor will be the lead clinician, developing a relationship with Mrs Salix and her family who live nearby. Her uncertain future is openly discussed, and the team set out on somewhat novel territory, supporting each other and the patient.

In a *deliberative* team, the discussions and decisions go beyond the patient's immediate priorities, to enter a more complex level. What are the contradictions in their aspirations? Are the patient's or family's wishes realistic or appropriate? Are the patient's 'highest interest or purposes' being served? This type of team will actively guide the patient in interpreting the possibilities, to see how the options relate to that individual's own life and values. In such a team uncertainty is accepted, even celebrated, and emotional expressions are accepted.

The deliberative team

The primary healthcare team are discussing the planned end-of-life care for Mrs Lily, a patient with end-stage dementia, who has had several major strokes, and who has chronic kidney disease and end-stage diabetes with heart failure. She is increasingly frail and largely bed-bound. Her retinopathy is so bad she has little vision and she cannot speak. She is developing bedsores in spite of the best efforts of the nurses at the home where she lives. Her son arrives from Australia demanding that 'more should be done for mother', saying 'She should be admitted to hospital.' The team recognise that she is close to death and that little more can be done. One of the doctors has a long and emotional discussion with the son, acknowledging his feelings of helplessness and grief. New goals are sensitively negotiated: that she should be pain free, nursed in familiar surroundings and with her son being there as much as feasible.

Organisational issues relating to teamwork uncertainty are also complex. Teams within larger organisations have to work with each other. This can mean that psychological processes of projection occur whereby difficult feelings from within a group are projected on to another group. We see this a lot across primary and secondary care; GPs can feel that hospital teams are remote, rigid, unfeeling and inflexible. Hospital teams find GPs to be inconsistent, unreliable, flaky and unavailable. The uncertainties or difficulties of the 'other' team are not seen as realistic or acceptable. These processes also reflect the impact that feelings of shame or embarrassment have in relation to others; such feelings are scarcely to be mentioned and are managed by suppression or deflection. Moreover, if a problem arises within a team, dealing with it means facing a real individual, and risks damaging the relationships within the team. In this situation it may be easier to pass the 'blame' on to another team or institution in a 'faceless', anonymous way. As no specific individual is named (just 'GPs' or 'the hospital'), no blame is attached to specific individuals and relationships are less likely to be disrupted. Uncertainty arising from teamwork conflicts is likely to increase as medicine becomes more complex, and as this comment suggests:

> *The pressure for diagnostic certainty and the push for therapeutic results at any price play themselves out in a world of limited resources but seemingly unlimited technological discoveries.*[13]

In this chapter, some of the psychological processes that underpin clinicians' reactions to uncertainty have been described. We know that some clinicians manage uncertainty better than others, which raises a crucial issue: can we train clinicians to be better at dealing with uncertainty?

That question brings us to Part IV 'Mapping uncertainty in training'.

References

1. Ofri D. *What Doctors Feel: how emotions affect the practice of medicine*. Boston, MA: Beacon Press, 2013.
2. Penrod J. Living with uncertainty: concept advancement. *Journal of Advanced Nursing* 2007; **57(6)**: 658–67.
3. Pimlott M. Managing uncertainty. *Canadian Family Physician* 2007; **53(6)**: 1000.
4. Croskerry P. Clinical cognition and diagnostic error: applications of a dual process model of reasoning. *Advances in Health Sciences Education: Theory and Practice* 2009; **14(1)**: 27–35. DOI: 10.1007/s10459-009-9182-2.

5. Hall K. Reviewing intuitive decision-making and uncertainty: the implications for medical education. *Medical Education* 2002; **36(3)**: 216–24.
6. Pelaccia T, Tardif J, Triby E, Charlin B. An analysis of clinical reasoning through a recent and comprehensive approach: the dual process theory. *Medical Education Online* 2011; DOI: 3402/meov1610.5890.
7. Frenkel-Brunswik E. Intolerance of ambiguity as an emotional and perceptual personality variable. *Journal of Personality* 1949; **18(1)**: 108–43.
8. Hamm R. Clinical intuition and clinical analysis: expertise and the cognitive continuum. In: J Dowie, A Elstein (eds). *Professional Judgment: a reader in clinical decision making*. Cambridge: Cambridge University Press, 1988, pp. 78–105.
9. Fox RC. Training for uncertainty. In: RK Merton, G Reader, PL Kendall (eds). *The Student-Physician: introductory studies in the sociology of medical education*. Cambridge, MA: Harvard University Press, 1957, pp. 207–41.
10. Merrill J, Camacho Z, Laux LF, *et al*. Uncertainties and ambiguities: measuring how medical students cope. *Medical Education* 1994; **28(4)**: 316–22.
11. Mizrahi T. Managing medical mistakes: ideology, insularity and accountability among internists-in-training. *Social Science and Medicine* 1984; **19(2)**: 135–46.
12. Biehn J. Managing uncertainty in family practice. *Canadian Medical Association Journal* 1982; **126(8)**: 915–17.
13. Gerrity M, Earp JA, DeVellis RF, Light DW. Uncertainty and professional work: perceptions of physicians in clinical practice. *American Journal of Sociology* 1992; **97(4)**: 1022–51.
14. Brashers D. Communication and uncertainty management. *Journal of Communication* 2001; **51(9)**: 477–97.
15. Personal communication. Geraldine Murphy highlighted this aspect of care. Notes are written to convey information about standards to other doctors, with an eye to preventing future criticism.
16. Collins M, Block SD, Arnold RM, Christakis NA. On the prospects for a blame-free medical culture. *Social Science and Medicine* 2009; **69(9)**: 1287–90.
17. Mizrahi T. Managing medical mistakes: ideology, insularity and accountability among internists-in-training. *Social Science and Medicine* 1984; **19(2)**: 135–46.
18. Katz J. *The Silent World of Doctor and Patient*. New York, NY: Free Press, 1984.
19. Light D. Uncertainty and control in professional training. *Journal of Health and Social Behaviour* 1979; **20(4)**: 310–22.
20. Ogden J, Fuks K, Gardner M, *et al*. Doctors' expressions of uncertainty and patient confidence. *Patient Education and Counseling* 2002; **48(2)**: 171–6.
21. Hofstede GH. *Culture's Consequences: international differences in work-related values*. Beverley Hills, CA, and London: Sage Publications, 1980.
22. Francis R. Report of the Mid Staffordshire NHS Foundation Trust Public Inquiry (3 vols). London: TSO, 2013, www.midstaffspublicinquiry.com [accessed 29 July 2015].

23. Gerrity M, DeVellis RF, Earp JA. Physicians' reactions to uncertainty in patient care. *Medical Care* 1990; **28(8)**: 724–36.
24. Janis IL. *Groupthink*. Boston, MA: Houghton Mifflin, 1982.
25. Whyte G. Groupthink reconsidered. *Academy of Management Review* 1989; **14(1)**: 40–56.
26. Emanuel EJ, Emanuel LL. Four models of the physician-patient relationship. *Journal of the American Medical Association* 1992; **267(16)**: 2221–6.

Resources

Gawande A. *Being Mortal*. London: Metropolitan Books, 2014.
Ofri D. *What Doctors Feel: how emotions affect the practice of medicine*. Boston, MA: Beacon Press, 2013.

Part IV

Mapping uncertainty in medical training

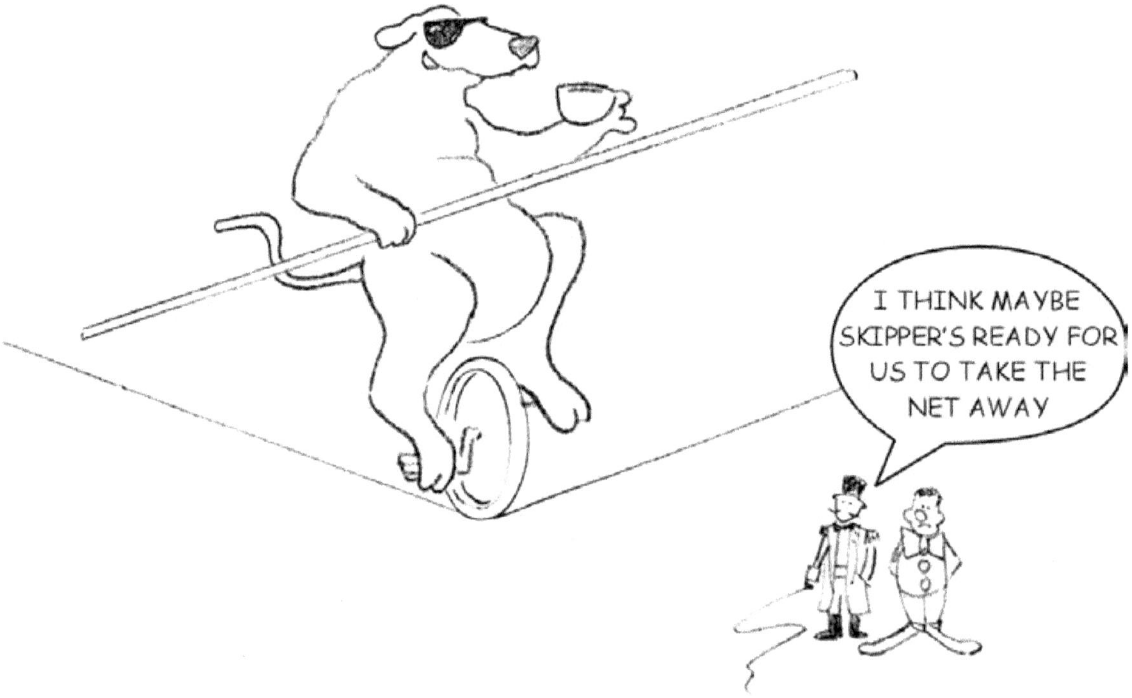
I THINK MAYBE SKIPPER'S READY FOR US TO TAKE THE NET AWAY

This part of the book considers how *educators* can use the explorations of uncertainty in Parts I, II and III of this book to incorporate effective teaching about uncertainty into training programmes.

Chapter 17 explores the educational aims of training for uncertain situations, including some of the difficulties in current training. **Chapter 18** considers how the MUM can be used to assess educational needs and define educational objectives. **Chapter 19** outlines effective educational methods for training for uncertainty and decision-making methods in uncertain situations. It also considers how such training can improve resilience. **Chapter 20** clarifies the educational skills needed to manage situations where the uncertainty is about trainees or underperforming colleagues. **Chapter 21** offers some suggestions for educators planning training sessions.

Chapter 17

Training clinicians to deal with uncertainty

> If a man begin with certainties, he will end in doubt; but if he will be content to begin with doubts, he will end in certainties.
>
> Francis Bacon

By now, it will be clear to readers that ALL clinicians face uncertainty and WDYDWYDKWTD questions in their work. Expertise lies in knowing what to do when you *do not know* what to do, being able to assess a situation and apply the appropriate skills. We hope that the preceding chapters will have helped clinicians think about what skills they themselves need to develop to move closer to higher levels of expertise. Any clinician facing a WDYDWYDKWTD situation can use the MUM algorithm (see p. 15) to identify the Quadrant that is causing a problem; the MUM will then help in the choice of relevant skills to unlock the uncertainty. Insights from Chapter 16 will enable clinicians to recognise the emotional, cognitive, relationship and organisational aspects of uncertainty, and approach uncertainty in a more nuanced way.

However, many clinicians are involved in the training or supervision of others and junior staff need to develop expertise in recognising and dealing with WDYDWYDKWTD situations. In one sense all clinical training is about managing uncertainty; the clinician starting out will have little knowledge, few skills and may have ineffective attitudes and values towards clinical work. The uncertainty of the novice is great, and also explicitly acknowledged. Learners are protected from some of the pressures of uncertainty because, while learning, others will be expected to make the decisions on which patient care depends. Once qualified, all clinicians will face uncertainty and may feel ill-equipped to cope with the complicated emotional, cognitive, relationship and organisational issues that follow. This chapter explores:

- difficulties in current training for uncertainty
- the educational AIMS of training for uncertainty.

Difficulties in current training for uncertainty

> *Doctors must be capable of regularly taking responsibility for difficult decisions in situations of clinical complexity and uncertainty.*
>
> General Medical Council[2]

This aspiration is echoed in other authoritative statements about how doctors should be able to manage uncertainty, such as the Royal College of General Practitioners (RCGP) curriculum.[3] So how do we currently 'train' clinicians to manage uncertainty?

It seems that some problems with uncertainty in training may start in medical school.[4] Medical students who are not comfortable with ambiguity, a hallmark of uncertain situations, choose more structured specialties (e.g. radiology), which suggests that they may retain this discomfort after training. Students who are particularly uncomfortable with ambiguous situations prefer to avoid the elderly, the addicted and other 'complex' patients.[5] Inherent personality traits of insecurity and tolerance seem to be significant, although the hope is that training in clinical reasoning will overcome these issues. Without this training, those who are intolerant of uncertainty manage it by 'over investigating, referring patients to other specialists and subspecialising to become an expert in a particular field'.[6]

This may be partly because some patients may be challenging; medical students naturally become anxious making decisions in uncertain situations and fear making mistakes.[7] This may have some advantages: those who are worried about mistakes have a strong driver towards conscientiousness and further learning. Such students are also more willing to disclose errors to patients, which accords with an attitude towards candour that is now widely endorsed in medical practice.[8] However, students may develop a sense of personal inadequacy in the face of uncertainty, rather than seeing uncertainty as inherent in medical practice, and their responses to uncertainty are very variable (like those of experienced practitioners), and are sometimes maladaptive.[9]

During training, approaches to uncertainty include:

- learning as much technical knowledge as possible
- observing supervisors' expectations of how to respond to uncertain situations
- approaching uncertainty in the same way as their supervisor to avoid sanctions and get positive reinforcement
- using collective solutions, talking to peers and subscribing to a 'school of thought' about particular issues.[9]

These approaches are strong components of the professionalisation of medical students, through adopting departmental or group 'norms', which cover many aspects of behaviour, including the approach to uncertainty. There is a strong element of modelling of the educator's behaviour; educators need to be 'aware of their own rules and the influence they may have on trainees'.[10] If educators are uncertain about uncertainty, they may model 'dysfunctional ways out'.

Specialisation, which limits the areas of knowledge to be mastered, is another strategy for limiting exposure to uncertainty. Those who can manage uncertainty are more likely to choose specialties such as family practice or psychiatry, where uncertainty is highly prevalent. Some writers consider surgery and gynaecology to encompass less uncertainty.[11] However, uncertainty exists in all areas of medical practice, and specialists in each field believe that their specialty is unique in its level of uncertainty. For example, both surgeons and psychiatrists highlight the extent of personal decision making and judgement in their roles. Surgeons recognise uncertainty from differences between patients (for example anomalies in anatomy), ambiguity or lack of information and factors arising from equipment or staffing issues. Surgeons observed that their strategies for managing these uncertainties were self-reliant: prioritising alternative approaches, revising the plan when the contextual clues changed, improvising and thinking creatively. Seeking advice was seen as a last resort when the other strategies did not work.[12]

Does an ability to manage uncertainty increase with increased training and experience? Since the 1970s it has been apparent that knowledge alone is not enough: 'In terms of training for control, this means that experience alone is considered to bring with it greater command over uncertainties than technical knowledge can provide.'[6]

That experience helps one cope with uncertainty seems confirmed by findings that those with lower workloads are less tolerant of uncertainty, presumably reflecting their reduced exposure to uncertain situations.[7] This has implications for staff in Less Than Full Time Training (LTFT) roles, or those who have 'portfolio' career paths. The ability to tolerate ambiguity varies with personality.[13]

As doctors become more experienced they develop 'treatment philosophies' that lead them to recommend treatments without question.[6] This is likely to represent a 'dysfunctional way out' by marginalising and minimalising complexity and uncertainty, making things more comfortable for the individual practitioner. However, when uncertainty is recognised and embraced, innovation or better solutions tend to follow. For example, surgeons encountering unexpected operative findings were able to develop innovative and helpful variations from standard practice.[12]

What characteristics make clinicians more likely to be effective in managing uncertainty, which can be considered one of the hallmarks of expertise? Trainees who make progress towards expertise are typically 'self-regulated learners'.[14] This means that they identify the scope of problems proficiently and seek feedback to check if their actions and ideas are relevant and effective. Their goals are about what they need to learn next ('learning goals', what is the 'next step' on the road to expertise) rather than the final standard they will need to achieve ('performance goals', such as passing a particular exam, or being able to do a certain procedure). Many non-self-regulated learners are unclear about what 'good performance' looks like.[14] Hitherto, there has been little definition of what 'good practice' in uncertainty might consist of, or how to teach or train for 'uncertainty'. We hope that the mapping approaches we have used in this book will overcome some of these difficulties, because the MUM and the examples in the chapters explain how 'effective practice' can be recognised, which behaviours are useful in different circumstances and how expertise can be built up through the acquisition of a series of learnable skills. Exploring what 'good practice' looks like facilitates discussions about appropriate professional attitudes and behaviours in uncertain situations. Effective partnership with patients, skilled teamwork and respectful networking matter crucially in situations of uncertainty.

Overall it seems that, although there is some recognition of uncertainty as a training issue, it is less clear that training is effective in this area. Uncertainty may not be directly addressed as a suitable subject for training in all clinical training programmes, although some would argue that it is crucial to dedicate training time 'to attend candidly to ambiguity and uncertainty as a formal part of every medical school curriculum'.[15]

The educational AIMS of training for uncertainty

Managing uncertainty requires sophisticated knowledge and skills[16] and commentators believe that adding uncertainty management to undergraduate and postgraduate curricula is now 'urgent'.[17,18] The professional role of a doctor is closely tied up with the ability to make judgements in situations of uncertainty, where rule-based approaches may not work very well. Both medical educators and their trainees need to be comfortable with managing uncertainties in clinical practice positively, using 'functional ways through'. The RCGP core curriculum statement 'Specific Problem Solving', advises Associates-in-Training (AiTs) to tolerate uncertainty and develop strategies that demonstrate this, without specifying in detail what these strategies might be.[3] Although uncertainty might be seen as the 'specialty of general practice',[19] clinicians in all specialties need tools for dealing with uncertainty. There have been different approaches to this in the past including using effective decision making[20] and improving existing models of the consultation.[10] Using evidence-based practice has also been recommended,[20] although uncertainty is just as likely to occur when clinicians find themselves drowning in 'evidence', 'guidelines' and 'pathways and protocols'.

The overall aim for training for uncertainty is to enable clinicians to recognise uncertainty, 'hold' uncertainty, and manage uncertainty. These aims are summarised in Box 17.1, classified into the knowledge, skills and attitudes needed. These considerations could underpin a formal curriculum for training in the area. Training for uncertainty should emphasise meticulous evaluation, methodical thinking about diagnosis and investigation, and establishing relationships of trust – with patients, within and between teams. This will enable shared decision making to occur,[10] and prevent some of the adverse effects of uncertainty that have been outlined in Chapter 16.

Box 17.1: Aims of training for uncertainty

KNOWLEDGE about uncertainty

- Recognition of uncertainty in practice (see Chapter 2).
- Classification of uncertainty into Analysing, Networking, Negotiating and Team-working categories.
- Identification of 'dysfunctional ways out' and 'functional ways through'.
- Recognition of the emotional, relationship, cognitive and contextual elements of uncertainty (see Part III).
- Knowledge of a range of decision-making methods for uncertain situations.

SKILLS for uncertainty

1. Using the MUM to identify types of uncertainty.
2. Selecting and using the relevant skills for different kinds of uncertainty.
3. 'Holding' uncertainty to allow careful decision making, avoiding too rapid decision making or 'dysfunctional ways out'.
4. Choosing and using appropriate decision-making methods for different types of uncertain situation.
5. Communication skills to enable uncertainty to be effectively discussed with patients.

ATTITUDES for uncertainty

1. Accepting uncertainty as being a crucial component of professional practice (see 'Conclusion: embracing uncertainty').
2. Willingness to discuss uncertainty with colleagues.
3. Willingness to discuss uncertainty with patients.
4. Willingness to recognise that managing uncertainty requires a range of learnable skills.
5. Willingness to support colleagues who are uncertain and willingness to learn appropriate training methods.
6. Treating uncertain colleagues skilfully, avoiding humiliation and 'blame and shame' approaches in training.

References

1. Bacon F. The advancement of learning (1605). In: E Knowles (ed.). *Oxford Book of Quotations*. (7th edn). Oxford: Oxford University Press, 2009.
2. General Medical Council. *Tomorrow's Doctors*. Manchester: GMC, 2009.
3. Royal College of General Practitioners. *Being a General Practitioner* (Core Curriculum Statement 1.00). London: RCGP, 2015, www.rcgp.org.uk/training-exams/~/media/Files/GP-training-and-exams/Curriculum-2012/RCGP-Curriculum-1-Being-a-GP.ashx page 14 specific problem solving skills [accessed 8 May 2015].
4. Luther VP, Crandall SJ. Commentary: ambiguity and uncertainty: neglected elements of medical education curricula? *Academic Medicine* 2011; **86(7)**: 799–800; DOI: 10.1097/ACM.0b013e31821da915.
5. Geller G, Faden RR, Levine DM. Tolerance for ambiguity among medical students; implications for their selection, training and practice. *Social Science and Medicine* 1990; **31(5)**: 619–24.
6. Light D Jr. Uncertainty and control in professional training. *Journal of Health and Social Behaviour* 1979; **20(4)**: 310–22.

7. Sarikaya O, Civaner M, Kalaca S. The anxieties of medical students related to clinical training. *International Journal of Clinical Practice* 2006; **60(11)**: 1414–18.
8. Nevalainen M, Kuikka L, Sjoberg L, *et al.* Tolerance of uncertainty and fears of making mistakes among fifth-year medical students. *Family Medicine* 2012; **44(4)**: 240–6.
9. Fox RC. Training for uncertainty. In: RK Merton, G Reader, PL Kendall (eds). *The Student-Physician: introductory studies in the sociology of medical education.* Cambridge, MA: Harvard University Press, 1957, pp. 207–41.
10. O'Riordan, Dahinden A, Aktürk Z, *et al.* Dealing with uncertainty in general practice: an essential skill for the general practitioner. *Quality in Primary Care* 2011; **19**; 175–81.
11. Gerrity M, Earp JA, DeVellis RF, Light DW. Uncertainty and professional work: perceptions of physicians in clinical practice. *American Journal of Sociology* 1992; **97(4)**: 1022–51.
12. Cristancho S, Apramian T, Vanstone M, *et al.* Understanding clinical uncertainty: what is going on when experienced surgeons are not sure what to do? *Academic Medicine* 2013; **88(10)**: 1516–21.
13. Budner S. Intolerance of ambiguity as a personality variable. *Journal of Personality* 1962; **30(1)**: 29–50.
14. Nicol D, Macfarlane-Dick D. Formative assessment and self-regulated learning; a model and seven principles of good feedback practice. *Studies in Higher Education* 2006; **31(2)**: 199–218.
15. Penrod J. Living with uncertainty: concept advancement. *Journal of Advanced Nursing* 2007; **57(6)**: 658–67.
16. Cassell EJ. *Doctoring: the nature of primary care medicine.* Oxford: Oxford University Press, 1997.
17. Lester H, Tritter JQ. Medical error: a discussion of the medical construction of error and suggestions for reforms of medical education to decrease error. *Medical Education* 2001; **35(9)**: 855–61.
18. Wellbery C. The value of medical uncertainty? *Lancet* 2010; **375(9727)**: 1686–7.
19. Pimlott M. Managing uncertainty. *Canadian Family Physician* 2007; **53(6)**: 1000.
20. Grol R. Implementing guidelines in general practice care. *Quality in Health Care* 1992; **1(3)**: 184–91.
21. Hunink MGM, Glasziou PP, Siegel JE, *et al. Decision Making in Health and Medicine: integrating evidence and values.* Cambridge: Cambridge University Press, 2001.

Chapter 18

Assessment using the Map of Uncertainty in Medicine

> Education is the path from cocky ignorance to miserable uncertainty.
>
> Attributed to Mark Twain

Training is more effective if it is matched to learners' specific needs; this implies a process of assessing exactly what those needs are. To promote professional development, accurate assessment of learning needs should be followed by defining what is to be achieved, the specific educational objectives (the intent of the teaching activity) and the specific learning outcomes (what learners will be able to do after the training). This chapter focuses on how to use the MUM to assess competency in understanding uncertainty and to set educational objectives. The next chapter will cover the training methods that are most effective in developing the ability to deal with clinical uncertainty.

This chapter covers:

- how to use the MUM in assessment
- assessing in the Analysing Quadrant
- assessing in the Networking Quadrant
- assessing in the Negotiating Quadrant
- assessing in the Team-working Quadrant.

How to use the Map of Uncertainty in Medicine in assessment

The MUM can be used in two ways to assess learners' needs and develop relevant educational objectives. First, in group training situations the Map can be used for the educator to help learners classify uncertainty for themselves, and to identify the kinds of skills they need to learn. More information about this approach can be found in Chapter 21. This chapter mainly addresses assessment of individual trainees. When a trainee 'doesn't know what to do', one simple solution used by teachers and trainers is to *tell* the trainee what to do. This is helpful in the short term and is a quick, low-effort, Type 1 thinking approach (see Chapter 3). However, in the longer term, trainees will have fewer opportunities to ask for advice, and with increasing experience they themselves will be the ones giving advice to others. If medical educators use a more analytical, Type 2 thinking approach, assessment of the learner's difficulty will become more precise and training can be more focused to the specific need of the learner.

Most opportunities to assess a learner's capacity to deal with uncertainty are likely to occur when she identifies a difficulty and asks for help from a senior. At this juncture, using the Situation Background Assessment Recommendation (SBAR) technique to assist in handover should be strongly encouraged (see Chapter 13 for full details). This refines and clarifies the question being asked and encourages self-reliance and commitment to attempts at decision making ('practice makes perfect', deferring decisions to others does not lead to development). Using the SBAR approach consistently is a 'cognitive forcing function' (see Chapter 5). This has the effect of consistently nudging the learner to get her thoughts in order first, which trains her to 'think about her thinking' ('metacognition' again). Another advantage of the SBAR method is that it encourages learners to 'have a go' and accept that failure to get it right first time is an acceptable part of training. Some highly conscientious clinicians think that they must get the 'right' answer all the time. This may result in excessive rumination, sometimes called 'paralysis by analysis'.[1] One crucial element of training for uncertainty is encouraging the acceptance that in some difficult situations there is no 'perfect' answer, only a range of possibly 'good enough' answers.

When an SBAR handover identifies a gap in knowledge or skill, the supervisor can direct training away from simply 'telling people what to do', and into a more coaching or training style of interaction. Often, the apparent WDYDWYDKWTD moment that the trainee is experiencing melts away when she approaches the situation systematically with her supervisor.

However, if uncertainty remains when the learner has explained his difficulty and made initial suggestions, the educator will need to assess the type of uncertainty that is present, and what needs to be learned next. The educator can use the WDYDWYDKWTD algorithm on p. 15 with the learner to identify which Quadrant of the MUM the learner is struggling with. Sometimes more than one Quadrant is involved. When the Quadrant causing the difficulty is identified, the educator and learner can turn to the relevant Quadrant (using this book as a reference) to decide what the educational need is. Is there an issue with knowledge in that Quadrant? If so, the trainer can direct the learner to appropriate sources of information. Is the issue one of a missing skill? Part II of this book identifies the skills that may be needed in different Quadrants of the MUM. When the 'gap' in skills is identified an educational objective can be set; in other words, a decision can be made about what needs to be learned next.

Sometimes, a trainee may be unwilling to commit to the Recommendation part of the SBAR tool in case he is wrong. This may reveal some important problems in how uncertainty is discussed. Uncertainty or error in juniors may still be greeted with humiliating remarks ('How could you think such a stupid thing?'), which will compound the shame and guilt experienced by the learner, sometimes to intolerable levels. Seniors need to model systematic ways to think through problems, seeing errors as learning opportunities, not as opportunities for 'education by humiliation'. Bullying restricts learning. Being wrong is mainly a problem if the learner fails to identify errors or learn from mistakes; if the training environment does not permit expressions of uncertainty or error trainees will simply tend to cover up their problems. This is not helpful. Encouragement can assist juniors to 'have a go' at making a decision, even if they then need help to get to a better decision. Errors are a strong motivator to active learning;[2] if no diagnoses or management plans are made (no action) then mistakes cannot be made either and some potential opportunities for learning will be lost.

Assessment using the MUM also offers opportunities to assess whether 'dysfunctional ways out' of uncertainty are used, helping to raise learners' awareness of how these approaches are not optimal.

A significant uncertainty for educators and trainers is summed up in Pilnick's phrase referring to the 'honest errors' of the inexperienced. Supervisors must avoid damaging the confidence, learning and experience of the trainee, while at the same time ensuring the quality of the patients' treatment.[3] Uncertainty will arise when educators are deciding how much a trainee can do, when to ask her to take on more challenging tasks, or when to reduce supervision to develop independent practice. Such uncertainties can only be resolved by explicit assessment and discussion of her capacities with the learner. The uncertainty of the educator about educational issues is covered in Chapter 20.

The process of using the MUM in discussion with learners is summarised in the training algorithm on p. 223.

The educational information revealed by assessment in each Quadrant of the MUM is summarised in the following sections; knowledge, skill or attitude deficiencies may contribute to difficulties in each Quadrant.

Assessing in the Analysing Quadrant

Does the trainee struggle to make an accurate diagnosis? Using the Analysing Quadrant can identify which skills are needed. Many trainees appreciate that they need knowledge, often from books or guidelines, about their work. The thinking skills used in diagnosis are just as important and are less often covered in written materials, usually being learned through practical experience. Making clinical reasoning methods more explicit can help trainees engage with the learning required.

A lack of skill in dealing with ambiguous or uncertain information may conceal an underlying discomfort with complexity or the muddled variety of daily medical practice. Is the trainee so uncomfortable with uncertainty that he tries to close off diagnostic avenues by focusing on one particular aspect of a problem? Premature closure (also called search satisficing) is a common cause of error and of frustrating consultations, because the patient's real problem is not fully identified. Some trainees seem over-confident. Perhaps they are denying or not recognising uncertainty? Or dealing with uncertainty by confidently, yet erroneously, referring on to others? This, together with a view that requires doctors to seem to be in control, is one of the predisposing factors behind over-treatment and iatrogenesis.[4] Creating awareness of how doctors' thinking skills affect error rates and risks of litigation or complaints can create strong motivation for learning in this Quadrant.[2]

What about communication skills? Accurate diagnosis also requires an effective partnership with the patient; the clinician must have the ability to pick up cues and respond to them. Without this skill, essential diagnostic information can be lost.

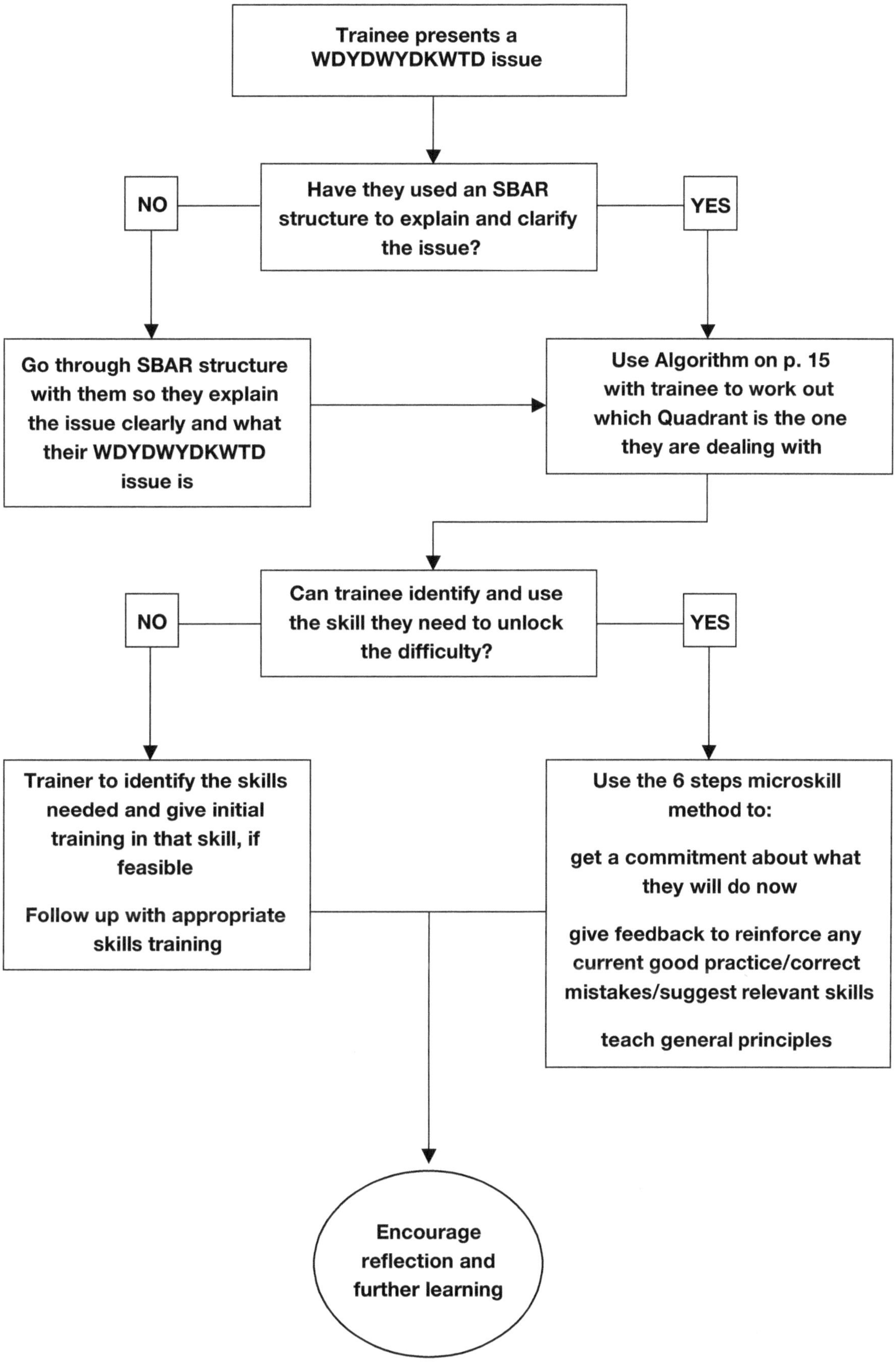

Helping a learner in a WDYDWYDKWTD situation

Assessing in the Networking Quadrant

Problems in diagnostic skills may also be revealed by issues in the Networking Quadrant. Does the learner refer onwards too often or too infrequently? Are their referrals valued, accepted and seen as being of good quality? Can they liaise informally to get useful advice? How are their relationships with laboratories, radiology departments and other teams or units? Can they contribute usefully to multidisciplinary team meetings, write a focused referral letter, or reply to a referral in a way that helps their colleagues? If not, review the skills of the networking chapter. Many team-working issues, such as handing over skills, are relevant here, and may not be explicitly learned or taught. Trainees making good progress often acquire these skills themselves by observing others and being willing to change. Trainees who are not progressing may need to be directed towards the networking competences they need, which they may not even recognise as being learnable skills. Educators can assess whether their learner can 'hold' uncertain situations temporarily, manage expectations of referral appropriately, and deal with unusual circumstances. Being able to 'break good news' and handle the many functional and somatising conditions that exist, without referral, is a key skill for doctors.

Assessing in the Negotiating Quadrant

If diagnoses are fine, is the trainee able to engage with an individual patient to plan her care smoothly? Are patients keen to see him again? Problems in the Negotiating Quadrant will appear as complaints, poor adherence to treatment plans by patients or the use of 'dysfunctional ways out' such as dismissing the patient's concerns. When negotiating skills fail, patients may seek help from elsewhere; discovering that patients frequently bypass a junior, seek help with another clinician or use another service within a short time-scale can indicate a lack of skills in this Quadrant. Exploring the attitudes that underpin the 'dysfunctional ways out' (e.g. 'blaming' the patient) will help learners to be open to the skills needed in the 'functional ways through'; better partnerships with patients will result. Enabling shared decision making or behaviour change needs specific skills from the doctor; identifying that such skills are important and may be lacking are the first steps to addressing the training need.

Assessing in the Team-working Quadrant

Most clinicians enjoy working in teams, yet the skills needed for effective teamwork may not be explicitly covered in all training programmes. The Team-working Quadrant offers ways to identify where teamwork skills are deficient, and to break these skills into several component parts that can be taught and learned incrementally. Problems in team-working may also highlight professionalism issues, such as the requirements to be available, meet obligations promptly and respect the contributions of other team members to the care of patients. Thoughtful reflections on the values and attitudes that underpin successful teamwork will help learners to make progress.

Using the MUM in this way will result in an overall assessment of how the learner is understanding and handling uncertainty. Used in combination with the information in this book, a curriculum for learning about uncertainty can be established, and the learner can learn the skills incrementally and in a way that focuses learning to the types of uncertainty arising in her daily work. For many learners, simply realising that uncertainty can be classified and understood, and that there are 'functional ways through' to deal with it, is an enlightening and encouraging experience.

References

1. Croskerry P. Context is everything or how could I have been that stupid? *Healthcare Quarterly* 2009; **12**: 171–17.
2. Lea A, Danczak A. Medical error: a dirty little secret or great learning opportunity? *Education for Primary Care* 2014; **25(2)**: 114–18.
3. Pilnick A, Hindmarsh J, Gill VT. Beyond 'doctor and patient': developments in the study of healthcare interactions. *Sociology of Health and Illness* 2009; **31(6)**: 787–802; DOI: 10.1111/j.1467-9566.2009.01194.x.
4. Gerrity M, Earp JA, DeVellis RF, Light DW. Uncertainty and professional work: perceptions of physicians in clinical practice. *American Journal of Sociology* 1992; **97(4)**: 1022–51.

Chapter 19

Educational methods for training for uncertainty

People learn in different ways, at different times and in different contexts. Learning about uncertainty can be promoted by using a variety of methods to suit the context. The use of the MUM for assessment was outlined in Chapter 18. The training algorithm (see p. 223) is a guide to use with trainees; the MUM helps to define the educational objective. However, while knowing the aims of training is crucial, and assessment will help to identify what is needed in a particular situation, effective education also requires the application of the right educational methods for the circumstances.

This chapter describes effective educational methods for training for uncertainty and covers:

- effective educational methods for training for uncertainty in different training settings
- training for uncertainty; can this improve resilience in practice?
- decision-making approaches for uncertain clinical situations
- learning about uncertainty in organisations and teams.

Chapter 21 has examples of teaching session plans.

Effective educational methods for training for uncertainty in different training settings

When a clinician is learning through *private study or reflection*, using the algorithm (see p. 15) will help direct attention towards the relevant Quadrant of the MUM. For some clinicians identifying which skill is needed will be enough. However, for others the skill will be unfamiliar; they will need to seek further training opportunities in that area, together with effective feedback. Educators who use this approach themselves will find that their skills in helping juniors cope with uncertainty will increase too as the process of analysing uncertainty becomes more familiar.

In *one-to-one training* situations (such as debriefing, juniors asking for help, regular tutorials), a crucial first step is to 'hold on' to the ambiguity, uncertainty or muddle for long enough to really think it through and reflect on it. This process of 'metacognition', which has been described earlier in the book, can be difficult for clinicians. Clinicians often feel so uncomfortable in uncertain situations that they 'jump away' to a decision, even if it's a premature one. Reflecting on 'dysfunctional ways out' (which can be explored while discouraged) as well as 'functional ways through' (which can be reinforced) will also help to demonstrate skills in 'holding' uncertainty.

When teaching one to one, uncertainty may first be assessed using the methods already outlined in Chapter 18. Initially, after working through the training algorithm/ MUM ask the learner what skill she thinks may unlock things (refer to the relevant Quadrant chapter for more detail). Clearly, at times, the difficulty is one of lack of knowledge, which must be rectified. However, dealing with uncertainty is often a matter of skill rather than knowledge. Learners *know about* topics or issues, without *knowing how* to bring that knowledge to good use in a particular situation. For many learners in a 'hot' clinical situation, identifying the right skill will be all that is required; they recognise the skill and can go off and use it. For other trainees the skill will be one that they have only a sketchy knowledge of, or have used infrequently, so they are unfamiliar with what is required. Then the trainer or supervisor may have to do some 'hot skills' teaching to manage the immediate problem.

Seniors can further help juniors develop these skills of metacognition, 'thinking about their thinking', in two ways. First, they can themselves identify and talk about uncertainty when they recognise it and model the skills they use to unpick the uncertainties in their own clinical practice. This demonstrates 'metacognition' in practice. Sometimes trainees observing expertise think only intuition and 'instant' assessment are involved, as the thinking processes are often hidden within the expert's head. Talking through solutions, perhaps also using the MUM, to demonstrate how thinking has evolved, will help learners to understand how apparently intuitive Type 1 thinking is usually the result of highly developed Type 2 analytical thinking, which develops into effective pattern recognition.[9]

Second, seniors can assist metacognition by training junior staff to ask for help in a structured way; this promotes learning of 'thinking skills' in action. This approach has been outlined in Chapter 18, on assessment methods using the Map of Uncertainty in Medicine. Handover skills, like the SBAR approach (see p. 150), also promote metacognitions by encouraging the learner to reflect on her problem thoroughly before asking for help.

It will usually be helpful to remind the learner to 'revisit' the issue later and learn about the skill in more detail, using the potential teaching and learning methods outlined at the end of each of the Quadrant chapters of this book.

Uncertainty is often avoided by clinicians because it feels challenging and uncomfortable. Exploring the painful emotions attached to uncertainty in a one-to-one situation needs sensitive handling and a supportive relationship; educators need to recognise their own discomfort with these issues. However, exploring the psychological aspects of clinicians' responses to uncertainty will pay dividends if trainees are then able to hold uncertainty more willingly, and reflect on their own thinking more. Developing 'holding skills' for uncertain situations is often more about the clinician understanding the psychological processes at work in difficult situations, than about straightforward clinical knowledge. Reflecting on these issues with an educator can help to develop a more nuanced approach.

Group teaching for uncertainty works best if the teaching methods encourage discussion, interaction and exploration of attitudes and values as well as knowledge and skills. This requires the group members to have developed trust in each other, and so may be more suited to a 'mature' group who know each other or who are skilled in group study methods. Teaching material about intuitive Type 1 thinking and how it interacts with complementary, analytical Type 2 thinking can be enlightening. In group situations, using real-life examples generated from the group discussion can be mapped against the Quadrants of the MUM, matching the uncertainties expressed with the possible skills needed.

For many groups, realising that uncertainty can be classified and understood is liberating, especially when there is an offer of useful skills to make uncertainty less painful. It is then useful for the cases to be discussed by participants who were not directly involved. They will usually recognise similar situations in their own experiences, which deepens the discussion. This can profitably be done in very small 'buzz' group of two to four people. These methods can reduce embarrassment and the potential for painful exposure of individuals' uncertainties or errors. At the same time the learning from error or uncertainty is maximised, by being openly discussed.[1]

Apart from case discussions and group debriefing, other activities can decrease the frustration, disillusionment and anxiety provoked by uncertainty. These include the use of Significant Event Analyses to examine uncertain situations, reflective writing and Balint or Schwartz rounds.[2] This can help to promote supportive relationships with other clinicians. Training needs to emphasise the relationship aspects of uncertainty, whether between doctors and their patients or between colleagues. Balint-style small group discussion, where the emphasis is on the doctors' relationships, can allow helpful exploration and acceptance of the difficult feelings engendered by uncertainty.[3] These issues are explored in Part III.

In *team meetings*, talking about uncertainty will benefit all members. If the senior members of the team share their uncertainties and also their methods of thinking, the team can become an evolving and more skilful group. This will also assist in the induction of new members who will 'acculturate' to a climate where uncertainty is accepted as a normal part of clinical practice.

These reflective approaches are endorsed by all medical educators but can be difficult for some learners to get used to. Reflection simply means being able to 'think critically about' an issue, something which most doctors will do quite naturally in discussion. Donald Schön proposes that learning to think critically about what you are doing after events have happened (reflection ON action) helps you to think critically about what you are doing in the heat of the moment (reflection IN action).[4] This critical thinking creates opportunities to choose appropriate strategies deliberately, rather than getting swept along by the uncertainties of difficult situations. This increases expertise, and makes uncertainty less uncomfortable.

Training for uncertainty; can this improve resilience in practice?

Resilience refers to a clinician's ability to keep going even when things are difficult. Modern medical practice is complex, multifaceted, with many different tasks and different options, and the expectations of medical teams are increasing all the time. This increases pressure on all decision making. Doctors who are constantly asking themselves 'Have I done the right thing?' or who are new to, or more vulnerable to, pressure or uncertainty, can readily get burnt out or develop mental health problems such as depression. Different clinicians respond to periods of uncertainty in different ways. For many, personal growth and an increased sense of confidence and control result from getting through a period of uncertainty. For other people, uncertainty simply accentuates the threats to their self-confidence and sense of control.[5] 'Black humour' may be a limited coping mechanism for dealing with the stresses of uncertainty. Such stress may manifest as indifference or poor performance, as has been seen in some recent scandals, and may also lead to doctors leaving the profession.

As long ago as 1957, in her extensive work on uncertainty Renée Fox catalogued adaptive coping strategies, used by more senior clinicians to deal with uncertainty:

> *Forming group bonds, commitment to each other, caring, informing and sharing with patients, honouring patients for their courage and dedication, telling success stories, trying new procedures or drugs, keeping meticulous records in hopes of discovering patterns in the uncertain swirl of events, turning to religion and finally accepting ignorance, uncertainty and death as part of life.*[6]

These are still relevant today, although the pressures of modern medical practice sometimes seem to limit the time available for group discussion and support.

Tolerating and dealing with ambiguity, and at the same time being expected to be 'right' and work to 'high standards', may create greater uncertainty for practitioners. Uncertainty arises not just because of the inherent uncertainties of medical practice ('This drug only works for 60% of people'), or solely from the difficulties of diagnosis or decision making, but also from the interpersonal aspects of negotiating, networking and team-working. This highlights the need for clinicians to develop interpersonal, conflict resolution, change management and motivational skills as well as purely medical diagnosis and treatment skills. This will enable uncertainty to be managed, coped with and tolerated more easily.

Mapping uncertainty will not eliminate this, although using the MUM can help to increase confidence and expertise. By highlighting a more holistic approach to uncertainty, and at the same time offering a way to subdivide skills into manageable parts, we hope that the MUM will be a tool to promote resilience to uncertainty in younger practitioners, and also help trainers or supervisors to increase their own skills in managing uncertainty. Training must also enable the recognition that uncertainty is an intrinsic part of the professional's role; this is discussed in more detail in the conclusion to this book.

Decision-making approaches for uncertain clinical situations

Planning for uncertainty will take different forms in different clinical situations. Having 'rational' approaches to uncertainty in different situations can help clinicians retain some sense of 'mastery' or control, even in trying circumstances. In this section, two approaches are described. First, decision-making approaches suitable for different types of clinical scenario are outlined. Second, approaches to uncertainty beneficial for organisational uncertainties are described. Seniors can talk through these approaches when helping juniors make decisions in uncertain situations. Modelling structured approaches gives a powerful message: that uncertainty is 'normal' and can be coped with, using learnable strategies. Uncertainty is discussed in organisational contexts outside medicine, and concepts such as the 'Stacey Matrix', which characterise the dynamics of complexity, can be helpful in a medical context also.[7]

It can be helpful to think of *clinical situations* as mapping along two axes. On one axis there is the degree of uncertainty, complexity or ambiguity in the clinical situation; on the other axis is the speed with which clinical situations are evolving (see Table 19.1).

Different types of decision making will help to manage the uncertainty in each Quadrant.

If the *speed of development of the clinical state is slow and complexity is low* (for example elective surgery), organisations can facilitate traditional planning methods, with fixed pathways. Uncertainty is minimised by excluding patients who cannot readily fit into a simple pathway, for example if they have comorbidity.

Table 19.1: Choosing decision-making strategies in uncertainty; rate of change versus complexity applied to clinical situations

Speed of clinical change HIGH Complexity or ambiguity LOW For example childbirth Use ALGORITHMS	Speed of clinical change HIGH Complexity or ambiguity HIGH For example an unstable patient in intensive therapy unit Use PATTERN RECOGNITION
Speed of clinical change LOW Complexity or ambiguity LOW For example elective hernia surgery Use PATHWAYS	Speed of clinical change LOW Complexity or ambiguity HIGH Comorbidity in ambulant care Use SCENARIO/OPTION PLANNING

Source: adapted from Devine and Syrett.[8]

If the *complexity is low but the speed of evolution is high* (for example abnormal labour and childbirth), then the organisational structure needs to facilitate the use of decision analysis techniques such as algorithms, to provide unambiguous measures of progress and outcomes, and the rapid availability of the relevant resources (for example theatre time or access to highly skilled senior staff) to manage the inherent uncertainty of a rapidly changing situation.

When *complexity is high but the pace of change is slow* (e.g. caring for patients with multiple stable comorbidities or end-of-life care in non-malignant conditions), then scenario planning, such as creating advanced care plans, creating and communicating options, partnership and collaboration between clinician, patients and teams become more relevant approaches for developing appropriate responses to uncertainty.

In situations of *high complexity and rapidly changing clinical situations* (e.g. in Accident and Emergency or intensive care units) pattern recognition, agility in care planning and clear communication will come to the fore in managing the emerging uncertainties.

An effective leader of a team or service can use these concepts to ensure that appropriate decision-making methods are used in different types of uncertain situation; articulating such strategies demonstrates that not all uncertainties need the same approach. Less experienced members of the team will be able to develop their understanding of uncertainty, to use relevant decision-making strategies and to develop a greater skill in managing uncertain situations. This will in turn create a sense of stability and support within the team.

Of course much of this is happening already in all kinds of clinical teams. However, from a training point of view, such approaches may not be identified as being about the 'management of uncertainty'. Making the use and purpose of such strategies explicit can help clinicians in training be more aware of different approaches to different types of uncertainty.

Learning about uncertainty in organisations and teams

Uncertainty, as we have seen in Part III, is subjective, occurs in relationships and in the ever changing organisational environment of clinical practice. Leaders of the teams and organisations in which clinicians work have the potential to help to contain and manage the inherent uncertainties of clinical practice. By articulating and modelling appropriate decision-making and leadership strategies in uncertain situations, educators can deepen understanding of how uncertainty can be coped with. Educators can work though organisational uncertainties in one-to-one or group teaching situations, exploring how the concepts outlined in this section can help make degrees of ambiguity and uncertainty understandable and tolerable. In the business world, the management of uncertain situations is accepted as requiring a specific set of skills: strategic anticipation, navigational leadership, agility, open collaboration and deep learning based on feedback.[8] How might this apply in clinical organisations?

Strategic anticipation means that the organisation or team leadership is 'clear enough' about what can be known, while also accepting that a range of outcomes is possible. This approach is especially useful when ambiguity or complexity is too great to plan for. In clinical terms, this may mean understanding and accepting that simple measures like length of stay or numbers of patients seen per clinic will not reflect quality in straightforward ways. If there is the prospect of reorganisations or organisational failures, this will generate many uncertainties for staff that will impact on the effectiveness of their work. Leaders need to ensure that staff can be well informed about the range of possibilities for the future. In purely clinical terms, this means promoting awareness that unstable patients, or those with a complex comorbidity, may not have linear or predictable clinical courses. This highlights the inherent uncertainty to the patient and to the staff involved. Accepting that a range of outcomes may occur can mean that uncertainty is less fearful, becoming a 'known unknown'.

Navigational leadership refers to having a collective sense of 'where things are up to' and the best ways to accept and approach uncertain issues. Seniors can model appropriate decision-making and planning strategies for uncertain situations. Seniors who recognise uncertainty and signal that this is a 'normal' state, with optimism that uncertainty can be 'weathered' rather than eliminated, help juniors to learn the skills needed to cope with uncertainty.

Agility means encouraging adaptability and flexibility in uncertain situations, reacting to new information or feedback. Many clinical situations require just this kind of adaptability; organisationally, new information or feedback needs to be readily available, for example by ensuring timely access to investigation results or senior input.

Open collaboration means that in uncertain situations it is helpful to work across usual boundaries, making new links or partnerships. Effective teamwork is part of this, as is the improvement of work between teams and, crucially, recognising the patient and family as 'part of the team'.

Continued learning means developing the capacity of 'deep learning', analysing patterns and learning about all aspects of care whether physical, psychological, social or organisational. This will help develop the capacity to anticipate disruptions from uncertain situations.

Chapter 21 outlines specific teaching plans for sessions dealing with uncertainty.

References

1. Lea A, Danczak A. Medical error: a dirty little secret or great learning opportunity? *Education for Primary Care* 2014; **25(2)**: 114–18.
2. Luther VP, Crandall SJ. Commentary: ambiguity and uncertainty: neglected elements of medical education curricula? *Academic Medicine* 2011; **86(7)**: 799–800; DOI: 10.1097/ACM.0b013e31821da915.
3. Balint E, Courtney M, Elder A, *et al. The Doctor, the Patient and the Group: Balint revisited*. London: Routledge, 1993.
4. Schön D. *The Reflective Practitioner: how professionals think in action*. London: Temple Smith, 1983.
5. Croskerry P. Context is everything or how could I have been that stupid? *Healthcare Quarterly* 2009; **12**: 171–17.
6. Fox RC. Training for uncertainty. In: RK Merton, G Reader, PL Kendall (eds). *The Student-Physician: introductory studies in the sociology of medical education*. Cambridge, MA: Harvard University Press, 1957, pp. 207–41.
7. Stacey RD. *Strategic Management and Organisational Dynamics: the challenge of complexity*. (3rd edn). Harlow: Prentice Hall, 2002.
8. Devine M, Syrett M. *Managing Uncertainty: strategies for surviving and thriving in turbulent times*. London: Economist Books, 2012.
9. Pelaccia T, Tardif J, Trilby E, Charlin B. An analysis of clinical reasoning through a recent and comprehensive approach: the dual process theory. *Medical Education Online* 2011; 16; DOI: 10.3402/meo.v16io.5980.

Chapter 20

Educational skills for uncertainty in training

When it is the *educator* who does not know what to do

In most situations, clinicians in training are open to learning the skills they need. Some direction from a trainer or supervisor, using the MUM as a guide, will be enough to move things forwards. However, sometimes, the trainer or supervisor is faced with a trainee whose lack of progress or whose difficulties mean that the *trainer himself* feels that, *as a trainer*, he 'doesn't know what to do'. Such WDYDWYDKWTD experiences in a training context can be unsettling. By definition, educators, trainers or supervisors are more senior than their trainees; they have succeeded in learning and progressed to the stage where they can train others. Educators are usually skilled and enthusiastic learners themselves. As a result, educators may find it difficult to develop insight into what makes learning difficult for some clinicians. This chapter considers uncertainty in training situations and covers:

- 'dysfunctional ways out' of uncertain educational situations
- a Map of Uncertainty in Medical Training (MUMT)
- mapping skills for educational uncertainty
- when the performance of a colleague causes the WDYDWYDKWTD experience.

'Dysfunctional ways out' of uncertain educational situations

As in most WDYDWYDKWTD situations there are 'dysfunctional ways out'. In educational situations these 'ways out' mirror the 'dysfunctional ways out' of the consultation, especially those of the Negotiating Quadrant. Much education and training is inevitably carried out by clinicians who are not necessarily trained as clinical teachers. Keen and enthusiastic learners can usually continue to obtain effective training even when their supervisors are not trained educators. However, not all learners are equally skilled at learning, and in all spheres of clinical work there are learners who have difficulty in progressing at the same speed as their contemporaries. The reasons for this are many and varied; being able to clarify what is needed to help a particular learner in difficulty is not always a straightforward task. Disruptions to training may arise when educators have not recognised the problems that some learners in difficulty are struggling with. As a result, when the educator experiences a WDYDWYDKWTD moment 'dysfunctional ways out' come into effect. 'Dysfunctional ways out' are less effective at producing change, but, if identified, can usually be overcome.

These 'ways out' include:

Blaming the trainee ('They are lazy, stupid, and oblivious to the need to change!'). This attitude to educational difficulty is effectively devolving the problem entirely to the learner. If training is not progressing, this is really a problem shared between the learner and the educator, the latter having a responsibility to create learning plans that will help all the learners they are responsible for, including the less effective learners.

Withdrawing support and bypassing them ('Ask the better trainee to do that procedure/see that patient'). Although this sorts out the short-term problem of getting clinical work done, the trainee in difficulty is likely to fall even further behind if she gets less experience and if her problems are not recognised and dealt with.

Not telling it like it is ('I don't want to tell them that they aren't doing well. They will get upset'). This situation can arise if educators are not secure in their assessment or feedback skills. Learners will get upset if unhelpful feedback is given. However, constructive feedback is usually welcomed. It is even more upsetting to reach the end of a placement or training programme and fail, having not been given feedback to aid improvement on the way.

Passing the problem on to others ('They scraped through this placement. Perhaps the next one will be better.' Or even worse: 'Thank goodness they are moving on soon'). This phenomenon sometimes happens because educators are unable or unwilling to give constructive feedback. Problems that are not dealt with tend to escalate.

Seeing the problem in isolation, rather than taking a team approach ('I should be able to deal with this issue by myself'). Most learners progress satisfactorily. When training is not going as well as it should, individual educators can easily take on the whole problem, worrying about what to do, trying things that do not work and becoming frustrated. Where there are major difficulties, educators will need to work with a wider educational team.

Applying training plans rigidly even if the individual has specific needs (a trainee with very sick parents gets an attitude of 'So what if your mother and father are both dying from cancer at the moment'). Some learners in difficulty are wrestling with multiple life issues, not just educational issues. Finding out what these issues are offers opportunities to ameliorate them, without resulting in educational failure, which is costly to all concerned.

Resorting to 'gossip' ('Watch out for that one. You will never guess what they did last week!'). Some learners get a 'reputation' that they are unaware of and this may prejudice subsequent educational encounters. As such, gossip is unrecorded and not accompanied by effective feedback. It is a 'dysfunctional way out'.

A Map of Uncertainty in Medical Training

To clarify a WDYDWYDKWTD situation in training, it can be helpful to consider the trainee holistically, using the same Quadrants as are used clinically, but focusing on the *educational skills* that the trainer needs to use to assess the learner, instead of the clinical ones. In this section each Quadrant is considered as part of an *educational* assessment, leading to an overall *educational diagnosis*. An educational diagnosis should clarify the nature of the problem.

The educational skills required are set out in the MUMT (page 240). This approach enables a fuller assessment if the trainer is having a *training* WDYDWYDKWTD moment. This may happen with a trainee whose progress is poor, or who does not respond well to the usual training methods, or even perhaps when a colleague's performance is causing concern.

Chapters 18, 19 and 21 describe how the four Quadrants of the MUM can be used as a training tool in 'usual' circumstances. When there is uncertainty about a training situation, a similar approach needs to be taken as to any WDYDWYDKWTD situation (i.e. use the MUMT to work out

Mapping Uncertainty in Medical Training (MUMT)

	TRAINER–TRAINEE DYAD	COLLEAGUES AND TEAM
DIAGNOSIS	**EDUCATIONAL ANALYSING** Using the educational methods of ASSESSMENT, RECORDING, and CALIBRATION to make an educational diagnosis • Work placed based assessments • Case based discussions • Observed consultations • Examination results • Skills assessments relevant to the trainee	**EDUCATIONAL NETWORKING** Using the educational methods of ASSESSMENT, MULTISOURCE FEEDBACK, HANDOVER, and RECORDING to extend the educational diagnosis • Triangulate assessments with colleagues • Obtain facts about professional behaviours from the observations of other teams, other units, other departments • Multisource feedback
MANAGEMENT	**EDUCATIONAL NEGOTIATION** Using the educational methods of FEEDBACK, NEGOTIATION, COACHING and MENTORING. • Feedback skills • Fill educational gaps • Address internal, external, emotional or practical issues • Clarify attitudes and expectations • Clarify what acceptable practice is like	**EDUCATIONAL TEAMWORK** Using the educational methods of HANDOVER, MANAGING MEETINGS, and LEADERSHIP. • Involve wider educational team, senior educators • Use handover skills • Manage meetings, • Record educational concerns appropriately • Leadership skills to manage difficult situations

which Educational Quadrant is relevant and work from there). The aim is to make an *educational diagnosis*, rather than a medical one, followed by an *educational prescription*. This is a plan of the actions that an educator and his learner will need to take to get training back on track.

In a training WDYDWYDKWTD moment, the first step is done directly by the trainer/supervisor and trainee working together, using the usual assessment tools relevant to the specialty (the Analysing Quadrant of the MUMT). If a clear educational diagnosis cannot be made with the educator and learner working together (a diagnosis should clarify what actions are needed), then a networking approach is needed, gleaning information from a wider network of those who interact with the trainee. This may yield enough information to be sure what the problem really is.

Next, consider how educational plans can be made to overcome the issues identified. Is the trainee receptive to change and further training? Can other factors getting in the way of training be dealt with using the Negotiating Quadrant of the MUMT? If so, all will usually be well. If not, then the wider educational team will need to be involved, using the Team-working Quadrant of the MUMT. This may include more senior educators, or deanery staff for medical trainees, or the responsible officer or senior colleagues, if the person in question is not in a training post. Each Quadrant of the MUMT is discussed in more detail in the following sections.

Mapping skills for educational uncertainty

When the educator is in a WDYDWYDKWTD situation, following a structured approach helps to clarify what the problem really is and what needs to be done next. Working through the training algorithm will identify which Quadrant of the MUMT is relevant, and the relevant educational skills for that Quadrant can be applied. Often learners in difficulty will have problems that require educational skills from more than one Quadrant to be used.

The MUMT algorithm (see p. 242) will clarify the process.

Educational Analysing Quadrant skills

Creating an educational diagnosis

When the educator 'does not know what to do', the first step is to create a useful 'educational diagnosis', a description of the learner's educational position and learning needs. Case-based discussions, workplace-based assessment and external examinations are all well-validated methods to assess progress. As training develops, a variety of other assessment tools will arise, and each specialty will have methods to assess specific areas of expertise.

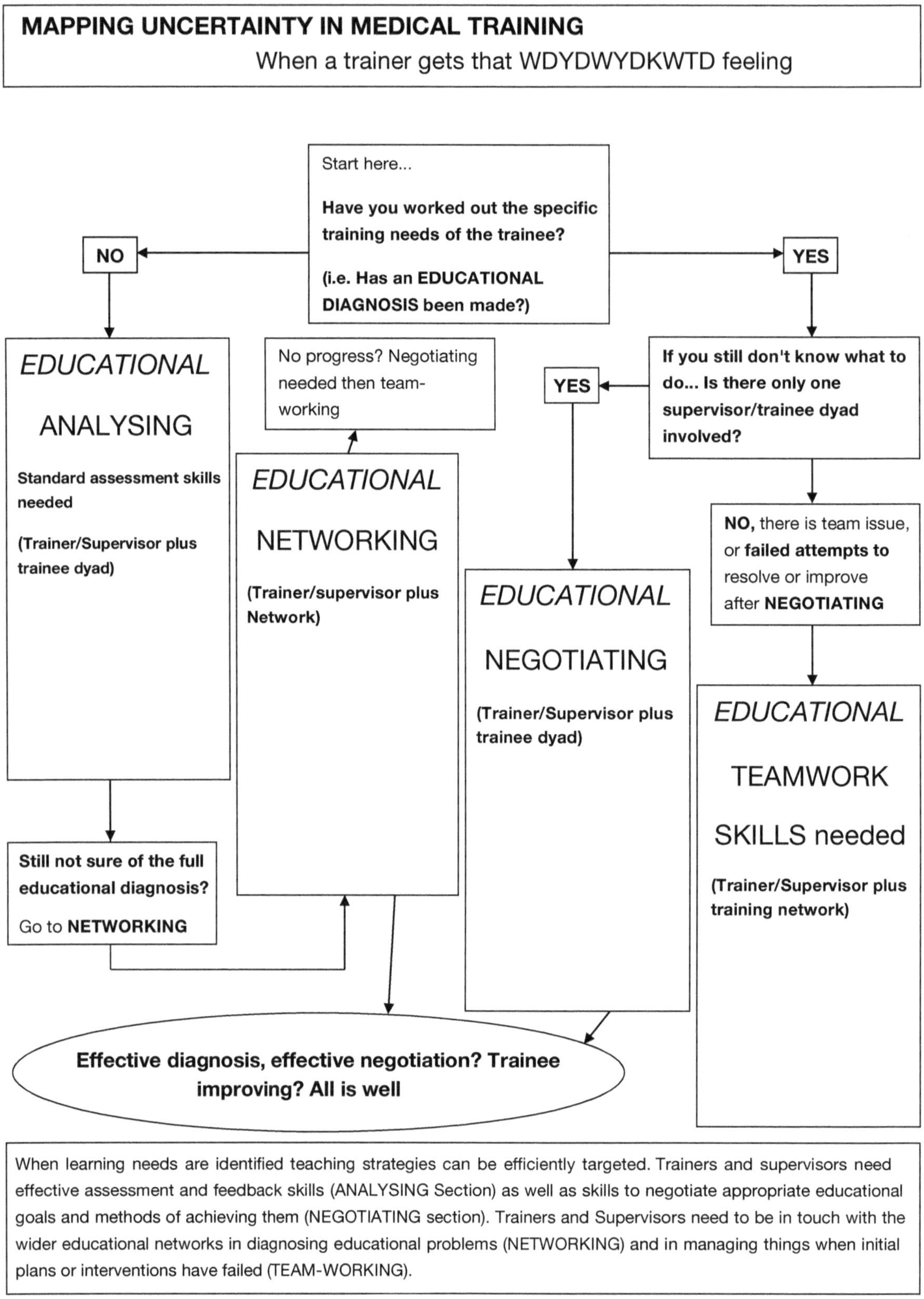

Assessment and calibration

The educational skills needed are those of assessment, calibrated against accepted standards of good practice, to make them fair, objective and based on facts, not opinions or prejudices. Assessors need to ensure that their assessments are calibrated against those of others in the same specialty, to ensure that the findings are objective and reliable. Educators can duplicate assessments, to ensure that there is reasonable agreement, or triangulate assessments, by getting feedback or observations from several sources. Sometimes it isn't possible to do this assessment just by interacting with the trainee alone. The RDM-p framework is useful here and focuses on:[1]

- R = Relationships (with patients and colleagues)
- D = Diagnostics (for patients and their own assessments of their learning)
- M = Management (of self, patients, others)
- p = Professionalism (attitude, honesty, integrity, trust).

An individual educator can use this together with the MUM to build up a picture of a trainee's strengths and weaknesses.

However, having done an assessment in the Educational Analysing Quadrant a trainer or colleague may *still feel uncertain* as to whether they need to do anything more, or what the exact nature of the problem is. If individual assessment is not enough to make a full educational diagnosis then use the Educational Networking Quadrant of the MUMT. Just as networking can help to make a clinical diagnosis, networking with colleagues can help to make an *educational* diagnosis.

Educational Networking Quadrant skills

Educational networking skills are helpful to make a more complete and rounded assessment of a trainee's learning needs.

Multisource feedback

Feedback from a variety of sources enables an educator to triangulate her own assessments with others and a fuller picture emerges. What professional behaviours have colleagues and team members observed? (Facts are friendly. Stick to the actions that can be observed.) How do colleagues in other departments view this trainee? Getting factual information rather than opinions or judgements can be difficult. It is a skill in itself to tease out objective descriptions from the observations of other team members. For example, a statement such as 'They are so lazy' needs to be clarified into discrete observations, such as, 'They arrived 20 minutes after the start of the clinic twice last week and left without seeing all the patients on the ward yesterday.'

Encouraging trainees to seek formal 'multisource feedback' is usual in most training programmes. To get a fuller picture of his attitudes, it can be helpful to ask the learner to reflect on his feedback and take the discussion further. Questions that may reveal issues in more detail include:

- 'Which aspect of your work with colleagues is the most difficult?'
- 'Which departments or teams are the most difficult for you to work with?'

Often this is enough to make a working 'diagnosis' of the problem or to reassure the trainer that all is well.

Handover and recording

Sometimes, deeper weaknesses or more complex training needs are identified, and referral to a wider educational network is needed (analogous to referring a patient). The skills of handover to others that have been discussed in the Team-working Quadrant (see Chapter 13) are just as relevant here. Furthermore, the assessment and reason for handover need to be properly and thoroughly recorded; this may be in a specific report or the electronic portfolio where relevant. Verbal handovers, without documentation of concerns or findings, can be ineffective and risk descending to the 'dysfunctional ways out' of gossip ('That trainee is not much use'), or blaming the trainee ('She never seems to learn').

To move forwards, all this needs to be fully discussed with the trainee using the skills of the Negotiating Quadrant of the MUMT.

Educational Negotiating Quadrant skills

Educational negotiating means knowing how to enact a suitable educational management plan. Knowing the diagnosis, as we have seen earlier in the book, is no guarantee that things will run smoothly. The initial process must be aimed at producing an accurate and jointly agreed assessment of the situation. A good relationship and a safe setting (not a meeting in a corridor!) need to be created to allow both parties' concerns to be heard and taken on board.

Feedback

The colleague who may be underperforming (whether trainee or experienced clinician) needs to receive feedback about his performance. This is not always easy to do, but is greatly improved if feedback focuses on observable behaviours and outcomes (facts are friendly) and is specific, non-judgemental, realistic and occurring soon after the events in question have occurred. The acronym SMART (specific, measurable, achievable, realistic and timely) is well known to most educators. Feedback needs to be set up and negotiated with the trainee ('Are you ready to discuss some feedback about your work?'). Anyone involved in training needs to develop their feedback skills thoroughly. A colleague who may be struggling with her work or with the feedback she has received needs support, as well as the challenge of the feedback, emphasising the relationship-building skills that are needed in this Quadrant.

In addition, throughout training, learners need to be taught how to *respond* to feedback. When offered feedback, however painful or however much we disagree with it, we all need to have a form of words to accept feedback graciously. Saying 'Thank you for giving me that feedback. That is something I need to think about' (or something along those lines) gives the listener time to digest the feedback. He can then move towards considering the feedback more seriously in relation to his learning needs. A clear understanding of what good practice is like may be required, including the helpful professional attitudes that underpin good practice.

Negotiation

Moving on from the feedback, possible solutions to problems need to be identified and plans made to act on them. There needs to be willingness from both parties to enter into discussion and dialogue, and to negotiate possible ways forwards. If there is a knowledge or skills gap, efforts need to be directed towards meeting those educational needs. The learner needs to be involved in planning how to address educational needs so that she herself gets 'ownership' of the problem. Sometimes the problem is different: not so much gaps in skills or knowledge, but that the trainee is not able or not willing to address the training need identified. This means that the influence of other factors may need to be addressed; this could include emotional issues, practical impediments to learning (such as having too long a commuting time) or internal issues like health problems. Sometimes past experiences such as bullying, or examination failure leading to demoralisation and expectations of failure, may be important too.

Taking a holistic view and understanding the constraints that may be impacting on training arising from personal, health, financial, language, visa or other difficulties can go a long way towards identifying possible solutions. Some issues can be resolved through negotiation, and a firm agreement to review and follow things up.

Coaching and mentoring

Coaching and mentoring skills are helpful in moving towards the completion of an effective educational prescription. One example of a structure that can be used is the GROW model (see Box 20.1). A full description of these skills cannot be given here but there are suitable resources at the end of this chapter.[2]

Box 20.1: The 'GROW' model of coaching to help learners develop

The mnemonic GROW helps to identify how a learner is going to move forwards once she has identified the problems in the discussion with her educator. It works like this:

G = GOAL

Ask the learner to clearly identify her *learning goals* ('I need to manage uncertain diagnoses by taking a more thorough history and examination rather than jumping straight to referral' or 'I need to learn how best to hand over patients properly to other team members') as well as their long-term *performance goals* ('pass my next set of examinations').

R = REALITY

Where is he now in relation to where he would like to be? What options are realistic for him now?

O = OPTIONS

What options are there for achieving the goals? This could include private study, having some supervised practice with feedback, observing a skilled practitioner and identifying what she is doing well.

W = WILL/WAY FORWARDS

What is his motivation to change what he is doing? How important is change to him? What would increase that? How confident is he that he can change things around? What would make him more confident? What are the immediate and subsequent steps towards the goal?

Source: Whitmore J. *Coaching for Performance*.[2]

If there are significant blocks to progress identified in the Educational Negotiating Quadrant, it is crucial to involve the educational team, using the skills of the Team-working Quadrant of the MUMT.

Educational Team-working Quadrant skills

Educational team-working skills relate to the wider educational context including senior trainers, specialty tutors or educational leads, as well as the director of postgraduate education and the deanery support structure. This means educators should not work in isolation when there is uncertainty about a training or performance issue. Supervisors, trainees and other clinicians need to fully understand their own network of training or performance management so that appropriate advice and support is sought at the relevant stage. Involving the local supporting structure is likely to lead to more productive ways forwards.

Recording and handover skills

When educators find themselves in a WDYDWYDKWTD situation, they will need to capture the progress of their learners accurately and objectively in writing, so that other people in the educational team can understand what is happening. Recording objective observations about behaviour makes it easier to negotiate change and develop a management plan for the educational diagnosis that emerges. Effective handover skills (SBAR for example; see p. 150) are also needed when working together with members of a wider educational team.

Chairing meetings

If a learner is struggling to the extent that a wider educational team needs to be involved, there will inevitably be meetings to discuss what should happen. Effective meetings will facilitate work with the larger educational team, and require the same skills as any other team meetings. Effective chairmanship, clear boundaries and effective reporting will help to create helpful relationships.

These twin approaches, using the MUM directly to assess the training needs in each Quadrant and then, if progress is blocked, to evaluate the whole educational experience of the trainee using the MUMT will usually move things forwards. Plans can be adapted to the realities of the individual trainee's situation, and the exact requirements of her educational or regulatory body. Having a structured approach helps educators to move things forwards, and helps the trainee in difficulty to feel that her problems are understood and being managed in a fair way.

When the performance of a colleague causes the WDYDWYDKWTD experience

The approach outlined in this chapter can also be used if a clinician finds herself concerned about the performance of a colleague rather than a trainee. Doubts about a colleague's performance can give rise to a troubling WDYDWYDKWTD feeling. The way forwards is not always clear and assessing performance is not as straightforward as with trainees; different clinicians may legitimately have different approaches and priorities. Analysing the problem using the frameworks suggested (MUM, RDM-p) can help to identify objective, observable behaviours that can be used to confirm or, indeed, refute an impression of underperformance. Are this clinician's diagnostics adequate? Are patients concerned or inadequately cared for? How does he work in teams? Does an assessment using the RDM-p approach identify areas of difficulty?

The uncertainty in training algorithm/MUMT can then help any concerned colleague to work out what they may need to do next. Does feedback lead to effective development? Who else needs to be involved? For doctors in non-training posts, senior clinicians or the responsible officer for their trust or primary care organisation will be able to help.

Completing such an assessment will help the doctor who 'doesn't know what to do' clarify her thoughts. Reflecting with her colleague, considering her willingness to engage with feedback, her ability to learn and resolve difficulties, will clarify whether remediation is required, and if so by what route it may be approached. Conversely, mapping uncertainty about a colleague's practice may also provide reassurance that concerns are not major.

References

1. Norfolk T, Siriwardena AN. A unifying theory of clinical practice: Relationship, Diagnostics, Management and professionalism (RDM-p). *Quality in Primary Care* 2009; **17(1)**: 37–47.
2. Whitmore J. *Coaching for Performance: GROWing human potential and purpose.* (4th edn). London: Nicholas Brealey Press, 2009.

Chapter 21

Learning about uncertainty

Teaching sessions

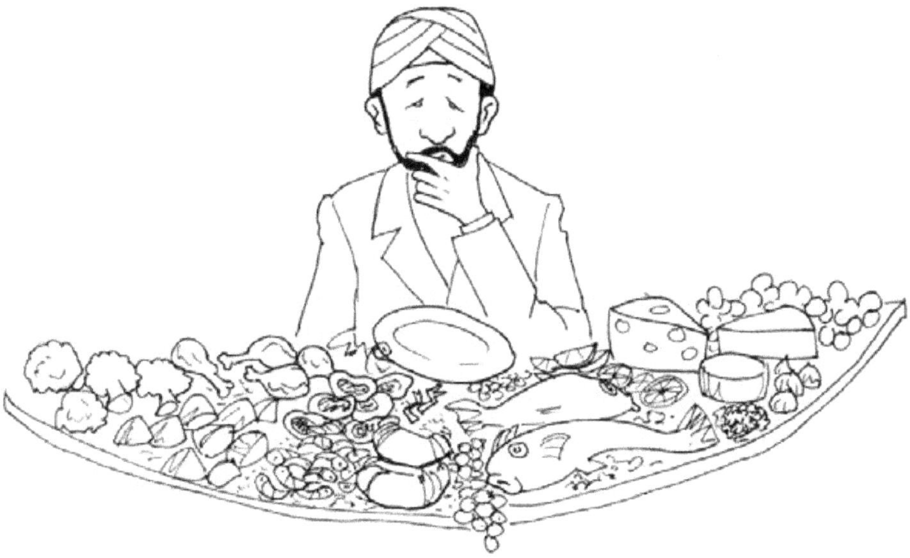

'Snack or five-course dinner?'

This chapter proposes some teaching sessions for helping clinicians to learn about uncertainty away from the 'hot' clinical setting. It is divided into sections that cover:

- setting the aims/objectives and intended learning outcomes of teaching sessions
- teaching plans for different situations
  - when you have five minutes
  - when you have an hour
  - when you have half a day
  - when you have a whole day.

Setting the aims/objectives and intended learning outcomes of teaching sessions

When planning education sessions concerned with uncertainty, educators will need to follow their usual practice of considering the three elements of the educational triangle: the aims of education; assessing the learners' current level and hence their learning needs; and finally choosing appropriate methods to achieve learning related to the aims in question.

The aims of training clinicians to deal with uncertainty are covered in more detail in Chapter 17 and can be summarised as being the knowledge, skills and attitudes that enable clinicians to:

- recognise uncertainty (knowledge)
- classify uncertainty, which will help to demystify it (knowledge)
- 'hold' uncertainty, which will encourage reflection on it (skills)
- choose the relevant skills to help them manage uncertainty (skills)
- value and create partnerships with patients to share decision making in uncertainty (skills and attitudes)
- accept that uncertainty is inevitable, which will help their resilience and overall professionalism to develop (attitudes)
- recognise uncertainty in colleagues and choose appropriate ways to support and develop others' skills using effective, non-judgemental approaches (attitudes).

Assessment in relation to uncertainty was covered in Chapter 18 and educational methods for uncertainty have been discussed in Chapter 19.

Thus, for all education sessions concerned with uncertainty, educators will need to consider what specific objectives and learning outcomes are required, what the starting point of their participants is, and what the appropriate educational methods will be.

The *specific learning objectives and intended learning outcomes* for teaching sessions will vary according to the level of seniority of the participants, the time available and how such training fits into a wider programme of learning and teaching. Clinicians from medical students to experienced consultants and GPs have participated in workshops dealing with uncertainty using the MUM, so we know that the material is adaptable to different needs.

The *starting point* should always be to establish where the participants are in their thinking and learning about uncertainty. This can be done successfully by asking participants to share their hopes for the session (what do they hope to learn?) and their fears for the session (what do they dread will happen?). Fears about exposure, having to do 'role play' or being criticised for not knowing things need to be acknowledged and addressed in the proper management of the group. Learners need to know that uncertainty is to be acknowledged and accepted, and that expressing uncertainty is encouraged, because it will enable the whole group to benefit from learning about it. Non-judgemental attitudes to uncertainty must be modelled by educators, and 'blaming and shaming' by participants discouraged.

The *education session* that follows this starting point should address:

- knowledge about uncertainty (using the material in the book as a resource)
- classification of uncertainty (using the MUM)
- exploration of the experiences of learners (using their own consultations and experiences).

Teaching sessions involving groups of clinicians will be more effective if participants are willing and able to share their own experiences, thoughts and feelings about the uncertainties they have faced. Talking about such matters will also bring clinicians close to considerations of what it is like to face possible errors. These are emotive and potentially threatening subjects for some clinicians, especially those who are not used to talking about their experiences, or who fear that they will face censure or ridicule. Thus, time spent in establishing a safe group environment is essential. Discussion should be explicitly required to be respectful, supportive and confidential. Smaller groups often enable people to talk more freely than large groups. In large group settings, breaking the group into smaller buzz groups of two to six participants may be the best way to get full participation, while providing protection when (as some participants may see it) embarrassing or uncomfortable material is discussed.

The learning objectives can be selected from those outlined below; the emphasis will need to vary according to the needs of the participants and the time available. Uncertainty will not be 'covered' in one training session. The knowledge, skills and attitudes needed will be built up through training and experience, provided there is time allowed for reflection after uncertain situations.

The *knowledge objectives* could include: defining uncertainty, identifying 'dysfunctional ways out', classifying uncertainty using the MUM, identifying the skills required.

The *skill objectives* could include: practising the skills identified in the different Quadrants, learning to 'hold' uncertainty and reflect on it rather than 'jumping' to a decision.

The *attitudinal objectives* could include: developing a willingness to discuss uncertainty, to accept and discuss the difficult feelings that uncertainty may generate, to accept that 'thinking about thinking' is a key skill for clinicians, to promote acceptance that uncertainty is an intrinsic and necessary part of having a professional role.

Teaching plans for different situations

When you have five minutes

This is 'hot' teaching in a clinical situation when a learner recognises that he is uncertain (see Box 21.1). Ask the learner to articulate how he recognised the uncertainty and ask him to use a structured handover (SBAR; see Chapter 13) to promote reflection on the problem. Show him how to classify uncertainty using the uncertainty algorithm and identify the skill he needs to move forwards. Empathise with his feelings of difficulty and inadequacy, and explain that managing uncertainty is the responsibility of the professional. Reinforce that uncertainty can be classified and managed with the appropriate learning. Ensure he follows up any learning needs identified after your discussion and report back to reflect on what he has learned. The 'One Minute Preceptor' model is a useful way to structure brief interactions.[1,iii]

Box 21.1: Useful opportunities for brief teaching on uncertainty

- Random case analysis (picking one patient at random to discuss, exploring the uncertainties).
- Debrief sessions (e.g. after ward rounds, emergency admissions, sharing the uncertainties others may have experienced).
- Reviews after specific activities (e.g. home visits, emergency procedures, meeting with relatives, reflecting on how uncertainties were coped with).

iii The 'One Minute Preceptor' teaching model was developed at the Department of Family Medicine at the University of Washington, Seattle.

When you have an hour

This teaching is likely to involve a group of learners, and the same approach can be used in a one-to-one tutorial.

Investigate their hopes and fears.

Ask learners to describe their experiences of uncertainty, initially one to one (if the setting is a tutorial) or in small buzz groups of three (if the setting is a group session) for about five to ten minutes. Debrief by asking what their thoughts AND feelings were in those uncertain situations, and what the relationships between the people involved in the uncertain situation were like.

Introduce the MUM algorithm (see Chapter 2) and ask them to classify the uncertainties they have been talking about into the Analysing, Networking, Negotiating and Team-working Quadrants. Divide the group into four smaller groups. Using prepared trigger case scenarios that relate to each Quadrant, ask the group to identify which Quadrant is involved using the algorithm and which skill they will need using the MUM (see Box 21.2).

Some of the scenarios in this book could make a good starting point. It works even better with scenarios developed to meet the circumstances of the group.

Pick one or two key skills from each Quadrant to discuss and/or to demonstrate.

Have a final debrief that goes back to the initial hopes and fears. Answer any learning needs that are outstanding at the end.

Box 21.2: Examples of trigger scenarios

Aisha is a 2-year-old child who started to become unwell around 10 a.m. with vomiting and fever. She has had diarrhoea once, and seems grizzly and irritable. Her mother has two other children at home; her partner is away on business. She is new to the area and has little social support. It is 2 p.m. when you see Aisha in general practice. What uncertainties in the Analysing Quadrant are there and what skills could be used to deal with them?

Mrs Bismuth is a 27-year-old woman with a history of belching, bloating and tiredness for three weeks. She attends Accident and Emergency with a friend because she has become very anxious that she has developed hypothyroidism (like her aunty), cancer of the ovary (like her neighbour) and severe anaemia (because she had a heavy period last month). What are the uncertainties here and what Networking Quadrant skills are appropriate?

Mr Calcite is a 56-year-old man with Type 2 diabetes, hypertension and Stage 3 chronic kidney disease who comes for an annual review. His blood pressure is 172/98, his weight is increasing and he now has proteinuria. He says he takes all his medications regularly, does not drink and can't see what all the fuss about his 20-a-day smoking habit is. What Negotiating Quadrant uncertainties may be occurring and what skills could be helpful?

Mr Diamond is 68 and lives alone in a small flat, which he never cleans and is full of rubbish and faeces from his small, yappy, dog. He needs dressings to an abdominal wound that became infected after he had a strangulated hernia repair. The nurses would like him to attend the clinic across the road from his house, because one of them was bitten by his dog. He refuses and calls the ward he was on three times a day to demand they send someone out to him, also calling the GP out-of-hours service several times each evening. What uncertainties in the Team-working Quadrant are there and how might they be resolved?

When you have half a day

Investigate their hopes and fears.

Using small groups, preferably with experienced small group facilitators, ask each group to reflect on the question 'What do you do when you don't know what to do?'

Emphasise that everyone faces this, and that this is not about 'looking up the dose of a drug' (because that means you know what to do), but where the situation is uncertain and the next step unclear. Encourage all participants to share experiences of uncertainty, which may be in their current practice or the past. Then develop the discussion by considering the following questions:

- 'What were you thinking then?'
- 'What did that feel like?'
- 'How did this affect your relationship with the patient?'
- 'How did your team/organisation help or hinder you with this situation?'

This process helps to focus the group to the subject matter and helps participants start to think clearly about what their own educational needs are in relation to uncertainty.

These discussions can be emotionally heartfelt and benefit from facilitators with educational group skills training or experience. Sharing uncertainty and associated difficult feelings can be cathartic and this can be a strong motivator for effective learning. Use the discussion to highlight 'dysfunctional ways out' that participants have experienced, helping them to recognise why such approaches are less than ideal.

Give participants some sticky notes or small cards. Ask them to summarise each uncertain situation on a separate card in a single sentence or two.

Create an empty MUM on a large wall chart, notice board or flip chart.

Explain the algorithm for classifying uncertainty and then populate the MUM with the situations that participants have described. This links uncertainty to one of the Quadrants. Some uncertainties cover more than one Quadrant.

Debrief the experience of classifying uncertainty in this way. Participants are often surprised and relieved to discover that other people have major uncertainties also, that uncertainty can be classified and therefore 'tamed', and that others have similar disturbing feelings, or face similar uncertainties, as themselves. A skilled facilitator can use this part of the session to explore the attitudinal objectives around uncertainty. How can participants develop and demonstrate their willingness to accept, discuss and explore uncertainty, and support others in a non-judgemental way?

Divide the group again into four groups, or small buzz groups of three or four. Ensure each group has a MUM to hand. Explain how the MUM works to classify uncertainty and to identify the relevant skills.

Either use the group's own cases or provide prepared scenarios for discussion. Take each case and work out which Quadrant it belongs to and which skills may be needed. If there is time, have a 'skills rehearsal'. Invite a participant to recreate the scenario she has struggled with by taking the role of the patient. Ask another participant to use the skill needed to explore what happens if a difficult approach is tried. Ask a third participant to give non-judgemental feedback about how the new skills were used.

Debrief the whole group by considering whether they have the relevant skills to 'unlock' the uncertainty in question and, if not, how can they acquire such skills? What effect does using a different skill have on the interaction with the 'patient'.

If there is time, ask them to consider situations where juniors have come to them with uncertainty, and go through how to do a 'hot skills' five-minute teaching on uncertainty (as in the section *When you have five minutes* on p. 252).

Finally, in twos, ask them to reflect on what it felt like to:

- recognise and talk about uncertainty
- classify uncertainty
- identify the skills.

Ask them how they will use MUM next time they reflect on an uncertain situation.

Finally debrief the group by going back to their initial hopes and fears. Answer any outstanding learning needs at the end.

When you have a whole day

Prior to the event, ask participants to bring a TYPED and therefore anonymised description of a situation in which they felt very uncertain and did not know what to do. Emphasise that these are anonymised (no names on them, and typed, so no handwriting recognition). Collect these at the start and shuffle them up so that when they are discussed later no one gets their own scenario to discuss.

Investigate their hopes and fears.

Using small groups, preferably with experienced small group facilitators, ask each group to reflect on the question 'What do you do when you don't know what to do?'

Emphasise that everyone faces this, and that this is not about 'looking up the dose of a drug' (because that means you know what to do), but where the situation is uncertain and the next step unclear. Encourage all participants to share experiences of uncertainty, which may be in their current practice or the past. Then develop the discussion by considering the following questions:

- 'What were you thinking then?'
- 'What did that feel like?'
- 'How did this affect your relationship with the patient?'
- 'How did your team/organisation help or hinder you with this situation?'

These discussions can be emotionally heartfelt and benefit from facilitators with educational group skills training or experience. Sharing uncertainty and associated difficult feelings can be cathartic and opens the way for effective learning.

Explain the MUM algorithm for classifying uncertainty (Chapter 2).

Create an empty MUM on a large wall chart, notice board or flip chart. Distribute the uncertain situations that participants have brought with them, ensuring that no one gets their own scenario to talk about. This enables a calm discussion, without individuals feeling exposed. Divide the group into groups of three or four and ask them to discuss the scenarios.

Ask participants to summarise several scenarios of uncertainty in one or two lines, each on a separate card or sticky note. Then populate the MUM with the situations that participants have described. This links uncertainty to one of the Quadrants. Some uncertainties cover more than one Quadrant.

To deepen understanding, present the Quadrants of the MUM formally, one by one in detail. This could be with an initial PowerPoint slide to trigger discussion and understanding. Discuss how uncertainties arise and the skills needed to unlock them. Involve the participants, inviting them to report on and discuss how this relates to any uncertain situations they have faced themselves.

Ask participants to identify and discuss 'dysfunctional ways out'. Allocate small buzz groups of two to four participants to discuss two each of these, from each Quadrant, in detail (i.e. so that all are discussed but each buzz group only discusses two, to get more depth): when do clinicians choose this way out? Why? What are the immediate benefits, the long-term effects, the alternative, more functional ways through? Debrief by exploring the general issues. What do 'dysfunctional ways out' offer to the clinician? How can we recognise any adverse effects? Are there any times when it is sensible, inevitable or necessary to use a 'dysfunctional way out'? Debrief the discussion by asking 'What issues come up?' Skilled facilitation will be needed to draw out the value of 'functional ways through', and the drawbacks of 'dysfunctional ways out', in a non-judgemental way.

Divide the group again into four smaller groups, or small buzz groups of three (depending on numbers). Ensure each group has a MUM to hand. Explain how the MUM works to classify uncertainty and to identify the relevant skills.

Either use the group's own cases (preferable) or provide prepared scenarios for discussion. Take each case and work out which Quadrant it belongs to and which skills may be needed. If there is time, have a 'skills rehearsal' where a participant recreates the scenario they struggled with by being the patient. Ask another participant to use the skill needed to see what happens if another approach is tried. Ask a third participant to give non-judgemental feedback about how the new skills were used.

Debrief the whole group by considering whether they have the relevant skills to 'unlock' the uncertainty in question and, if not, how can they acquire such skills?

After lunch

Go back to the feelings they expressed in the first part of the workshop and introduce *mapping the psychology of uncertainty*, identifying the emotional, cognitive relationship and organisational aspects of uncertainty. This could be a formal presentation, with interactive discussion from the group, inviting them to comment on occasions when they have experienced the psychological processes in question.

Divide participants into four groups. Allocate each group one of the Quadrants and with a facilitator ask them to work though the emotional, cognitive, relationship and organisational aspects. Ask each group to identify two ways to manage the psychological impact of uncertainty differently in their own setting. Ask each group to identify two ways to improve their team or organisational approaches to uncertainty.

To explore the patients' perspectives, get participants to use their iPads or smartphones. Search for 'uncertainty' on some patient websites (give them the best ones) and ask them to report back what they have found. What do patients experience? Map that if possible also on the wall chart.

Uncertainty in training

Introduce the MUMT (see Chapter 20) and ask them to reflect on what to do with a colleague or trainee whose performance they have been concerned about. Use the training algorithm in the same chapter to work out the issues. Where do the problems lie? What needs to be done?

Finally debrief the group by going back to their initial hopes and fears. Answer any outstanding learning needs at the end.

References

1. Neher JO, Gordon KC, Meyer B, Stevens N. A five-step 'microskills' model of clinical teaching. *Journal of the American Board of Family Practice* 1992; **5(4)**: 419–24

Resources for uncertainty in training

Epstein RM, Hundert EM. Defining and assessing professional competence. *Journal of the American Medical Association* 2002; **287(2)**: 226–35.

Montgomery K. *How Doctors Think: clinical judgement and the practice of medicine*. New York, NY: Oxford University Press, 2006.

O'Riordan, Dahinden A, Aktürk Z, *et al*. Dealing with uncertainty in general practice: an essential skill for the general practitioner. *Quality in Primary Care* 2011; **19(3)**: 175–81.

Schön D. *The Reflective Practitioner: how professionals think in action*. London: Temple Smith, 1983.

Devine M, Syrett M. *Managing Uncertainty: strategies for surviving and thriving in turbulent times*. London: Economist Books, 2012.

Part V

Exploring uncertainty from the patient's perspective

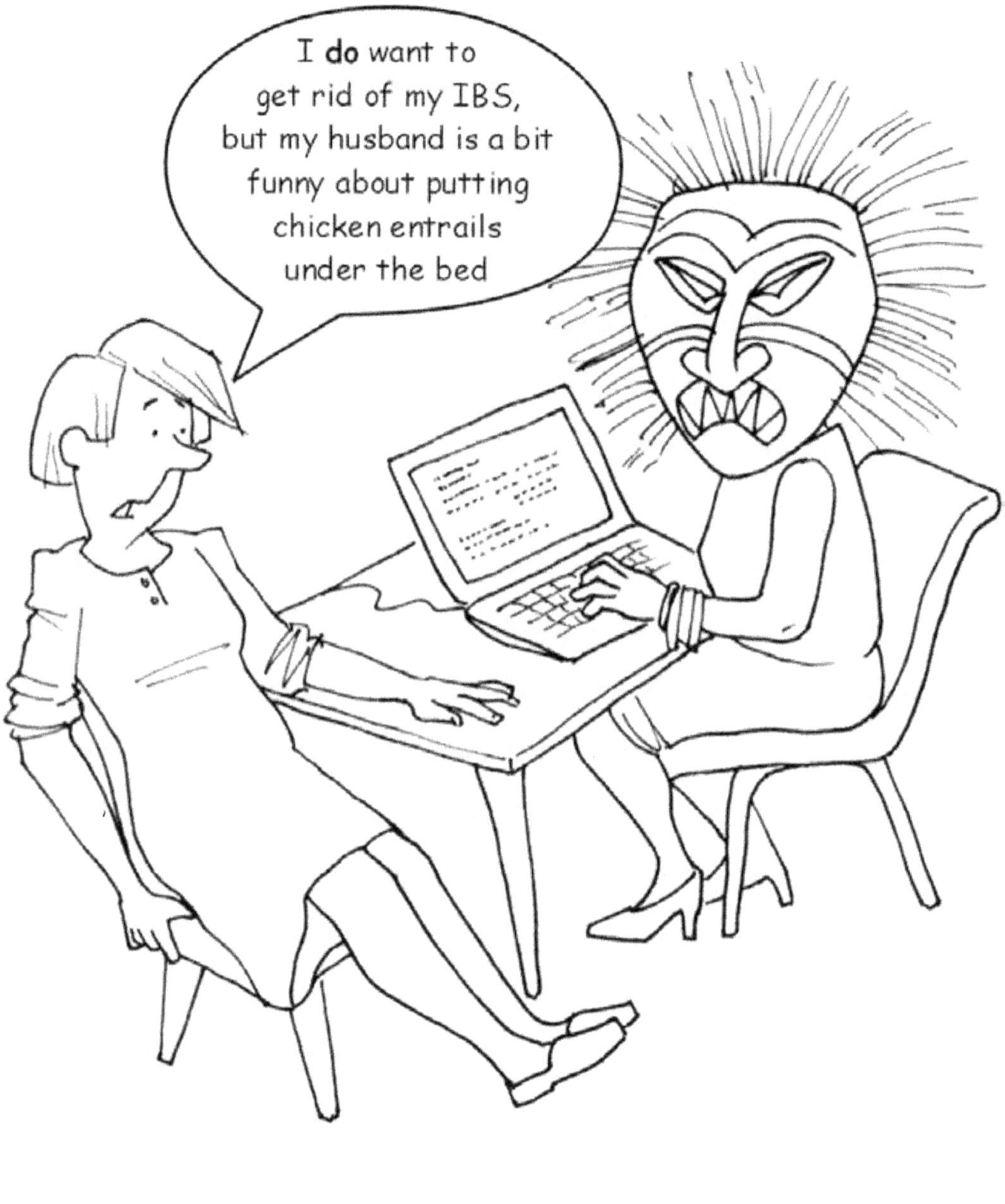
I **do** want to
get rid of my IBS,
but my husband is a bit
funny about putting
chicken entrails
under the bed

> The answers you get depend on the questions you ask.
>
> Thomas S. Kuhn

This part of the book looks at uncertainty from the point of view of the patient. **Chapter 22** highlights the impact of uncertainty on patients. **Chapter 23** is concerned with mapping uncertainty from the patient's perspective against the Analysing, Networking, Negotiating and Team-working Quadrants.

Chapter 22

The impact of uncertainty on patients

> Ignorance more frequently begets confidence than does knowledge.
>
> Charles Darwin[1]

Clinical practice has become very complex, with many treatments available, some of uncertain effectiveness, especially for life-threatening illnesses such as cancer. This means that clinicians may end up dealing with more difficult and more uncertain situations. However wisely clinicians try to deal with such problems, patients may be left with troubling uncertainties. Are patients ready for this? What does uncertainty in medicine feel like for patients?

This chapter considers:

- uncertainty in a complex situation
- does modern medical practice actually increase uncertainty for patients?
- how patients respond to uncertainty in their clinicians
- do patients have their own 'dysfunctional ways out' or 'functional ways through'?

Uncertainty in a complex situation

Box 22.1 summaries some distressing events that involved great uncertainty for senior clinicians caring for children with recurrent, complicated cancer. It quotes the mother of a child whose death was linked to stem-cell treatment.

It seems that, for this mother, uncertainty is unacceptable 'in this day and age', implying that she has high expectations of certainty and predictability in healthcare matters. Is this a general view held by patients? Do

Box 22.1: Uncertainty for clinicians facing a painful dilemma

At a leading children's hospital in London, a technique for freezing stem cells had been used successfully for ten years. In 2013, children having the stem cell treatment for advanced cancer were found not to be responding as anticipated, and some died unexpectedly. Their doctors were faced with a dilemma: should they stop the treatment and risk patients' lives from under-treatment while things were investigated? As one doctor was reported to have said, 'cancer won't wait'. These were very sick children. After eight adverse outcomes the procedure was abandoned and the problem investigated. Unfortunately, it remained impossible to identify the problem with the technique; there had been no changes in the methods that had worked well for the previous ten years. Investigation resulted in the coroner remarking that the treatment may have contributed to a child's death, but that is was 'unclear', that 'we don't know why the treatment stopped working' and that 'there was no consensus'. In spite of this uncertainty, the problem has been treated as a medical failure, an error, and therefore blameworthy. The child's mother is quoted by the BBC as saying, 'It's a lot of "don't know, we don't know why", which to me is not good enough, not in this day and age.'[2]

patients reject the idea that the clinicians caring for them may be uncertain about what to do? On the other hand, are patients perhaps perfectly aware that life itself is uncertain, that we don't know all the answers and that medicine itself is a complex, evolving and unpredictable business? Is it reasonable, from a patient's perspective, for clinicians to find themselves having WDYDWYDKWTD moments?

Perhaps it will come as no surprise, in a book about uncertainty, to find that the answers to these questions are, well ... somewhat uncertain. In preparing this chapter we had many questions about what the patient's view of uncertainty might be. These are summarised in Box 22.2.

We expected to find answers to these questions. Clinicians have been pondering and writing about uncertainty for decades, and if uncertainty is troublesome to clinicians then it can be agony for patients whose very life and existence is at stake. Patients' attitudes to uncertainty, and what elements of uncertainty matter to patients, must surely be at the forefront of our minds. However, it seems that this is an under-researched area. We know a little about how patients understand uncertainty. We know far less than we need to know about how they understand or respond to the uncertainties *of their*

Box 22.2: The patient's view of uncertainty

1. Do patients recognise WDYDWYDKWTD moments in themselves or in their clinicians?
2. What do patients think when the clinician doesn't know what to do?
3. What do patients think when the clinician says the diagnosis is uncertain?
4. What do patients think when the clinician refers for tests/discusses with colleagues to find the diagnosis? What if the diagnosis remains uncertain?
5. What do patients think when their clinician is uncertain about the best plan of action?
6. What do patients experience when the GP (or another clinician and/or family members and/or another healthcare professional) are not in agreement or have opposing views to a plan of action?
7. What if the patient himself has opposing views to others involved in his care?

clinicians. Uncertainty is perceived as uncomfortable, even threatening, by clinicians and patients alike, and we make strenuous efforts to reduce it. In this part of the book, the patient's point of view about uncertainty is brought into focus. Using the mapping approach from the patient's perspective enriches our understanding of uncertainty in medicine, and offers insights into how we can move forwards in partnership with patients. Clinicians and patients each have important contributions to make: the patient has unique expertise in understanding her own life and needs; the clinician can offer expertise that interprets medical information so that shared decisions can be made.

Does modern medical practice actually increase uncertainty for patients?

The success of modern medical practice has had two contrary effects. Admiration for the scientific aspects of medicine and a trusting belief in the power of medicine to improve our lives are probably greater than they have ever been. In the UK, at least, we are less likely than ever to die from previously common causes such as childbirth, accidents or catastrophes such as heart attacks and strokes. Indeed, so strong is this belief in the power of medicine that many areas of human life are becoming 'medicalised':

problems are seen as issues that can and should be diagnosed, given names, treated and managed by clinicians. Problems such as bereavement, learning difficulties or relationship problems that perhaps used to be considered as normal features of life are increasingly expected to be 'diagnosed' and treated by clinicians. The reasons for this are likely to be due to a complex interplay between the subjects clinicians find interesting (ever expanding), the pressure from Pharma interests (to widen the uses of medication) and increasing expectations in society in general (that difficulties will find a name and a solution). Only a few conditions make it the other way, to being 'un-medicalised'. Homosexuality, which used to be regarded as pathological or even criminal, is now seen as normal, at least in Western medical discussions. Increasing medicalisation may be a part of the way that patients can project a powerful persona onto their clinician, with hope that the clinician will deal with all life issues.

As one patient remarked, 'Doesn't matter if he is young or old, as far as I am concerned he is a genius to be a doctor and he knows everything about everything.'[3]

Perhaps this patient is really offering a strategy for their own WDYDWYDKWTD moment: it is likely to be more comforting to have a doctor who 'knows everything about everything'. If the doctor on this pedestal turns out to have feet of clay, then the patient would have to hold on to the uncertainty instead of the clinician.

Less often mentioned is that the development of this powerful scientific element to modern medicine itself derives from the acceptance and examination of uncertainty. Scientific ideas and hypotheses are always incomplete, partial and subject to change. The enquiring scientist's mind has an attitude of doubt and questioning, even of apparently established concepts and methods; only by accepting this uncertainty will we proceed. When patients become aware of this kind of uncertainty, they may see it as unsatisfactory or confusing. For example, as our understanding of healthy eating develops, recommendations tend to change; this evolution is often ridiculed in the press, although, scientifically, evolution and changing ideas are the norm. Health matters, like everything else, are also subject to 'fads and fashions', which creates further uncertainty about what is the 'best' way forwards.

An emphasis on scientific development also drives a pressure for clinicians to concentrate on the 'technical, rational' aspects of practice. Yet the practice of medicine is not truly a science, relying solely on objective findings, but is a system of practice that encompasses subjective issues in every aspect. The patient's subjective experience is fundamental to all clinical work. Clinicians also work with their own subjective experiences as they assess, form relationships with and support patients though the process of illness. This inevitably involves what is usually called the 'art' of medicine, the ability to relate to patients and colleagues in an empathic way, being alive to the nuance of a given individual's needs and responses. This is what makes for truly effective care overall.

The power of modern medicine to preserve life might be expected to reduce uncertainty about health and enable us to face illness with equanimity. Yet, paradoxically, patients are more anxious about their health, seek medical advice more often (consultations with GPs have nearly doubled over the last 15 years) and seem more angry with clinicians and health services in general. Like the mother quoted at the beginning of this chapter, people seem to want certainty more than ever. In less developed times or places the uncertainty of life ('Will mother and child survive childbirth?') had to be acknowledged and endured in the absence of any alternatives. Sophocles put this succinctly when he said 'Chance rules our lives, and the future is all unknown' and even 'Call no man happy until he dies'.[4]

Renée Fox's view of uncertainty is summed up as having three components:

> *The first results from incomplete or imperfect mastery of available knowledge. No one can have at his command all skills and all knowledge of the lore of medicine. The second depends on limitations in current knowledge. There are innumerable questions to which no physician, however well trained, can as yet provide answers. A third source of uncertainty derives from the first two. This consists of difficulty in distinguishing between personal ignorance or ineptitude and the limitations of present knowledge.*[5]

Both patients and clinicians can be uncomfortable with the awareness that medical science is so vast that no one can know it all. From the patient's perspective the uncertainty is not usually about the limits of scientific knowledge, but rather 'What if my doctor just doesn't know enough and has got it wrong?'

How patients respond to uncertainty in their clinicians

How do patients respond when their clinician is having a WDYDWYDKWTD moment? Clinicians tend not to share their bewilderment explicitly, especially in the earlier part of their careers. If a clinician makes a remark such as 'I have not got a clue what is happening here', patients may expect referral for a more senior opinion, especially if the clinician seems inexperienced. Younger clinicians often perceive uncertainty as a failing in themselves, a limitation of knowledge or skill (which obviously plays a part). Referring upwards is an acceptable way to resolve this uncertainty and will usually be accepted by patients, even if they become frustrated by delays or by the fact that different clinicians will end up with differing opinions of what to do next. If referral is not offered, or if patients perceive the clinician to be unsure, this can lead to dissatisfaction with the consultation, on the part of both clinician and patient.

Clinician uncertainty has, in the past, resulted in patients being kept in the dark with regards to investigations, likelihood of diagnosis and success of treatment. There appears to have been a perception among clinicians that sharing uncertainties with patients results in unnecessary anxiety and loss of trust.[6] This paternalism denies patients the chance to make properly informed decisions about their health. When a clinician feels uncertain about an outcome or risk there is a tendency to talk in 'possibilities' or 'probable outcomes' rather than giving exact numbers, despite the fact that this could be construed in many different ways by the patient.[7]

In contrast, senior clinicians report that they often say 'I don't know' to patients, and this is more readily accepted than the same message from less experienced colleagues. There may be a difference between 'not knowing' (a diagnosis for example) and 'not knowing what to do'. Without having a diagnosis it is still possible to have a safe and effective management plan. For example, a patient distressed because of a failing marriage may come to his clinician with typical non-cardiac chest pain. The clinician does not really know whether the pain originates in the chest muscles, ribs, peripheral nerves or indeed in the pain perception processes in the patient's brain. However, the treatment will be the same: empathetic understanding of his problems, an empowering explanation of the pain, symptomatic treatment and appropriate follow-up and safety netting. In the wake of scandals about poor performance such as the Bristol Inquiry, a *British Medical Journal* editorial commented that the trust between clinicians and patients will never be the same again, 'but that will be a good thing if we move to an active rather than a passive trust, where clinicians share uncertainty'.[8]

Although the diagnostic and treatment uncertainties of clinicians have been identified in this book, there are other uncertainties in the discussions that clinicians and patients have about illness and health. An interesting Health Foundation report called *When Doctors and Patients Talk: making sense of the consultation* explores the implicit, unvoiced uncertainties that arise in the interactions between doctor and patients.[3] The nature of the problems at stake, the differing cultural expectations of the consultation, the underlying fears and anxieties that clinicians and patients have, and the awareness that each party has of the complexity and uncertainties of medical practice all influence how patients respond to any uncertainty about their health.

The report's authors refer to the idea that there are 'tame' problems, which are readily defined and exist in a stable environment. For example, building an office block is a complicated and essentially solvable problem if the right expertise is brought to bear. A health-related example would be the treatment of pneumonia. If the clinician and patient share priorities for action, then they 'coordinate' a plan together. If they have competing priorities, they may find themselves in 'competition' to decide the plan, for example if the patient wants to go to hospital for her treatment and the clinician considers that it would be more appropriate for the patient to be treated at home.

In contrast, 'wicked' problems are more complex and the outcomes may be unpredictable, emergent properties that occur as the situation evolves. For example, solving the problem of the best way to bring up a child has no ideal solution; things will change as the child grows and circumstances fluctuate. A medical example would be working out how best to care for someone taking 20 medicines daily, for five or more diseases; how that individual's overall health will develop is hard to predict, yet this is a common situation. If the patient and clinician have differing priorities they can move forwards only by 'negotiation', whereas if they can work out some shared priorities then 'co evolution' of plans occurs.[3]

Such clinician/patient interactions are influenced by many variables and uncertainties about how the interaction will proceed. Individuals vary in their knowledge of what health care can offer and the different roles and responsibilities of the professionals they encounter. Different individuals and their clinicians vary in their expectations of what will be discussed and whether uncertainty can be openly acknowledged, and this will change over time as a relationship develops between individual clinicians and patients. This will also be influenced by other variables including the presence of third parties such as parents, interpreters, carers and varying cultural norms that affect the approach to the consultation. External pressures such as clinical or public health guidance intended to change clinician behaviour or people's lifestyles, or media attention to particular medical issues, will bring further uncertainties to the way individuals communicate.

So it is clear that from the patient's point of view these complexities are almost bound to raise uncertainties about what to do. This is intensified by other uncertainties in the clinician–patient consultation that are rarely openly acknowledged. These can be summarised as different kinds of fear, parallel but different, in clinicians and patients. Clinicians fear that they will make a career-threatening error, whereas patients fear a life-threatening illness. Clinicians fear that they will not be able to keep up with patients' needs and demands, whereas patients fear that they won't be heard or acknowledged properly. Clinicians worry that they will face censure for using too many resources, whereas patients wonder whether they are really ill enough to take up a clinician's time. Such underlying fears may inform the behaviour of clinicians or patients, without being overtly apparent. The people involved may not appreciate or understand the fear driving the other party to the consultation, which can make for difficult interactions. These uncertainties, rarely voiced explicitly, weave through many consultations that clinicians have with their patients.

Further uncertainty from the patient's perspective occurs because of the complex 'power relationships' in the consultation. It can sometimes seem as if doctors, in particular, are almost 'trained to be arrogant'. This is a cruel shorthand to express the way in which clinicians sometimes fail to find a way of being that balances confident decision making (without being 'bossy'), a willingness to take on responsibility (without narcissism or egotism), and yet face disease, suffering and death with equanimity. 'Arrogance' is sometimes the outcome, as clinicians try to remain in control of difficult situations. Yet within individual consultations the clinician does have more knowledge, not only of medical practice but also even of how the consultation is to be structured, and this can also be a cause of uncertainty to patients, who may not know exactly what to expect or how to respond, and who may feel bewildered or disempowered by the experience:

- "'When I go to the GP I always forget what I have gone for'"
- And "'Sometimes I have gone out of the surgery and thought I haven't necessarily told them everything I should have done … I think I am going to tell them something but if they are not … if they don't put me at ease then (I don't)'".[3]

Finally, a clinician's focus may well be on the past, on the story that the patient is telling, because this will usually lead to the diagnosis, a lessening of uncertainty for the clinician. The clinician's attention may also be on the present, as decisions are made about possible management plans. However, patients are just as likely to be focused on the future. 'What is going to

Table 22.1: Clinician's and patient's reciprocal uncertainties

Dimension considered	What patients may be thinking about	What doctors may be thinking about	What effects this may have when things are uncertain
Patient has a 'tame' problem	Can I get my own priorities met?	What are the medical priorities?	Coordination when doctor and patient share priorities; competition when they don't share priorities
Patient has a 'wicked' problem	Can I identify my priorities?	Can medical and patient's priorities be aligned?	Negotiation when priorities compete, coevolution when they align
Cultural context	Different views of the doctor; on a pedestal or peer to peer?	How to achieve all the tasks of the consultation and ensure trust and confidence	Increased uncertainty or mismatch between expectations of the doctor's role and actual behaviour
What is feared	Am I going to die? Will I be heard and understood? How difficult will the treatment be? Am I entitled to consider myself as deserving to take up time?	Will I miss something and risk my career? Will I be overwhelmed by the patient's needs? Will I be criticised for not following the guideline, budget, etc.?	Miscommunication can happen if these fears are not acknowledged
Structure of the process	Invisible to patients	Embedded in doctor's training	Structure may be lost, ineffective or bewildering to patient
Where is the focus in time?	On the future: what will happen to me?	Focus on the past to inform diagnosis	Doctor and patient focusing on different things, dysfunctional actions

Source: derived from Fischer M, Ereaut G. *When Doctors and Patients Talk: making sense of the consultation*.[3]

happen to me?' is a question that creates fear for many. The dimensions of this and the effects of uncertainty are summarised in Table 22.1.

Do patients have their own 'dysfunctional ways out' or 'functional ways through'?

Patients have their own WDYDWYDKWTD moments in relation to their health and wellbeing. What do *patients* do when they don't know what to do? In other chapters we have identified 'dysfunctional ways out' that clinicians often use when uncertain and have tried to identify more 'functional ways through'. Patients have their own strategies for trying to deal with a WDYDWYDKWTD situation relating to their health. Clearly some strategies work better than others and some patients are just as good at 'metacognition' and working out what to do as clinicians are. Overall, however, the strategies patients use are simply described, rather than being judged as 'functional' or 'dysfunctional'. Clinicians are the professionals, with certain expectations placed on them that make it easier to consider whether their actions are functional or not. Such judgements seem inappropriate to apply to patients struggling to make sense of illness.

Patients who are not sure how to respond to symptoms, a diagnosis or a treatment plan may take different approaches. Conversations with friends, family or neighbours often precede any decision about whether, or when, to consult a professional about worrying symptoms. On seeing the clinician, other variables affect how patients behave in situations of uncertainty. Do they assume a sickness role or insist on their independence despite their safety being in question? Do they accept a diagnosis and comply with medication or do they listen to a friend or neighbour who recommends an alternative that worked for them? Do they come to their own diagnostic conclusions or trust the clinician? If they disagree do they seek further opinions, by repeatedly seeking medical care, 'going private', or seeing practitioners who are not part of the mainstream, such as complementary therapists of various kinds?

The attitude the patient takes will depend on several intertwined components: his interaction with the clinician, how credible he finds the diagnosis, his prior knowledge of the disorder, and his previous experience of that clinician and of medicine as a whole. Ultimately if he gets better, is more able to cope with his symptoms or has his expectations met, he is more likely to place trust in future encounters.

In the next chapter, patients' responses to uncertainty will be mapped against the four Quadrants of the MUM.

References

1. Darwin C. *The Descent of Man*. 1871, http://infidels.org/library/historical/charles_darwin/descent_of_man/introduction.html [accessed 25 August 2015].
2. Great Ormond Street stem cell freezing 'may have led to death'. BBC News, 25 November 2014, www.bbc.co.uk/news/uk-england-london-30193466 [accessed 25 August 2015].
3. Fischer M, Ereaut G. *When Doctors and Patients Talk: making sense of the consultation*. London: Health Foundation, 2012.
4. Sophocles. *Oedipus Rex*, https://en.wikiquote.org/wiki/Sophocles [accessed 8 September 2015].
5. Fox R. *Essays in Medical Sociology*. New Brunswick: John Wiley & Sons, 1979.
6. Katz J. Why doctors don't disclose uncertainty. *The Hastings Center Report* 1984; DOI: 10.2307/3560848.
7. Knoll SM, Johnson JL. Uncertainty and expectations: taking care of a cardiac surgery patient at home. *Journal of Cardiovascular Nursing* 2000; **14(3)**: 64–75.
8. Smith R. All changed, changed utterly. British medicine will be transformed by the Bristol case. *British Medical Journal* 1998; **316(7149)**: 1917–18.

Chapter 23

Mapping uncertainty from the patient's perspective

This chapter maps patients' uncertainties against the Analysing, Networking, Negotiating and Team-working Quadrants, and the sections are illustrated by the words of the people most concerned, that is, patients themselves. These quotations are from publicly available sources such as healthtalk.org (a site where patients talk about their own experiences of health care), listed in the resources section at the end of this chapter. The issues covered are:

- the patient's perspective on uncertainty in the Analysing Quadrant
- the patient's perspective on uncertainty in the Networking Quadrant
- the patient's perspective on uncertainty in the Negotiating Quadrant
- the patient's perspective on uncertainty in the Team-working Quadrant.

The patient's perspective on uncertainty in the Analysing Quadrant

> *It's very hard because you want the clinicians to give you a sign that things are getting better. Looking back I can see why they can't give you that answer; it's really trying to accept that they don't know.*
>
> (Woman describing her experience of her mother being in an intensive therapy unit (ITU), healthtalk.org)

As many clinicians know, getting a diagnosis, a 'name' for their condition or problem, can be very helpful in enabling patients to cope with the uncertainties of what comes next. A patient's comment illustrates this:

> *We are still in the process of getting an accurate diagnosis for J, which makes life really uncertain. In a way, it is this uncertainty that is the hardest thing to live with.*
>
> (Parent, epilepsy.org.uk).

Uncertainty in diagnosis is keenly felt by clinicians and patients. However, the impact of uncertainty is very different for the patient. If a firm diagnosis can be arrived at, uncertainty for the clinician is likely to reduce, as the options for care of the patient are narrowed down, being strongly determined by the presumed diagnosis. However, for the patient a firm diagnosis is just the beginning of other uncertainties. If the diagnosis is minor and treatment and cure assured, uncertainty will diminish for the patient also. But what if the diagnosis is a serious one such as cancer, dementia or organ failure? The individual will then encounter many troubling uncertainties, the impact of which is likely to be underestimated by clinicians, whose attention can become distracted by the demands of getting appropriate treatment plans in place.

However, in some situations, this new uncertainty seems to help things. A positive HIV test result is a piece of serious and even life-threatening information. Some men tested for HIV initially refused to get the test result. However, they had less mood disturbance after subsequently finding out they were HIV positive. Knowledge, although bringing uncertainties about prognosis and treatment, seemed to allow a greater sense of control and less anxiety.[1]

For patients, questions go beyond the diagnosis and the 'name of the condition' to include questions of a more existential nature, which are perhaps less easy to answer. Cecil Helman, who worked as a GP and medical anthropologist, considered that patients were interested in six important questions. What has happened? Why has it happened? Why has it happened to me? Why now? What would happen to me if nothing were done about it? What are its likely effects on other people (family, friends, employers, workmates) if nothing were done?[2] These questions and uncertainties may be even more difficult or troubling when the patient needs to face the issue of a long-term condition such as multiple sclerosis or diabetes, or a debilitating mental health problem such as schizophrenia.

The anguish of a firm diagnosis is illustrated by these comments about cancer:

> *I was fortunate in so far as I only had a lumpectomy with clear margins but I feel the problem here is dealing with the psychology of being diagnosed. I truly feel we have been changed forever and cancer will always be at the back of our minds!*
>
> (Macmillan)

An apparently successful diagnosis and treatment has left a permanent state of uncertainty about cancer in its wake. Another patient's experience illustrates the agony of waiting, and how threatening the final diagnosis was:

> *My husband almost died while they were trying to figure out what kind of cancer he had – took FOREVER – and the cancer was insanely aggressive. At the last minute they found … melanoma and started a targeted treatment that worked wonders. He came back from the brink. … The clinicians weren't very specific about his future.*
>
> (Macmillan)

This individual and his family, having faced uncertainties about diagnosis and even survival, as the patient came 'back from the brink', now have painful uncertainty about the future, in a context where the clinicians concerned struggled even to make a diagnosis at all. The clinicians' uncertainty may only have been partly recognised by the patient and his family, yet the impact of that uncertainty will surely have been greater for the patient than for the clinicians involved.

This quotation also illustrates other aspects of diagnosis from the patient's perspective. First, the making of a diagnosis is rarely a linear process, proceeding through orderly steps, towards a clear-cut answer. Making a diagnosis is often iterative, especially where serious illness is concerned, and the diagnostic process is distributed between specialists, laboratory services and other diagnostic processes such as radiology. This can mean frightening uncertainty for patients trying to navigate the process and this is discussed further in the Networking section of this chapter. Second, diagnosis is not merely a cognitive task, managed in the clinicians' thoughts and discussions. Diagnosis involves relationships, between clinician and patient, and also between the members of the clinical team. Both of these relationships can cause uncertainty for patients, and yet diagnosis inevitably involves a cooperation between patient and clinician, with the human story evolving alongside the medical one, as patients 'practise telling their stories'.[3]

So what about situations where either the clinician, or the patient, or even both of them, remain uncertain about the overall diagnosis? Patients think about these kinds of uncertainties in different ways. Some recognise that the situation is uncertain and that even specialists may disagree or remain unclear.

> *I've brought this up in rheum and neuro appointments but not got anywhere. ... In clinical (sic) today I said that I think you could put three consultants together and they could argue about me.*
>
> (A patient with comorbidities, healthunlocked.com)

Other individuals may be considerably more disturbed by uncertainty than their clinicians:

> *I haven't been diagnosed with anything. I have a swollen lymph node on my neck ... have had blood tests (all fine), an ultrasound ... confirmed it was a swollen lymph node. ... I am really glad the clinician is not worried ... there is nothing in the ultrasound to suggest anything sinister ... she just thinks ENT should look again at the node ... but I am also very itchy ... so when I'm not very busy and getting on with my very happy full life, I can't help but dwell on it being lymphoma – then I tell myself off for being stupid and wishing I'd never read about symptoms or googled enlarged lymph node! ... Feeling very silly for thinking this.*
>
> (Cancer Research UK)

This patient feels 'silly' and 'tells herself off' in the face of these uncertainties, which echoes the sense of shame and guilt felt by clinicians facing uncertainty, explored more fully in Part III 'Mapping the psychology of uncertainty'. Uncertainty can be especially difficult for patients when the clinician and the patient do not have a shared understanding of what the diagnosis really is. Such uncertainty can arise in a variety of situations including:

- disorders where the issue is of the function rather than the structure of the body (IBS and muscular back pain are common examples)
- where the diagnosis is a contested one such as 'multiple chemical sensitivity' or 'Gulf War syndrome', where clinicians disagree about whether the label is a true phenomenon

- where the medical diagnosis of bodily distress (which may go by various names such as medically unexplained symptoms, somatisation, Bodily Distress Disorder) is not accepted by the patient
- when clinician and patient both remain uncertain about the diagnosis. Some American physicians refer to this as 'diagnostic limbo', a situation that is extremely difficult for patients to tolerate.[4]

When the patients' view of their illness is not endorsed by a formal medical diagnosis the uncertainty experienced can be painful. They may struggle to get social legitimacy for their experiences: friends, family and professionals may not be as ready with support or sympathy as with 'conventional' illness.[5] Patients may respond with feelings of shame, guilt and secrecy, or may 'shop around' different clinicians or alternative practitioners until they receive a diagnosis that they can accept. Many clinicians feel that treating the patient symptomatically is a reasonable approach in such situations, but this does not meet the need that most patients have for a diagnosis that can explain and give meaning to their experiences and symptoms.

If patients' responses to the uncertainty expressed by clinicians vary, to what extent can clinicians safely express their uncertainty about diagnosis, and does this affect patients adversely? It seems that patients are less tolerant of uncertainty about diagnosis expressed by female clinicians than male clinicians.[6] A study in general practice as long ago as 1987 showed that if the clinician was positive and definite about the diagnosis and prognosis, then symptoms resolved more quickly, although this was usually in the context of less serious illness.[7] A later study, again in general practice, found similar results but the authors warned:

> *It may be difficult to be positive if the clinician is genuinely uncertain about the diagnosis, which is often the case in primary care when patients present with early disease. Nevertheless, clinicians should be aware that airing their uncertainties about diagnosis and prognosis might reduce satisfaction and empowerment.*[8]

Most studies show that patients want more information from their professionals than they are actually given, and yet it is clear that sharing uncertainty may have adverse effects in some situations. This places clinicians in a potentially awkward position; should they be open and honest, and risk harming a patient or should they exhibit certainty, which can be empowering and even lead to faster recovery? Perhaps the answer in the Analysing Quadrant lies in the communication skills by which uncertain diagnoses are disclosed. Explaining the clinical reasoning while remaining patient centred, recognising and incorporating the patient's own views, building a partnership with the patient and taking steps to ensure a health promotion approach are likely to be the best way forwards. Uncertainty in diagnosis expressed in a positive way, with positive comments about what will happen next and assurance of the clinician's continuing concern for the individual, is likely to help patients manage the uncertainties in the Analysing Quadrant.

The patient's perspective on uncertainty in the Networking Quadrant

This Quadrant refers to the situation where, to achieve a diagnosis, the clinician–patient dyad need the services of a wider diagnostic network. This could include referral for diagnostic tests, such as X-rays, laboratory tests or scans, or could mean referral to another clinician whose expertise is thought to be more relevant to the problem at hand. We have explored how clinicians may find themselves in a WDYDWYDKWTD situation in the Networking Quadrant. However, patients also find themselves in that predicament. Patients and their families are often excluded from important discussions and left feeling in the dark about how their problems are being managed and how to navigate the overwhelming array of diagnostic and treatment options available to them.[9]

So do we know anything about how patients respond to uncertainty in this Quadrant?

Uncertainty in the Networking Quadrant is very common for patients. Before patients see their clinicians, they have usually already done some networking of their own to decide whether or not to consult a medical professional about their problem. This may be friends, family or neighbours. Patients frequently consult the internet ('Dr Google' brings great benefits in terms of information, in terms of wisdom perhaps not so much) or even phone Apps, which may help explore, diagnose or assess conditions like diabetes. Some patients may not be as keen on referral or investigation as clinicians think, just as patients may not be as keen on prescriptions for antibiotics as clinicians think. The Health Foundation report quotes a patient who says:

> *Yeah, they're like, "go for a blood test", no problem, "go for an x-ray", no problem. You do have other things going on.*[10]

Perhaps this patient's priorities for their care had not been discussed, or perhaps the referral was really a 'dysfunctional way out' for a clinician who was herself having a WDYDWYDKWTD moment. If the patient does not agree that investigation is the key next step, he may use his own strategy for expressing this; failing to go for the blood tests or X-rays, or failing to return for follow-up. Patients' responses to referral may also reflect that they literally 'don't know what to do'; patients who are illiterate or who do not speak English may not understand their appointment letter. Referral may pose dilemmas for patients who have competing priorities as carers, employees or parents; accessing time or resources to get to a referral appointment may require difficult choices between their obligations. Perhaps the patient who does not take up a referral needed time to talk, to have their concerns dealt with and have a reasonable explanation, rather than more time-consuming and inconvenient tests. Even attending the out-patient part of the care network can be fraught and frustrating. One clinician comments:

> *well every patient is very important to us but sometimes you have to prioritise a very sick patient, you need to go yourself and see them … but sometimes [the out-patient] won't appreciate that and they think you have abandoned them and that makes it awkward to restart [the consultation] … again.*[10]

Interruptions and discontinuities, a feeling of being temporarily 'abandoned' during a pivotal consultation, can only compound the stress of the patient's uncertainty. In a fascinating description of her own progress though a complex diagnostic approach, requiring multiple imaging processes and discussions with clinicians, Mildred Blaxter comments that her own experiences end up being seen as less important than what the images show, even to the extent of 'the possible disappearance of the person behind the images'.[11]

Interestingly, some of the imaging helped her to feel that she was getting to know her own body in a different way and the lung function testing relieved some uncertainty: 'Although not altogether understood, the numbers provided some very welcome "certainty" about the body's functioning.'[11]

Even when the diagnostic network is proceeding in its inexorable way, patients are experiencing great uncertainty while waiting for results or treatment. Living with the uncertainty is painful:

> *unsettled because today there have been sad moments of us both crying as my husband is scared of what oncologist will say on Monday about scan result.*
> (Macmillan)

Sometimes procedures have to be delayed because of diagnostic developments or the availability of resources. This reinforces the huge uncertainties patients face. In this exchange from the Macmillan website, a patient 'in limbo', when new information delays her operation, gets a response from a fellow website user that seems to recognise that the medical staff may be trying to resolve their own uncertainties about what to do, by having a multidisciplinary team meeting to discuss things:

> *I was supposed to be having a RC & Hysterectomy this morning but on Friday they told me it's been cancelled due to a problem with my lymph nodes shown in a PET scan. So I'm back in limbo land waiting again … don't these people understand that they need to look after their patients' mental health too?*

A fellow forum member replies by saying:

> *I guess they'll be having an MDT meeting to decide what the next best step should be. As you say, it's the stress of uncertainty & waiting for results etc that's so hard.*
>
> (Macmillan)

These remarks also show how hard it is for professionals' uncertainty about the way forwards to be fully shared with patients. Inevitably the stress is greater for the patient who is facing an important challenge to his health, or, in the case of serious illness, a threat to his existence.

These kinds of uncertainties are managed by patients in various ways, including the use of complementary therapies to address their emotional needs:

> *A lot of people think Hypnotherapy is just Paul McKenna type stuff but it's much more than that. Hypnotherapy is like receiving an injection of positive thoughts. During the session you are put into a deep state of relaxation. It's really helped me deal with my anxieties.*
>
> (Cancer Care UK)

This highlights that patients may use networks beyond conventional health services; diagnosis and support may come from family, friends, church, colleagues, complementary practitioners and the internet. Many guidelines for care recommend referral to relevant patient support groups or sources of information such as websites run by organisations that advocate for patients (e.g. Diabetes UK). Many such groups provide valuable information and support and may help patients access the right care. However, patients' uncertainty and anxiety may increase if such organisations create pressure for certain kinds of care, which may not be available or endorsed by the services concerned.

Cultural and individual differences in how patients expect medical problems to be managed can compound uncertainty. Many clinicians will try to contain problems that seem to be ill defined, lacking serious implications or which have been investigated already, by continuing management in their own setting. This happens in general practice especially. Patients who continue to feel uncertain about their diagnosis may then press for further referral, may use private services or even travel abroad to places where there is no gatekeeping for scans or other investigations. Patients may use the influence of family members to expedite referral or exaggerate symptoms to get referred more quickly.

International differences can play a part in patients' uncertainty about the need for referral. The same diagnostic information would lead American clinicians to recommend surgery twice as often as UK-based surgeons,[12] and there are similar differences in the rate of diagnostic testing and referral for other specialist opinions. In the USA, rates of investigation are high, sometimes revealing data about abnormalities of very uncertain significance, which can give rise to difficult decisions about what to do for patients and clinicians alike.[13] Such differences compound uncertainty if patients believe that there is a 'right answer' in medical practice. Not only do patients have access to such differing opinions via the internet, but in this age of international travel they may also even have direct experience of a clinician in one country recommending an investigation or treatment of which another clinician in a different place disapproves.

Clinicians' and patients' fears and uncertainties are at odds in these situations. The clinician may be fearing criticism or professional censure if she refers too much, uses too many services and 'wastes' NHS money. This is an anxiety about entitlement ('Can I refer when the patient doesn't fit the guidelines?'). The patient's anxiety is likely to be much more existential in nature ('If I am ill might I get worse and die?'). Patients may resolve this by pressing for the conclusion they trust the most. The threat of litigation may drive different investigation or treatment practices, particularly if there is poor understanding of the inherent uncertainty in health care, and the way that there may be more than one legitimate approach.

The patient's perspective on uncertainty in the Negotiating Quadrant

> *I have had the tests in order to confirm or not whether I have it. No other things were found and the neurologist clinician has offered to put me on medication for this. I have been given a few months to consider this … I know it's up to me, but the only advice I've been getting is from people who aren't all that aware of the illness.*
>
> (Epilepsy UK)

This quotation describes the experience of a patient facing uncertainty about the best way to treat or manage his illness. There are many such examples on patients' forums and websites across the internet. What can we glean from research about how patients themselves view the uncertainties in their care?

Sometimes the uncertainty in this Quadrant arises because the clinician has not fully clarified the reason for the consultation. This can lead to him feeling frustrated and uncertain of how to proceed. This in turn leads to further uncertainty about the problem for the patient also. Clinicians do not always verbalise the uncertainty they are experiencing, which means it cannot be discussed with the patient openly. Reflecting on the difficulty may help: 'Do I fully understand the patient's reasons for the consultation? Do I know what kind of help the patient expects from me? Is it really possible to help this patient?'[14]

Many analyses of the conversations between clinicians and patients emphasise the patients' contribution to the meanings that emerge.[15] There are intricate interactions between what patients say, what kinds of information clinicians try to elicit from the conversation and what kinds of subjects are seen as 'acceptable' subjects for discussion. These complexities can give rise to a lot of confusion and uncertainty for the patient.

Many, if not most, treatments have a failure rate as well as a success rate; no treatment plan will be expected to work 100% of the time in 100% of patients. However, in some situations this is readily accepted by both parties, especially if, on balance, the benefits to be expected far outweigh the risks of side effects or failure. In some fields of medicine there has been an increasing willingness to share this information about the risks and benefits of interventions with patients, which may raise uncertainty for patients about whether to accept treatment. Having a greater involvement in decision making brings new responsibilities for patients, who may construe their illness or make decisions in different ways from their clinicians.[16]

The attitude of the clinician to the patient in this decision-making, negotiating aspect of care has been described as being one of four kinds by Linda and Ezekiel Emanuel.[17]

Clinician knows best. This is when the clinician takes a paternalist position and makes the decisions about the best care. Although this attitude has a bad press, most people accept the need for this when the situation is life threatening and the action needed is clear cut. No one expects clinicians to do anything other than make decisions when dealing with a multiply injured patient in an emergency department.

The informant clinician promotes 'informed choice'. This clinician avoids instructing patients and presents them with lots of information to help *them* make an informed choice. The patient quoted at the start of this section has experienced this approach.

The interpretative clinician shares information with the patient, but goes beyond leaving the patient to make a choice herself, guiding the decision making by using expert knowledge while also incorporating the patient's values and priorities. This latter approach is usually called 'shared decision making' and thus has important differences from 'informed choice'.

The deliberative clinician goes beyond what the interpretative clinician does by helping the patient to explore and examine the health-related values 'that can be realised in the clinical situation', and which of those values are 'more worthy and should be aspired to'.[18] In this situation the clinician is acting more like a teacher or friend, engaging in a dialogue about what values are most important to the patient at the time, and even indicating what decision about medical care would be 'admirable'.

How do patients experience these different approaches when there are uncertainties in play?

The paternalist clinician is well recognised by patients:

> *It's like being back at school...or going to a lawyer or something...they're big and you are small, they have authority. And they must know what's wrong or they know the fixes, know more than you.*[10]

> *You have to just go through the hoops or you'll get nowhere ... they've got a way of working ... you fit in ... get the business done, that's it.*[15]

The approach of the clinician here is to 'know best' and take responsibility for all decisions. This might be comforting if all goes well or in the face of immediate life-threatening problems with unequivocal decisions to be taken. Those situations are actually unusual; most clinician/patient encounters are less clear cut.

When the 'authority' of a paternalistic clinician fails or comes into question the disappointment can be huge. The mother quoted at the start of Chapter 22 could not accept that the clinicians involved in her child's care did not know why things went wrong, even though the coroner recognised that they had made strenuous efforts to find out. Clinicians and patients who initially share the attitude that 'clinician knows best' may find uncertainty almost too painful to deal with openly. If clinicians express uncertainty in this context patient satisfaction is reduced. When clinicians were observed advising about antibiotics for patients' heart murmurs, patient satisfaction was markedly reduced if clinicians expressed uncertainty, even if they then resolved that uncertainty by consulting a reference text or computer resource.[19] So perhaps it would be better to avoid the 'clinician knows best' approach from the outset and give patients more involvement in the process.

At first sight, the informant clinician giving patients an 'informed choice' seems to respond to current ideas that more information is better and that choice is a good thing. However, having choices in itself increases anxiety (there are more details about this in Part III 'Mapping the psychology of uncertainty'). Offering information, but no guidance, could lead to a sense of abandonment for patients facing difficult choices. For example:

> *I was told my husband could die if he didn't have the operation or he could die during the operation … obviously the choice was mine.*
>
> (Should her husband have an amputation after a heart attack? healthtalk.org)

The clinicians here were not saying they 'knew best', and the patient's wife was left with the uncertainty of which decision to take. The following carer's experience at the end of life suggests that firmer decision making by the physicians could have been helpful.

> *The lack of clarity about whether he is dying, the feeling that everyone is waiting for an infection to take him away but in the meantime keep him*

> *in what he describes as himself as "hell" reluctant to make any decision is wearing me into the ground.*
>
> (Macmillan website)

How do the other approaches (the 'interpretative clinician', or 'deliberative clinician' who enables 'shared decision making') affect patients in uncertain situations? In all areas of medicine there is an expressed wish to 'involve patients in their care' and to involve patients in 'shared decision making'. This is usually held to be most relevant where the outcome of a treatment is uncertain, or only works for some but not all patients, or when there is 'equipoise' in the decision making, such that there is no clear-cut 'best' way forwards in the treatment.[20] We know that patients want to be consulted more about their care, and in particular to be involved in significant decisions. Some decisions will involve significant uncertainty about the outcomes for individual patients, significant uncertainties about the risks and side effects that an individual patient may experience, and even uncertainties about the costs of treatment. In spite of these uncertainties when researchers ask patients, they generally say they want increased involvement in decision making. The phrase 'no decision about me without me',[21] captures this idea.

However, a true shared approach does not abandon the patient to making difficult decisions alone. The professional involved has specific expertise that enables *problem solving*; this is at least partly a technical matter requiring skills to elucidate the problem, the possible solutions and knowledge about what is entailed. The patient brings *specific expertise about their own situation*. It is the combination of these things that enable a second process, which is that of *shared decision making*, once the problem has been clarified.[12] How do patients see uncertainty in this context?

The answer is, again, 'it depends'. In a study of patients making decisions about ischaemic heart disease about 40% of patients came to a decision they were happy with, but 40% had increased anxiety and 77% still cited their physician as being the most important factor in decision making.[12] Patients making decisions about whether to accept high-risk cardiac surgery (with a real possibility of death with or without surgery) were prepared to talk about the risks and face the possible consequences. However, their final decisions reflected their 'unconditional trust' in the clinician offering the treatment, and their disinclination to face a 'fading away'.

Clinician: *The prerequisite is that you are willing to take a somewhat greater risk than normal.*
Patient: *I'll sign right away.*[22]

The patient and clinician accepting the risks of surgery may also be avoiding facing a different, more challenging uncertainty about the approaching end of life. In the USA in particular, clinicians offer choices about heroic treatments in end-stage disease 'in case' there is a 'small chance' of improvement. This may not give patients opportunities to think through more important choices about their own end-of-life care, or to face their impending death with the support and accompaniment of a physician who can help them and their families. In his book *Being Mortal*, Atul Gawande describes the uncertainty and difficult decisions that his father encountered when he developed a major spinal tumour.[23] His decisions were not just about his medical care, but also about what kind of life and what kind of death he wished to espouse: how much risk, when to stop treatment, when to gracefully accept that death was approaching. These are existential and moral uncertainties as much as medical ones, and such issues are not always part of the discussions that patients and clinicians have together.

Some patients seem to be able to achieve a more equal relationship with their clinicians:

> *If I go to see my GP it's very much … it's almost peer to peer, I'm not affected by them in any way, I say "right this is the problem, this is what I want" and they generally do it.*[10]

And another comments:

> *I thought "wait a minute" [laughs], "you're not a magician"! So I do ask the questions and I do challenge and I always, always ask, "why are we doing it this way and we're not doing it another way?"*[10]

These glimpses suggest that there could be situations in which there is more partnership between patients and clinicians, with patients feeling empowered to become involved and shape their care. Patients and carers are not only affected by decisions concerning treatment. In planning what to do, they have many other decisions to make, some of which are discussed in the team-working section of this chapter below. In the following example it seems to be the oncologist who is not prepared to accept a risk that the patient is proposing, when considering whether to take a respite break to a much loved holiday destination:

> *And today despite R … being still well the oncologist said we should not go and if we did it would be against medical advice.… We'd go the easy way on Eurostar … friends to pick us up then home to our little corner of heaven. I've said it's his choice … if he wants to go then we'll go.… What do you think we should do?*
>
> (Macmillan website)

Another writer on the same site gave conflicting advice too, acknowledging the uncertainty and sense of responsibility of the oncologist:

> *I think you should go, but if I had the same choice I don't really know. The oncologist will not give their blessing because it could cause problems for them if anything happened.*
>
> (Macmillan website)

Some patients are very articulate about what is gained and what is lost with an approach that involves patients fully in decision making:

> *We've gained [today] in that we're wiser and we can challenge and when something's wrong, we can take it further, etc., etc. But what we've lost is that permission for it not to be all on our shoulders, "clinician says, therefore it must be correct". Now everything's on our shoulders, which is good, but bad.*[10]

The patient's perspective on uncertainty in the Team-working Quadrant

> *As to the recovery they don't know … we just didn't know and as a family that was the worst thing to deal with.*
>
> (Uncertain recovery after brain injury, healthtalk.org)

Patients face many uncertainties in the Team-working Quadrant. These may be uncertainties about what to make of the information they are given, about the processes of care, and also about many issues that are not strictly 'medical' but can have a large impact. A patient's 'team' is wider than the network of professionals involved with them, and includes family and other supporters, and they also struggle with the impact of uncertainty:

> *My dad has been told there is an 85% chance he has cancer in his neck/throat.... We are now waiting for results.... I can't think of anything more terrifying than sitting in that clinician's office.... I've pretty much accepted that there will be a cancer there ... but the results of the CT terrify me. The possibility of metastases just doesn't bear thinking about. People have told me to concentrate on the 15% chance it's not malignant. Not sure how this is possible.*
>
> (Macmillan)

Sometimes the uncertainties inherent in care, or the uncertainties of the professionals involved, were recognised and accepted:

> *flushing him with this drug that we were told ... is a poison, is not good but ... it was probably the best course of action rather than operating and risking a low recovery rate. But with head injuries they don't know, they just don't know. It could go either way ... there is no rule of thumb.*
>
> (healthtalkorg)

In contrast, the unwillingness of clinicians to disclose information merely served to increase uncertainty for this family:

> *From what I can tell, French oncologists prefer to keep their patients in a kind of murky fog, telling them what they need to know and not much else.*
>
> (Macmillan)

Uncertainty in the process of care is difficult, as vividly described here:

> *it has been such a tremendous rollercoaster ... yesterday Hammersmith rung to say ... liver op had been postponed and they would let us know next week when it would be, So why phone at all it just unsettles.*
>
> (Macmillan)

Trying to navigate the way into the best type of care can be traumatic and patients have their own 'what do you do when you don't know what to do' moments, such as these:

> *The thought had crossed my mind that maybe I should call an ambulance, but I didn't … listened to my answer phone … telling me to go straight to A&E because my haemoglobin (Hb) was 5.2 grams per decilitre. … I had no idea what this meant but I called a cab and, strangely, I felt a sense of relief after being told that something was wrong and that I wasn't going mad.*
>
> (Leukaemia Care)

Trying to work out how to use health services for the best, and the unpredictability of visits by staff, gave this carer a bad time. She ends up 'begging' for a hospice admission in a traumatic WDYDWYDKWTD experience:

> *Emergency ambulance at 6 am … poor man looked and felt dreadful. … Ambulance said wait and see GP, don't go to hospital too many infections around. Try and get him to a hospice. District nurse due this morning didn't turn up. GP due 2pm ish. Then … fell over. Arm black and blue desperate for the loo. … Terrible mess black and tarry. Back to bed still in a mess now can't breathe … second emergency ambulance … very unwell GP turned up. The point to this story is in 48 years I have never had to clean up after my husband and I cried and cried. The young and beautiful lady Clinician and the paramedic gently cleaned him and helped me to change him into clean clothes and make him comfortable how wonderful is that!! … I begged for him to go the hospice.*
>
> (Macmillan)

The difficulties that carers have in doing such tasks are also experienced by professionals: 'District nurses felt like cowards, and also experienced meaninglessness, uncertainty, shame, irresolution, and insufficiency in the trying situations.'[24]

Many uncertainties in the Team-working Quadrant relate to the difficulties carers have and the way that professionals do not appreciate the impact of what is happening at home. This carer is struggling to manage the care for a relative with severe dementia. A colonoscopy has been proposed. The carer seems to accept that without question but says:

> *The actual colonoscopy itself is not my worry, I am rather selfishly wondering how the prep is to be managed. I can't get MIL to drink 75ml of liquid so how am I going to get her to drink 5000ml. … As for not eating … It's going to be 24 hours plus of raging and crying and running round to the neighbours, and calling the police, and saying we're abusing her. … Her*

bedroom is upstairs and the loo is downstairs so she probably won't be able to go to bed and sleep … and what if she falls down the stairs because of hunger or dehydration or trying to get to the downstairs loo?

(Alzheimer's Society)

Difficult decisions about future care sometimes left family members feeling isolated:

I personally feel it's time to think about a care home, but how do we persuade him? It's such a big step, daunting for us all. We just need some friendly advice as no one seems to help from his clinic.' [and] 'Social Services won't answer the question about what flags or behaviours need to be demonstrated before they consider moving him in to residential care. Social Services keep fobbing us off.

(Alzheimer's Society)

This last quote shows how uncertainty is mirrored in both professionals and families. It is likely that the Social Worker is also having a WDYDWYDKWTD moment trying to manage extremely limited resources and budgets, balancing the needs of different families and under pressure from time constraints. Yet the shared uncertainty seems not to be voiced. Sometimes carers even felt isolated by their relatives:

My husband has just been diagnosed with lung cancer, a week ago by GP & radiologist … had CT done on Wednesday. … He is refusing to talk about it. & I am feeling frustrated about him not wanting to find out anything or to chase an appointment. How long should we have to wait do you think?

(Macmillan)

Much care outside hospital is carried out by family members, who are not necessarily acknowledged as part of the 'team'. Such caregivers have to be very vigilant in monitoring progress and knowing when to involve other staff such as nurses. Such tasks are stressful, create uncertainty and carers often feel that the rest of their lives is 'on hold'.[24] Uncertain carers and family members retain feelings of guilt and fear. This heartfelt comment on the Macmillan website was entitled 'never any certainty':

What am I missing? What if I'd paid more attention two or three years ago to his vague complaints of ill-health and pressed for him to get a scan instead

> *of focusing on my own concerns? … what if I researched another treatment or did another search or went to another patient conference? What if I got a juicer and made him drink raw kale juice? … There has to be something I can do … but there isn't really. Or is there?*
>
> (Macmillan)

Other uncertainties may not be appreciated fully by health service staff:

> *I am currently on statutory sick pay from my employer. I have been told this stops after six months – what happens then? Where do I apply after the six months? … I am so worried about our finances.*
>
> (Macmillan)

One carer trying to make sense of their entitlements wrote in a forum:

> *Can anyone on here understand this nonsense?*
>
> (Alzheimer's Society)

Uncertainty for patients does not come to an end when treatment is finished, and again there is a sense of isolation from professionals in this comment:

> *I'm struggling with the uncertainty. The focus of getting through the treatment has gone and I'm now frightened for the future. How long have I got? Will it spread? When will it return? Last week I desperately wanted the oncologist to say everything will be ok but of course nobody can say that. I'm struggling knowing that there is no full stop to this nightmare.*
>
> (Macmillan)

The discussion threads that patients use when turning to the internet seem to be a potent source of comfort in uncertain situations as these comments show:

> *It is often a comfort to know you are not alone in the uncertainty and the condition and that although it may be a long time coming there is light at the end of the tunnel.*
>
> (Epilepsy UK)

> *We may all be strangers to each other BUT we care about each other and try to support wherever we can. I do so hope something can be done for J. … BUT obviously, at the moment, we are all in the dark. We know in many ways we shouldn't intrude but you initially invited us – so here we all are!!*
>
> (Macmillan)

Being aware of the realities of uncertainty from the patient's perspective is important for professionals. Patients have to face many of the same issues as clinicians: uncertainty, complexity, trying to predict an uncertain and frightening future, facing a sense of failure. Although it is not the task of patients to support professionals themselves, perhaps knowing that these uncertainties are shared can help professionals be more empathic towards those they care for. Training for uncertainty should incorporate improved understanding of the shared experiences of clinicians and patients, develop communication skills and encourage clinicians to learn about patients' experiences. Multidisciplinary team meetings could offer opportunities to discuss and process the emotional work of caring for patients in extreme or uncertain situations. Being open about our own fears and uncertainties, and empathising with those of our patients, will make for more sensitive and effective care, while providing support for professionals themselves.

> *I have no experience of cancer on a personal level, but work with people in this awful situation every day. It's very different on the other side.*
>
> (Macmillan)

References

1. Brashers D. Communication and uncertainty management. *Journal of Communication* 2001; **51(9)**: 477–97.
2. Helman CG. Diseases versus illness in general practice. *Journal of the Royal College of General Practitioners* 1981; **31(230)**: 548–52.
3. Wen L, Kosowsky J. *When Doctors Don't Listen: how to avoid misdiagnoses and avoid unnecessary tests*. New York, NY: St Martin's Press, 2013.
4. Goldstein Jutel A, Dew K (eds). *Social Issues in Diagnosis: an introduction for students and clinicians*. Baltimore, MD: Johns Hopkins University Press, 2014.
5. Nettleton S. 'I just want permission to be ill': towards a sociology of medically unexplained symptoms. *Social Science and Medicine* 2006; **62(5)**: 1167–78.
6. Cousin G, Schmid Mast M, Jaunin-Stalder N. When physician-expressed uncertainty leads to patient dissatisfaction: a gender study. *Medical Education* 2013; DOI: 10.1111/medu.12237.

7. Thomas KB. General practice consultations: is there any point being positive? *British Medical Journal* (Clin Res Ed) 1987; **294(6581)**: 1200–2.
8. Little P, Everitt H, Williamson I, *et al.* Observational study of effect of patient centredness and positive approach on outcomes of general practice consultations. *British Medical Journal* 2001; **323(7318)**: 908–11.
9. Barry MJ, Edgman-Levitan S. Shared decision making: the pinnacle of patient-centered care. *New England Journal of Medicine* 2012; **366**: 780–1; DOI: 10.1056/NEJMp1109283.
10. Fischer M, Ereaut G. *When Doctors and Patients Talk: making sense of the consultation*. London: Health Foundation, 2012.
11. Blaxter M. The case of the vanishing patient? Image and experience. *Sociology of Health & Illness* 2009; **31(5)**: 762–78; DOI: 10.1111/j.1467-9566.2009.01178.x.
12. Frosch DL, Kaplan RM. Shared decision making in clinical medicine. *American Journal of Preventive Medicine* 1999; **17(4)**: 285–94.
13. Welch G. *Less Medicine, More Health: 7 assumptions that drive too much medical care*. Boston, MA: Beacon Press, 2015.
14. Arborelius E, Bremberg S, Timpka T. What is going on when the general practitioner doesn't grasp the situation? *Family Practice* 1991; **8(1)**: 3–9.
15. Pilnick A, Hindmarsh J, Gill VT. 'Beyond doctor and patient': developments in the study of healthcare interactions. *Sociology of Health and Illness* 2009; **31(6)**: 787–802; DOI: 10.1111/j.1467-9566.2009.01194.x.
16. Elwyn G, Edwards A, Kinnersley P. Shared decision-making in primary care: the neglected second half of the consultation. *British Journal of General Practice* 1999; **49(443)**: 477–82.
17. Emanuel EJ, Emanuel LL. Four models of the physician-patient relationship. *Journal of the American Medical Association* 1992; **267(16)**: 2221–6.
18. Croskerry P. Clinical cognition and diagnostic error: applications of a dual process model of reasoning. *Advances in Health Sciences Education: Theory and Practice* 2009; **14(1)**: 27–35; DOI: 10.1007/s10459-009-9182-2.
19. Johnson CG, Levenkron JC, Suchman AL, Manchester R. Does physician uncertainty affect patient satisfaction? *Journal of General Internal Medicine* 1988; **3(2)**:144–9.
20. Elwyn G, Edwards A, Kinnersley P, Grol R. Shared decision making and the concept of equipoise: the competences of involving patients in healthcare choices. *British Journal of General Practice* 2000; **50(460)**: 892–9.
21. Coulter A, Collins A. *Making Shared Decision-Making a Reality: no decision about me, without me*. London: King's Fund, 2011.
22. Schaufel MA, Nordrehaug JE, Malterud K. 'So you think I'll survive?': a qualitative study about doctor–patient dialogues preceding high-risk cardiac surgery or intervention. *Heart* 2009; **95**; DOI: 10 11 36/hrt 2008.164657.
23. Gawande A. *Being Mortal*. London: Metropolitan Books, 2014.

24. Pålsson MB, Isovaara S, Norberg A. Meeting cancer patients. Interviews with Swedish district nurses. *Scandinavian Journal of Primary Health Care* 1995; **13(1)**: 68–73.

Resources

Gawande A. *Being Mortal*. London: Metropolitan Books, 2014.

Emanuel EJ, Emanuel LL. Four models of the physician-patient relationship. *Journal of the American Medical Association* 1992; **267(16)**: 2221–6.

Many patients' experiences and stories can be accessed online and make for interesting and highly educative reading for clinicians. The following websites are particularly useful. There are many others, devoted to specific conditions:

- Alzheimer's Society, www.alzheimers.org.uk
- Cancer Care, www.cancercare.org.uk.
- Epilepsy Action, www.epilepsy.org.uk.
- HealthTalkOnline, www.healthtalk.org.
- HealthUnlocked, www.healthunlocked.com.
- Leukaemia CARE, www.leukaemiacare.org.uk.
- Macmillan Cancer Support, www.macmillan.org.uk

Chapter 24

Conclusion

Embracing uncertainty

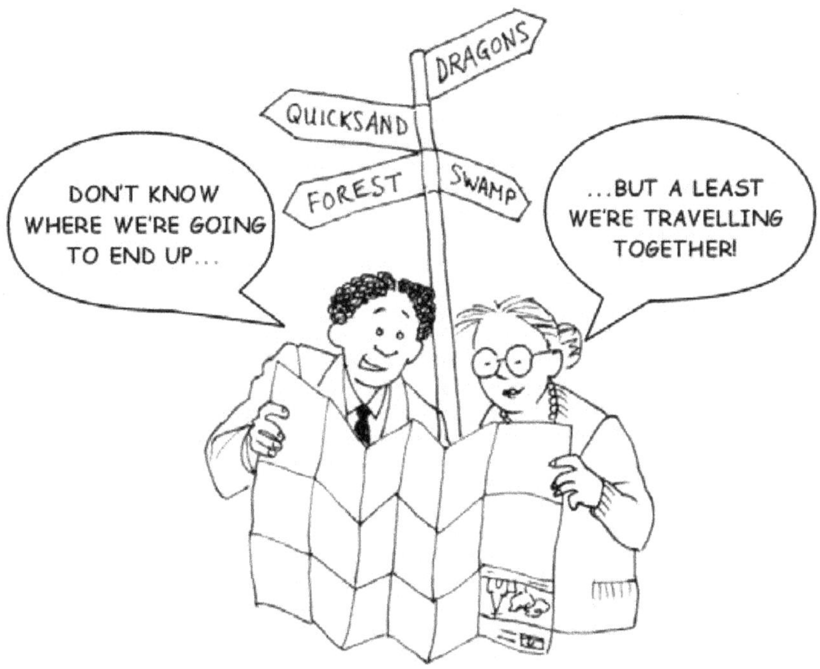
DRAGONS
QUICKSAND
FOREST
SWAMP
DON'T KNOW WHERE WE'RE GOING TO END UP...
...BUT A LEAST WE'RE TRAVELLING TOGETHER!

> This glorious twilight zone of uncertainty.
>
> K. Dew[1]

> Only because we do not understand everything and because we cannot control the future is it possible to live.
>
> Iona Heath[2]

This conclusion reflects on the themes of this book and includes acknowledgement that:

- uncertainty is inevitable
- uncertainty is necessary
- uncertainty can be shared with patients
- uncertainty is the defining characteristic of professional practice.

Most of this book has been about understanding uncertainty and proposing strategies to reduce or manage uncertainty more effectively. If we learn the right skills and think a bit harder, will uncertainty go away? Will this mean that we can or should get rid of uncertainty in medical practice? Clearly that is never going to happen; uncertainty is an inevitable part of human life and can never be eliminated in situations of illness, clinical care or death.

Uncertainty is inevitable

Although many clinicians do recognise that uncertainty is inevitable in clinical work, the roots of discomfort with the uncertain state run deep. For clinicians, the fear of error or professional loss of face can combine with a reductionist approach that values instrumental, 'scientific' knowledge above all else. Such knowledge, which allows us to control or manipulate disease states, may be viewed as reliable, desirable and powerful. Uncertainty may then be seen as a deficient state, similar to failure. However, a purely 'biological' approach to medical care excludes other important forms of knowledge that are crucial in understanding and caring for patients, and which cannot be bound down to measurable phenomena. We can engage with patients more deeply if we use the deep understanding of the human condition obtained from non-scientific sources to inform clinical work; the social sciences, literature and art all have potential parts to play. A more extended biopsychosocial model of illness, familiar to primary care clinicians, allows an understanding of patients' individual personal experiences and their social context to influence medical care, so that it becomes nuanced to the individual's needs. Each patient is unique and their individuality cannot be objectively described, measured, predicted or controlled. With such wider perspectives, uncertainty is not failure, but rather an irreducible reality.

Uncertainty is necessary

If the inevitability of uncertainty is accepted, we can go further and recognise that uncertainty is necessary for effective clinical practice. At one level, this is because a 'jumping away' from uncertainty into premature conclusions can create fertile ground for error (if decisions are made too rapidly), poor performance (if intolerance to uncertainty leads to over-confidence) or excess anxiety (if uncertainty is not tolerated). Thus, being able to recognise and 'hold' uncertainty is a necessary part of clinical work.

At a more profound level, when a broader intolerance to uncertainty is underpinned by a fear of death (shared by clinicians and their patients), such fear can result in distorted views of reality.[3] This may include magical thinking ('The doctor can always fix me'), denial ('If I don't acknowledge my diabetes it cannot change my life') or moralistic views of health and illness ('If you do the right things, eat well, exercise, stop smoking, you will be protected from illness or even death'). Such thinking tends to create the illusion that everything can be controlled, predicted or understood and tends to overvalue the power of medicine to influence disease and defeat death. Modern medical care has many spectacular successes, and this can easily promote a passivity in patients who may develop unrealistic expectations of what clinicians can deliver. Many illness trajectories owe as much to the intrinsic healing powers of the patient as to the treatment. Many treatments are poorly supported by evidence and although death may be delayed, or the course of a disease modified, we cannot protect individuals from disease (at some point in their lives) or death (which remains inevitable). If we seek out certainty and technological or medical 'fixes', our ability to face death is compromised. If we deny the uncertainty and inevitability of death we will over-use technological solutions at the end of life and be 'doomed to failure, frustration and dehumanization':[3]

> *The transformation of death from a personal, family oriented, human experience to a technologically dominated ritual masks its mystery and deprives many patients and families of the opportunity to experience and explore the spiritual significance of this profound event.*[3]

Accepting uncertainty as a necessary part of practice, acknowledging the 'mystery' and uncertainty of death with patients, can open the way for humane, flexible and attentive care, rather than a simple, and sometimes futile, pursuit of 'cure'.

Uncertainty can be shared with patients

Although many patients would prefer their clinicians to be certain about everything, and some may be unhappy when their clinicians share uncertainties, we cannot assume that offering certainty to patients is the best long-term strategy. Uncertainty can be uncomfortable for clinicians. That is nothing compared with the pain and breach of trust felt by a patient expecting that medical care will have predictable and helpful results, but who finds himself the unlucky one for whom treatment fails or complications ensue.

To be able to share uncertainty with patients, clinicians need to be secure and grounded in two things: their own expertise, and their willingness to openly discuss uncertainty and share decision making with patients. Clinicians' expertise is not just about theoretical knowledge. It also comprises the clinical skills they use in practice and above all the communication skills they will use to build relationships with patients, to cope with the various uncertainties that have been outlined in the Quadrant chapters of this book and to share decision making effectively. An open partnership with patients is attainable, when certainty is not always possible. Where clinicians cannot be certain of outcomes they can ensure robust processes of decision making, in partnership with patients.

One consequence of modern life is that patients have similar access to information, via the internet, as do clinicians. Indeed many patients have more time to research their care and most will have a strong motivation to access information about the right care. If clinicians and patients can work together, such approaches will be beneficial as patients will become aware of the inherent uncertainty of illness and care trajectories. However, in sharing decision making with patients, clinicians must also be prepared to share their ethical imperatives and codes of conduct. Such drivers of equity in care and the effective use of limited resources constrain clinicians in ways that may make for complex conversations if patients are not willing to consider these wider issues.

In the past, much uncertainty in clinical practice was absorbed by clinicians, without patients having to face uncertainty directly. In effect, clinicians were also expected to be 'supermen and superwomen' whose personal needs were subsumed in their work; they were supposed to be certain about everything but not supposed to become tired, hungry, bad tempered or in error. If we become more open about uncertainty and error, perhaps clinical practice can be a more mutual enterprise. If care is organised to promote the development of effective and long-term relationships between clinicians and patients, a more trusting acceptance of the iterations of medical care is likely to occur.[2] Patients may then be enabled to recognise the unpredictability and uncertainty of clinical work, which is not a science, but rather a caring practice, informed but not defined by scientific understanding. Clinicians should be able to acknowledge their humanity and its attendant frailties.

Uncertainty as the defining characteristic of professional practice

It is unreasonable to expect clinicians to be certain all the time. In a complex world, with many constraints operating, including a lack of time or resources, certainty is not merely impossible; expecting certainty can even militate against good practice. Clinicians may be unable to enact 'good enough' practice if they are aiming for perfection, wanting to be certain of the 'right answer'. Desire to be certain can lead to intolerable burdens for clinicians, who may burn out under the pressure of expecting to be correct all the time. Paradoxically, more senior clinicians may experience even more uncertainty than their junior colleagues, as their workload becomes dominated by more complex, ambiguous or difficult situations referred to them by others. Expertise usually increases alongside this, but managing increasing uncertainty can be stressful.

One response is a culture of defensiveness in medicine, sometimes called 'medical excess', causing over-investigation and over-treatment. The harms to patients that follow such excess are rarely well understood, even within the professions; patients and journalists generally have little appreciation of the risks of over-diagnosis or over-treatment, although campaigns are starting to rectify this. Conversely, the pressures of limited resources (especially time), may pressurise some clinicians into abbreviated assessments or management plans that are incomplete. The inherent uncertainty in medical practice will be managed slightly differently by different people. There is no 'right' way to deal with uncertainty in all situations.

Rather than aiming for certainty, sharing ideas about 'good enough' practice, 'safe enough' practice or 'acceptable practice in the prevailing circumstances' might be more appropriate. When patients are medically complex, their care may be a negotiated 'reasonable compromise', which will inevitably give rise to ambiguous or uncertain judgements at times. The reality is that all clinical practice can be ambiguous and uncertain, and no amount of pretending or litigation will make it any the less likely that clinicians will be uncertain or even in error. The main issue is how clinicians respond to uncertainty and error: do they shrug or do they think harder? It is better to ensure rigorous 'thinking' processes are in place and accept that clinicians cannot guarantee the outcome, than it is to aim for 'pseudocertainty'. Being able to integrate different kinds of information and different competencies to manage ambiguity and uncertainty is difficult and requires high-order skills.[4] Clinicians should be proud to assert that accepting uncertainty is an acceptable part of professionalism.

Donald Schön goes further: he considers that having to deal with 'unstructured and indeterminate zones of practice' is precisely what *defines* a professional.[5] These ambiguous areas are in stark contrast with the world of algorithms and protocols that imply structure and clarity in practice. Schön contrasted two faces of professionalism, 'professional artistry' and 'technical rational' approaches, which promote an acceptance and understanding of uncertainty and ambiguity. These are illustrated in Table 1.

We increasingly seem to sign up to a technical rational notion of how clinicians should behave, closely tied up with the idea that there is a 'right answer'. This can lead to the conclusion that, if things go wrong, it must be because a clinician 'got it wrong'. However, all clinicians and many patients recognise that clinicians must act with flexibility and the ability to work creatively in complex situations that cannot be captured in a simple set of rules. Professional skill, often called 'clinical judgement', means being able to balance competing claims, for example guidelines and protocols versus respecting patients' wishes, the ethical imperatives of autonomy versus justice, beneficence versus non-maleficence, the unusual needs of an individual patient versus the requirements of regulatory bodies for consistency. At the same time, clinicians must maintain an ability to critically appraise all their actions. Experienced clinicians recognise that this balance is what the *practice of medicine truly is.* It is not a 'science' as such, but more an *interpretive* task, whereby clinicians have to work out how biomedical information applies to each individual patient, one by one. The skills required have been well described as:

> *a flexible cast of mind, steady attention to the methods of practice, the habit of questioning and a willingness to learn from others; observing, refining ideas, comparing notes.*[6]

Table 1 'Technical rational' and 'professional artistry' models of professional behaviour

Technical rational	Professional artistry
Routines and protocols dominate	Frameworks guide but do not dictate practice
Inspection and external accreditation are necessary	Self-regulation is appropriate
Professional activity is masterable. Efficiency is demanded	Professional judgement is central to practice
Standards must be fixed	There is room to be wrong

Source: derived from Schön.[5]

These *feel* like scientific methods, although they are also shared with all kinds of other investigators. Such methods would be just as readily recognised by naturalists, historians, detectives, novelists or social workers as by clinicians. It must now be time to develop a medical culture where uncertainty is accepted and discussed, where patients involved in shared decision making are helped to understand the uncertainty attached to the harm/benefit profile of many treatments, and where we abandon a 'blame and shame' approach. Perhaps it really is time to challenge 'technical rational' ideas in medicine: ideas such as 'more is better', 'information is power', 'technology can solve all our problems' and even that 'death is optional'.[7]

Uncertainty and failure are inevitable, as is error. This means accepting that, in medicine, success may come only after trying a few things and failing, or may not come at all. Increasing dialogues about uncertainty, about the pressures that impinge on diagnosis, decision making and teamwork, help us to develop the concept that best care is often an evolving and iterative enterprise, involving many different aspects of medicine and many personnel who have to be linked together. The developing field of 'improvement science' will drive these developments in appropriate ways: away from 'name and shame' and towards better systems. Many clinicians work in circumstances that are less than ideal, perhaps with too many patients to see, not enough time to reflect or research the best treatment for each individual, or under pressure to meet targets. As funding for health care ceases to expand at the same rate as it has done in the past, and medical complexity increases, technical rational 'fixes' can only go so far.

As the possibilities of medicine increase, the uncertainties will necessarily increase alongside, because there will be more options and increased complexity. Concepts of 'safe enough' or 'good enough' decision-making processes must take into account not just the outcomes, but also the honest efforts by clinicians to get it right. When clinicians find ways to share uncertainty with each other and with their patients, the way forwards, although no less complex or demanding, will have less conflict between clinicians and patients and be more rewarding for both:

> *Exploring the unique meaning that the illness and its associated uncertainty hold for the patient can create a strong bond between patient and clinician. This understanding is often a major source of reassurance and comfort.*[3]

Perhaps clinicians and patients are ready for a different, more profound perspective. Uncertainty need not be seen as a deficient or undesirable state.

Rather, a radical acceptance of the inevitability of uncertainty in professional practice allows for more intellectual interest in clinical work, stimulates professional growth and develops deeper and more rewarding partnerships with patients. If clinicians and patients can both be released from the illusion that everything can be predicted and controlled, a more humane and realistic professional practice can emerge.

References

1. Dew K, Dowell A, McLeod D, *et al.* 'This glorious twilight zone of uncertainty': mental health consultations in general practice in New Zealand. *Social Science and Medicine* 2005; **61(6)**: 1189–200.
2. Heath I. Role of fear in overdiagnosis and overtreatment. *British Medical Journal* 2014; DOI: 10.1136/bmj.g6123.
3. Quill TE, Suchman AL. Uncertainty and control: learning to live with medicine's limitations. *Humane Health Care* 2009, www.humanehealthcare.com/Article.asp?art_id=440.
4. Epstein RM, Hundert EM. Defining and assessing professional competence. *Journal of the American Medical Association* 2002; **287(2)**: 226–35.
5. Schön D. *The Reflective Practitioner: how professionals think in action*. London: Temple Smith, 1983.
6. Montgomery K. *How Doctors Think: clinical judgement and the practice of medicine*. New York, NY: Oxford University Press, 2006.
7. Hoffman JR, Kanzaria HK. Intolerance of error and culture of blame drive medical excess. *British Medical Journal* 2014; **349**: g5702; DOI: 10.1136/bmj.g5702.

Index

- Alzheimer's Society 293–4, 295, 298
- ambiguities
  - ambiguous symptoms *79*
  - ambivalence and, maintenance of state of 181
  - in decision-making, acceptance of 190
  - discomfort with 212
  - time and resolution of 79
  - uncertainty and 176
- analysis *12,* 13, 15, 25, 27–68
  - anchoring bias *38*
  - anxiety, feelings of 188
  - ascertainment bias *38*
  - assessment and teaching methods for uncertainty in 65–8
  - assessment of learning needs in 222
  - 'automatic pilot', working on 33
  - availability bias *38*
  - bandwagon bias *38*
  - clinical guidelines, use of 41, 52–4
  - clinical settings, management of uncertainty in 63–4
  - clues, handling of 55
  - cognitive bias, types of *38*
  - cognitive processes 189–90
    - emotional reactions and 188–9
  - decision-making
    - acceptance of ambiguity and 190
    - psychological research on 29
  - diagnosis, clinician's judgement about 38–9
  - diagnostic safety netting 41, 44–8
  - dysfunctional responses 28, 34–8
  - educational skills in 241–3
  - emotional content of the consultation, exploration of 41, 54–6
  - emotional intelligence 189
  - emotional reactions 188–9
  - expert thinkers 30–1
  - exploration 27–8
  - external factors leading to failure in 29
  - favourite diagnosis, selection of 36
  - focus lock 37–8
    - avoidance of 58–9
  - functional symptoms, explanation of 41, 59–61
  - functional ways through uncertainty in 41–61
  - gambler's bias *38*
  - guidelines, limits of 189–90
  - guilt, power of 188
  - heuristics 189–90
  - hypothetico-deductive reasoning using 'restricted rule out' 41, 42–4
  - information, availability of 190
  - information transmitted by emotions 189
  - institutional support, availability of 190
  - internal factors leading to failure in 28–9
  - interpretation of illness narratives from patients 38
  - intuition 189
  - investigation 35
  - key skills 25
    - functional ways through uncertainty in 41
  - malpractice claims 190
  - medicine, practice of 27
  - negative emotions, effects of 188, 189

normality, awareness of bias towards 58
omission bias *38*
opting out of diagnosis 36–7
organisational setting 190
patient factors leading to failure in 29
patient perspective on uncertainty in 277–82
pattern recognition 189
pitfalls of analysis 34–8
positive emotions, effects of 188–9
premature closure *38*
premature reassurance 28, 35
previous diagnosis, sticking with 37
psychological components of uncertainty in 187–90
referral 36
reflection-in-action, Schön's concept of 30
relationship building 60
relationship issues 190
resources for 68
ruling in or ruling out 41, 44–8
same sex, referral to GP of 35
satisficing bias *38*
sharing clinical reasoning process with patient 41, 50–2
situational awareness skills 41, 56–9
symptoms
  explanation of physiological origins of 60–1
  useful phrases for explanation of *61*
teaching methods for uncertainty in 65–8
thinking strategies 30
time, availability of 190
trust and verify (Russian military proverb) 41, 48–50
Type 1 (intuitive) thinking 30–1, 33–4, 37
  comparison with Type 2 thinking *32*
  development of 33
Type 2 (analytical) thinking 30, 33–4
  comparison with Type 1 thinking *32*
  development and impact on diagnostic process of 33–4
unconscious incompetence 28
WDYDWYDKWTD, application of thinking types to 31–2
widening the view 41, 59–61
anxiety
  anxiety transfers 80
  in both doctor and patient, increases in 75
  feelings of 188
  perfection seeking, anxiety of 142, 183–4
  uncertainty and 177
  of 'what if' questions 181
Associates-in-Training (AiTs) 215

Bacon, Francis 211
Baggini, Julian 34
Balint group/Schwartz round-style discussion 128, 230
BATHE technique 125–7
behaviour change, motivational interviewing and 106, 118–22
Being Mortal (Gawande, A.) 290
Berne, Eric 118
blaming
  others in team-working 141
  patients 103, 195–6
  the system 103
  trainees in education 238
Blaxter, Mildred 283
boundaries, management of 143, 154–9
brain systems 177
breaking good news 77, 86–9
British Medical Journal 270
burnout 141–2

cancer, uncertainty about 279
Cancer Care UK 284, 298
Cancer Research UK 280
Care Quality Commission 197
carers, difficulties for 293–5
Cates plot *116*
certainty
  diagnostic, pressure for 203
  educational, mapping skills for 241
  pressures on clinicians for 184
  pseudo 7
  total, downside of 177–8

cognitive processes 189–90, 191–2, 195, 198–9
  for dealing with uncertainty, development of 179–80, 183
  emotional reactions and 188–9
cognitive uncertainty 176
complex problems, engagement with 106, 123–4
Covey, Stephen R. 101, 106–7

Darwin, Charles 265
death
  fear of 182
  intolerance to uncertainty and fear of 301
decision-making
  acceptance of ambiguity and 190
  anxieties about 212
  clarity in identification of decision to be made 113
  collective 198
  decision scales for patient's ability to change 120
  decision talk 114–15
  encouragement in 221
  explaining complexities of 102
  involvement in 286–7
  patients and, skills of involvement 73
  processes of, embracing uncertainty in 305
  psychological research on 29
  shared 106, 112–15, 289–91
  trying but failing to share with patient 104
defensive omnipotence 181–2
delegation
  effective delegation, pathways to 160
  skills in 159–61
  of tasks within teams 138
depersonalisation 141–2
Dew, Kevin 299
Diabetes UK 285
diagnosis
  clinician's judgement about 38–9
  conceptual approaches to, understanding differences in 79
  development and impact on diagnostic process of Type 2 thinking 33–4
  diagnostic certainty, pressure for 203
  diagnostic complexities 102
  diagnostic network, involvement of 71–2
  diagnostic safety netting 41, 44–8
  diagnostic services, array of 72
  differential 5
  educational 239–40
    creation of 241
  favourite diagnosis, selection of 36
  firm diagnosis, anguish of 279
  naming a diagnosis, problem of 278
  opting out of 36–7
  over-diagnosis 191–2
  over-reliance on tests and investigations for 74
  patient perspective on process of 279–80
  previous diagnosis, sticking with 37
  time as a diagnostic tool, use of 192
  uncertainty in 278

Eddy, David M. 5
educational skills for uncertainty in training
  analysis, educational skills in 241–3
  assessment, calibration and 242–3
  blaming the trainee 238
  coaching 246
  dysfunctional ways out of uncertain educational situations 238–9
  educational diagnosis 239–40
    creation of 241
  educational prescription 240
  feedback 244–5
    responses to 245
  'gossip', resorting to 239
  'GROW' model of coaching *246*
  handover, recording and 244
  Mapping Uncertainty in Medical Training (MUMT) *240*
  mentoring 246
  multisource feedback 243–4
  negotiation, educational skills in 244–6
  networking, educational skills in 243–4
  not telling it like it is 238

'ownership' of problems 245
passing problems on to others 238–9
RDM-p framework 243
recording and handover skills 248
rigidity in application of training plans 239
seeing problems in isolation 239
SMART (specific, measurable, achievable, realistic and timely) 245
solutions, identification and negotiation of 245
team-working, educational skills in 247–8
WDYDWYDKWTD
experiences in training context 237, 241, *242*, 247
performance of colleague as cause 249
withdrawing support, bypassing trainees and 238
Emanuel, Linda and Ezekiel 287
embracing uncertainty 299–306
balance in practice, skills needed for 304
death, intolerance to uncertainty and fear of 301
decision-making processes 305
error, inevitability of 305
failure, inevitability of uncertainty and 305
'good enough practice', sharing ideas about 303, 305–6
illness trajectories 301
inevitability of uncertainty 300, 306
investigatory methods 304–5
medical excess 303
necessity of uncertainty 300–1
openness on uncertainty 302
over-investigation 303
professional behaviour, models of *304*
professional practice, uncertainty as defining characteristic of 303–6
security in expertise 302
sharing uncertainty with patients 301–2
unstructured and indeterminate zones of practice, Schön's concept of 304
emotional content of consultation, exploration of 41, 54–6
emotional difficulties in consultation 75–6
emotional intelligence 189
emotional reactions 188–9, 191, 194, 197
emotional uncertainty 176
empathy
BATHE technique for 125–7
with impact of symptoms *88*
Epilepsy UK 286, 295, 298
error
'honest errors' of inexperience 221–2
inevitability of 305
potential wrongdoing, fear of 180–1
uncertainty and, relationship between 180–3
'wrong decisions' 180
evidence-based practice 107, 215
expectations, management of 77, 80–2
expert thinkers 30–1
explanation
skills in 106–9
using language effectively in *108*

fairness and justice 91–3
false-positives (and false-negatives) 5–6
feedback 244–5
multisource feedback 243–4
responses to 245
The Fifteen Minute Hour (Stuart, M. and Lieberman, J.) 125–7
focus lock 37–8
avoidance of 58–9
Fox, Renée 178, 231, 269
Francis Report on Mid-Staffordshire Hospital 138, 197

Games People Play (Berne, E.) 118
Gawande, Atul 175, 290
General Medical Council (GMC) 180–1, 212
'good enough practice' 143, 160
sharing ideas about 303, 305–6
see also practice examples
groupthink 199
'GROW' model of coaching *246*
guilt 194
power of 188
shame and 191

handover
  recording and 244
  risks to patients in 72–3
  skills in, SBAR and 143, 149–53
Harvard Business Review 6
Health Foundation 270–1, *273,* 282
healthtalk.org 288, 291, 292, 298
HealthUnlocked 298
Heath, Iona 299
Helman, Cecil 278
helpfulness 161–2
heuristics 30, 32, 49, 189–90, 195
holding skills 77, 78–80
How to Communicate Basically Brilliantly (McDonnell, D.) *108*
humiliation, education by 191
hypothetico-deductive reasoning 41, 42–4

iatrogenic harm, over-treatment and 192
informed choice, clinician and 287, 288
intra-team boundaries 155–7
intuition 19, 29, 39, 189–90, 195, 228
  see also Type 1 (intuitive) thinking
investigations 35
  investigatory methods 304–5
  uncertainty and 191–2

justice, fairness and 91–3

key skills
  analysis 25, 41
  negotiation 100, 106
  networking 70, 73, 77
  team-working 136, 143
Kuhn, Thomas S. 263

learning about uncertainty
  attitudinal objectives 252
  brief teaching on uncertainty, useful opportunities for *252*
  dysfunctional ways out, identification and discussion of 257
  education session content 251
  group sessions 251
  hopes and fears, investigation of 254
  intended learning from teaching sessions 250–2
  knowledge objectives 251
  mapping the psychology of uncertainty 258
  outcomes of learning 250, 251–2
  setting aims/objectives 250–2
  skill objectives 252
  specific learning objectives 250
  starting point 250–1
  teaching plans for different situations 252–8
    five-minute sessions 252
    half-day sessions 254–6
    hour-long sessions 253
    whole-day sessions 256–8
  trigger scenarios, examples of *253–4*
  uncertainty in training 258
Less Than Full Time Training (LTFT) roles 214
Leukaemia Care 292–3, 298

McDonnell, David *108*
Macmillan Cancer Support *157, 159, 202,* 279, 283–4, 288–9, 291–2, 293, 294–6, 298
Map of Uncertainty in Medicine (MUM) 7–8, *12,* 16–17, 18–19
  analysis, assessment of learning needs in 222
  assessment of learners' specific needs using 219–25
  decision-making, encouragement in 221
  group training situations 220
  'honest errors' of inexperience 221–2
  identification of difficulty, seeking help and 220
  individual trainees, assessment of 220
  metacognition 220
  negotiation, assessment of learning needs in 224
  networking, assessment of learning needs in 224
  Situation Background Assessment Recommendation (SBAR) technique 220, 221
  systematic approaches to situations 220
  team-working, assessment of learning needs in 225

WDYDWYDKWTD
helping learners in situations of *223*
identification of difficulty with 221
see also analysis; negotiation; networking; team-working
Mapping Uncertainty in Medical Training (MUMT) *240*
Marinker, Marshall 43, 79
medical training, uncertainty in 7, 209
assessment of learners' specific needs with MUM 219–25
educational skills for uncertainty in training 237–48
learning about uncertainty 249–58
training for uncertainty, educational methods for 227–35
uncertainty, training to deal with 211–16
meta-ignorance 176, 195
meta uncertainty 179
metacognition 220
negotiation 127
networking 73
training for uncertainty and 228, 229
uncertainty and 14
mind map *124*
motivational interviewing 106, 118–22
multidisciplinary teams *12, 15,* 29, 65, 137, 201, 224, 284, 296
multisource feedback 243–4

negotiation *12,* 13, 15, 99–100, 101–33
affirmation 120
agreement on way forward, difficulties in reaching 112
arguments and conflicts 103–4
assessment and teaching methods for uncertainty in 132–3
assessment of learning needs in 224
Balint group/Schwartz round-style discussion 128
BATHE technique 125–7
behaviour change, motivational interviewing and 106, 118–22
blaming the patient 195–6
blaming the system 103
Cates plot *116*
choice, anxiety of 195
clarity in identification of decision to be made 113
clinical settings and management of uncertainty in 131–2
cognitive processes 195
complex problems, engagement with 106, 123–4
conflicts, arguments and 103–4
counter-transference 128
decision-making
clarity in identification of decision to be made 113
explaining complexities of 102
trying but failing to share with patient 104
decision scales for patient's ability to change 120
decision talk 114–15
deferring decisions to another time, place and preferably another doctor 103
diagnostic complexities 102
doctor–patient interaction 101–2
dominant relationship 196
dysfunctional responses 102–4
educational skills in 244–6
effective use of 'but' in explanation *108*
emotional reactions 194
empathy, BATHE technique for 125–7
explanation
skills in 106–9
using language effectively in *108*
functional ways through uncertainty in 105–28
future, patient concerns relating to *111*
game of 'why don't you' and 'yes, but ...' 104, 106, 117–18
guilt 194
'heartsink' 102
key skills 100
functional ways through uncertainty in 106
management of 'non-medical' problems 106, 125–7
matching patient's style to explanation *108*

medical reasoning, explaining complexities of 102
meta-ignorance 195
metacognition 127
mind map *124*
motivational interviewing 106, 118–22
negotiation, skills in 106, 108–12
negotiation of uncertainty, frustrations of 102
'non-medical' problems, dealing with 106, 125–7
OARS (open questions, affirmation, reflection, summarisation) 119–21
open questions 120
opening questions *122*
option talk 114
organisational factors 196–7
past, patient concerns relating to *111*
patient perspective on uncertainty in 286–91
patient's concerns, examples for dealing with *111*
patient's own concerns, linking to *108*
patronising relationship 196
pitfalls of negotiation 102–4
placement of 'when' effectively in explanation *108*
positive BATHE technique 126–7
positive language, use of *108*
present, patient concerns relating to *111*
projection 128
psychological components of uncertainty in 194–7
psychosocial issues in doctor–patient relationship 106, 127–8
rapport, achievement of *108*
reflection/rolling with resistance 120–1
relationship issues 195–6
resources for 133
risk, skills in talking about 106, 115–17
shared decision-making 106, 112–15
summarisation 121
talking about risk 106, 115–17
teaching methods for uncertainty in 132–3
team talk 113
transference 128
transferring responsibility entirely to patient ('blaming the patient') 103
trying but failing to share decision-making with patient 104
uncertainty avoidance 196–7
'why don't you' and 'yes, but ...', game of 104, 106, 117–18

networking *12,* 13, 15, 69–70, 71–97
ambiguities, time and resolution of 79
ambiguous symptoms *79*
anticipation of results 82
anxiety in both doctor and patient, increases in 75
anxiety transfers 80
assessment and teaching methods for uncertainty in 96–7
assessment of learning needs in 224
autonomy 91
beneficence 90
breaking good news 77, 86–9
care after referral, continuity in *93*
clinical settings and management of uncertainty in 96
cognitive processes 191–2
conceptual approaches to diagnosis, understanding differences in 79
confusing symptoms *79*
contempt for others 191
continuing care after referral 77, *93*–4
diagnostic network, involvement of 71–2
diagnostic services, array of 72
dialogue with patient, aim for *88*
dysfunctional responses 73–6
educational skills in 243–4
effective referrals, informal strategies to assist *84*
emotional difficulties in consultation 75–6
emotional reactions 191
empathy with impact of symptoms *88*
ethical issues in consultations 89–90
exceptional circumstances, dealing with 77, 89–94
excess referral, resources and 73

expectations of referrals or investigations in advance, management of 77, 80–2
fairness and justice 91–3
fragmentation of health services, problem of 76
functional ways through uncertainty in 77–94
good news, transmission of *88*
guilt, shame and 191
handover, risks to patients in 72–3
harm caused by network misuse or overuse, examples of *97*
holding skills 77, 78–80
humiliation, education by 191
iatrogenic harm, over-treatment and 192
interpretation of results in light of previously expressed concerns 88
investigations and uncertainty 191–2
justice, fairness and 91–3
key skills 70, 73
    functional ways through uncertainty in 77
'Medically Unexplained Symptoms' 81
metacognition 73
network misuse or overuse, examples of harm caused by *97*
non-maleficience 90
organisational factors 193–4
over-diagnosis 191–2
over-reliance on tests and investigations for diagnosis 74
patient perspective on uncertainty in 282–5
patients and decision-making, skills of involvement 73
pitfalls of networking 73–6
planning for breaking news 87, *88*
positive language, use of *88*
psychological components of uncertainty in 191–4
purposes of referral 83–4
referral, handover and 72–3
referral letters, informal approaches as supplements to 85
referral network, understanding about 77, 83–5
referral or investigation, resolving uncertainty by 192
relationship issues 193
resources for 98
shame 191
signalling good news 87–8
Situation Background Assessment Recommendation (SBAR) 84
symptoms likely to cause uncertainty *79*
teaching methods for uncertainty in 96–7
tests, mismatch between doctor and patient in understanding purpose of 74
time as a diagnostic tool, use of 192
timely referral 84
training, uncertainty in 193–4
Type 1 (intuitive) thinking 73
under-appreciation of frequency of 'functional' conditions 74
undifferentiated early symptoms *79*
vulnerabilities, exceptional circumstances and 92–3
neurological systems 177
'non-medical' problems, dealing with 106, 125–7
normality, awareness of bias towards 58

OARS (open questions, affirmation, reflection, summarisation) 119–21
Ofri, Danielle 181
open questions 120
opening questions *122*
option talk 114
organisational factors
    meetings and 145–7
    negotiation 196–7
    networking 193–4
    team-working 203
Osler, William 183
outcomes
    guilt and 181–2
    learning outcomes 250, 251–2
over-diagnosis 191–2
over-investigation 303

passing the buck 140–1, 238–9

paternalism
  paternalist clinician 287–8
  paternalistic teams 200–1
patient's perspective, uncertainty from 263, 265–74, 277–96
  analysis, patient perspective on uncertainty in 277–82
  attitudes of patients to uncertainty 274
  cancer, uncertainty about 279
  carers, difficulties for 293–5
  clinician knows best attitude 287, 288–9
  clinician's and patient's reciprocal uncertainties *273*
  conversations between clinicians and patients, analyses of 286
  cultural differences, influence of 285
  decision-making, involvement in 286–7
  deliberative clinician 287, 289
  diagnosis
    patient perspective on process of 279–80
    uncertainty in 278
  equality in clinician–patient relationship 290–1
  existential questions 278
  firm diagnosis, anguish of 279
  future care, difficult decisions about 294
  health matters, fashions in 268
  informed choice, clinician and 287, 288
  international differences, effects of 285
  internet and uncertainty 295–6
  interpretative clinician 287, 289
  interruptions and discontuities, problems of 283
  living with uncertainty, pain of 283–4
  medical practice and uncertainty for patients 267–9
  multidisciplinary team meetings 296
  naming a diagnosis, problem of 278
  negotiation, patient perspective on uncertainty in 286–91
  networking, patient perspective on uncertainty in 282–5
  paternalist clinician 287–8
  patient–clinician interactions, influences on 271–3
  patient disempowerment 272
  patient networks 284–5
  patients' responses to uncertainty in clinicians 269–74, 281–2
  patient's view of uncertainty *267*
  power relations, uncertainty and 272
  problem solving, expertise and 289
  questions and answers, Kuhn on 263
  realities of uncertainty from patient's perspective, awareness of 296
  reciprocal uncertainties of clinicians and patients *273*
  referral, dilemmas for patients in 283
  scientific medicine 268
  shared decision-making 289–91
  sharing uncertainty with patients, problems of 284
  social legitimacy 281
  'tame' problems 271
  team-working, patient perspective on uncertainty in 291–6
  technical aspects of practice, focus on 268–9
  training for uncertainty 296
  treatment failure rates 286
  trust between patient and clinician 270
  trust in clinician 289–90
  uncertainty
    for clinicians facing painful dilemmas *266*
    clinicians pondering and writing about 266–7
    in complex situations 265–7
    Fox's components of 269
    patients' responses to 274
    situations making for 280–1
  WDYDWYDKWTD moments in patients 274, 292–3
  When Doctors and Patients Talk (Health Foundation, 2012) 270–1, *273*, 282
  'wicked' problems 271
perfection seeking, anxiety of 142, 183–4
pitfalls
  of analysis 34–8
  of negotiation 102–4

of networking 73–6
of team-working 140–2
positive BATHE technique 126–7
positive emotions, effects of 188–9
positive language, use of *88, 108*
power relations, uncertainty and 272
practice examples
boundaries, management of 155, 156–7
breaking good news 88–9
clinical issues in teamwork 149
complex problems, engagement with 124
creation of a good team 145
decision tools, use of 54
delegation, skills in 161
diagnostic safety netting 47–8
emotional context of consultation, exploration of 56
exceptional circumstances, dealing with 92, 94
expectations, management of 82
explanation 108–9
functional symptoms, explanation of 61
handover skills 152, 153
holding skills 80
hypothetico-deductive reasoning 43–4
negotiation 110, 111
non-medical problems, dealing with 127
organisational issues in teamwork 147
psychosocial issues 128
referral network 85
risk, talking about 116–17
shared decision-making 115
sharing clinical reasoning 52
situational awareness 59
stressful situations, management of 162–3
team and turf issues 158
trust and verify 50
'why don't you … ?' 'yes, but …' 117–8, 122
premature reassurance 28, 35
psychological components of uncertainty in
analysis 187–90
negotiation 194–7
networking 191–4
team-working 197–203
psychology of uncertainty 173, 175–84, 187–203
ambiguity and uncertainty 176
ambiguity or ambivalence, maintenance of state of 181
analysis, psychological components of uncertainty in 187–90
anxiety, feelings of 188
anxiety and uncertainty 177
anxiety of 'what if' questions 181
blaming the patient 195–6
brain systems 177
certainty, pressures on clinicians for 184
choice, anxiety of 195
choice and uncertainty 177
clinicians' thoughts about uncertainty 178–80
cognitive processes 189–90, 191–2, 195, 198–9
emotional reactions and 188–9
cognitive processes for dealing with uncertainty, development of 179–80, 183
cognitive uncertainty 176
collective decision-making 198
collective 'norms', danger of 198–9
conceptual uncertainty 179
contempt for others 191
death, fear of 182
decision-making, acceptance of ambiguity and 190
defensive omnipotence 181–2
definitions and psychological elements of uncertainty 176–8
deliberative teams 202
denial of uncertainty 180
diagnostic certainty, pressure for 203
disease and death, daily contact with 182–3
dominant relationship 196
emotional intelligence 189
emotional reactions 188–9, 191, 194, 197
emotional uncertainty 176
error and uncertainty, relationship between 180–3

evolutionary aspects of uncertainty 177
'existential' issues, uncertainties of 180–3
failure, belief in own publicity and 184
fault, facing up to 181
fear of error 180–1
Francis Report on Mid-Staffordshire Hospital 197
groupthink 199
guidelines, limits of 189–90
guilt 194
  power of 188
  shame and 191
heuristics 189–90
humiliation, education by 191
iatrogenic harm, over-treatment and 192
illness, disability and death, uncertainties of 180–3
incomplete or imperfect mastery of available knowledge 178
information, availability of 190
information transmitted by emotions 189
informing teams 201
institutional support, availability of 190
interpretative teams 201–2
intuition 189
investigations and uncertainty 191–2
key themes 180–3
'lucky escapes' 181
malpractice claims 190
medical knowledge, limitations of 178
meta-ignorance 176, 195
meta uncertainty 179
negative emotions, effects of 188, 189
negotiation, psychological components of uncertainty in 194–7
networking, psychological components of uncertainty in 191–4
neurological systems 177
organisational components of uncertainty 176
organisational factors 193–4, 196–7, 203
organisational setting 190
outcomes, guilt and 181–2
over-diagnosis 191–2
'overwhelmingness' of disease and death 182–3
paternalistic teams 200–1
patronising relationship 196
pattern recognition 189
perfection seeking, anxiety of 183–4
personal responsibility, sense of 199
personal uncertainty 179
positive emotions, effects of 188–9
potential wrongdoing, fear of 180–1
psychological components of uncertainty 175–8
referral or investigation, resolving uncertainty by 192
relationship issues 190, 193, 195–6, 199–202
relationships, uncertainty and 176
relationships and resilience to uncertainty 183–4
research, limitations of 178
resilience to uncertainty, strategies for maintenance of 183–4
responsibility and uncertainty 181–2
rigidity of protocol of guideline, insistence on 197
shame 191
subjective experience of uncertainty 176
team-working, psychological components of uncertainty in 197–203
technical uncertainty 179
time, availability of 190
time and uncertainty 176
time as a diagnostic tool, use of 192
total certainty, downside of 177–8
training, uncertainty in 193–4
trust, patient-clinician relationship of 182
Type 1 (intuitive) thinking 177
Type 2 (analytical) thinking 177
uncertainty, experiences of 175
uncertainty avoidance 196–7
uniformity, pressures for 199

questions and answers, Kuhn on 263

RDM-p framework 243
referral 36
  dilemmas for patients in 283
  handover and 72–3
  networks of 77, 83–5
  referral letters, informal approaches as supplements to 85
  resolving uncertainty by 192
reflection-in-action, Schön's concept of 30, 230
relationships
  dominant relationship 196
  equality in clinician–patient relationship 290–1
  error and uncertainty, relationship between 180–3
  patronising relationship 196
  power relations, uncertainty and 272
  relationship building 60
  relationship issues 190, 193, 195–6, 199–202
  resilience to uncertainty and 183–4
  between teams 139
  trust, patient–clinician relationship of 182
  uncertainty and 176
risk
  handover, risks to patients in 72–3
  skills in talking about 106, 115–17
  uncertainty and 8
Royal College of General Practitioners (RCGP) 79, 212, 215

Schön, Donald A. 30, 68, 230, 304
scientific medicine 268
sharing
  of clinical reasoning process with patient 41, 50–2
  of decision-making 106, 112–15, 289–91
  of uncertainty with patients 301–2
    problems of 284
Shipman, Harold 182
signalling good news 87–8
Situation Background Assessment Recommendation (SBAR) technique 84, 220, 221
  team-working and 150–3
situational awareness skills 41, 56–9
Skills for Communicating with Patients (Kurtz, S. and Silverman, J.) 81, 107
SMART (specific, measurable, achievable, realistic and timely) 245
Specific Problem Solving 215
Spence, Sir James 27
symptoms 5
  empathy with impact of *88*
  explanation of physiological origins of 60–1
  functional symptoms, explanation of 41, 59–61
  likely to cause uncertainty *79*
  'Medically Unexplained Symptoms' 81
  useful phrases for explanation of *61*

talking about risk 106, 115–17
teaching methods for uncertainty in
  analysis 65–8
  negotiation 132–3
  networking 96–7
  team-working 167–9
teaching plans for different situations 252–8
  five-minute sessions 252
  half-day sessions 254–6
  hour-long sessions 253
  whole-day sessions 256–8
team-working *12,* 13, 15, 135–6, 137–63
  affiliation, promotion of 139
  ask 'X' to do it, failure of 140
  assessment and teaching methods for uncertainty in 167–9
  assessment of learning needs in 225
  attachment, promotion of 139
  behavioural complications 139
  benefits of team-working 137–8
  blaming others 141
  boundaries, management of 143, 154–9
  bullying leadership, failure of 140
  burnout 141–2
  cameraderie 137
  clinical issues, meetings and 147–9
  clinical settings and management of uncertainty in 165–7
  cognitive processes 198–9

collective decision-making 198
collective 'norms', danger of 198–9
communication within teams 139
creating a good team 143, 144–5
deferring decisions (and hence actions too) 140
delegation, skills in 159–61
delegation of tasks within teams 138
deliberative teams 202
depersonalisation 141–2
diagnostic certainty, pressure for 203
difficult situations, management of 143, 161–3
dysfunctional responses 140–2
educational skills in 247–8
effective delegation, pathways to 160
emotional reactions 197
failure of team-working 138
fluid memberships 139
focusing groups 146–7
Francis Report on Mid-Staffordshire Hospital 138, 197
frustrations of team-working 138–9
functional ways through uncertainty in 143–63
'good enough practice' 143, 160
groupthink 199
handover skills/SBAR 143, 149–53
helpful actions 162
helpful people, identification of 162
helpful thoughts 161–2
informing teams 201
interpretative teams 201–2
intra-team boundaries 155–7
key skills 136
  functional ways through uncertainty in 143
leadership 139
line management, boundaries and 156
making meetings work, including skills in chairing meetings 143, 145–9
mobilisation of groups 147
multiple perspectives, benefit of 138
organisational factors 203
organisational issues, meetings and 145–7
passing the buck 140–1
paternalistic teams 200–1
patient perspective on uncertainty in 291–6
patients and families, interactions with teams 139
perfection seeking, anxiety of 142
personal–professional boundaries 154–5
personal responsibility, sense of 199
pitfalls of team-working 140–2
professional issues in boundary management 154–5, 155–7
psychological components of uncertainty in 197–203
relationship issues 199–202
relationships between teams 139
relevance of boundaries 156–7
resources for 169
retreat in face of difficulty 141
rigidity of protocol of guideline, insistence on 197
roles and capacities of members, effective use of 140
Situation Background Assessment Recommendation (SBAR) 150–3
teaching methods for uncertainty in 167–9
team and turf issues in boundary management 157–9
team failure 138
team framework 144
uniformity, pressures for 199
uniting groups 146
unkindness 141–2
thinking strategies 30
  see also Type 1; Type 2 thinking
time
  availability of 190
  as diagnostic tool, use of 192
  timely referral 84
  uncertainty and 176
training for uncertainty
  aims of *215–16*
  patient's perspective, uncertainty from 296
training for uncertainty, educational methods for
  adaptive coping strategies, Fox's work on 231

agility 234
ambiguity, toleration and dealing with 231
Balint or Schwartz rounds 230
case discussions 229–30
clinical situations, axes of change and complexity in 232–3
continued learning 235
decision-making, choice of strategies for *232,* 233
decision-making approaches for uncertain clinical situations 232–3
educational methods in different settings 227–30
group debriefing 229–30
group teaching 229
holding skills, development of 229
'hot skills' 228
learning, different ways of 227
learning about uncertainty in organisations and teams 233–5
metacognition 228, 229
navigational leadership 234
one-to-one training situations 228
open collaboration 234
pattern recognition, development of 228
planning for uncertainty 232
private study, learning through 227–8
reflection, learning through 227–8
reflection-on-action, reflection-in-action and 230
reflective writing 230
resilience in practice, training and 230–1
Significant Event Analyses 230
skills, identification of needs in 228
Stacey Matrix concept 232
strategic anticipation 234
structured approaches, modelling of 232
team meetings 230
thinking about thinking 228
thinking skills, promotion of 229
Type 1 (intuitive) thinking 228
Type 2 (analytical) thinking 228
uncertainty, situations making for 231
uncertainty avoidance 229
trigger scenarios, examples of *253–4*
trust
  in clinician 289–90
  between patient and clinician 270
  patient–clinician relationship of 182
  verify and (Russian military proverb) 41, 48–50
Twain, Mark 219
Type 1 (intuitive) thinking 30–31, 33–4, 37
  comparison with Type 2 thinking *32*
  development of 33
  networking 73
  psychology of uncertainty 177
Type 2 (analytical) thinking 30, 33–4
  comparison with Type 1 thinking *32*
  development and impact on diagnostic process of 33–4
  psychology of uncertainty 177

uncertainty
  awareness of 13–14
  classification of 14–16
  for clinicians facing painful dilemmas *266*
  clinicians pondering and writing about 266–7
  cognitive uncertainty 176
  in complex situations 265–7
  decision-making under conditions of 8
  dysfunctional responses to 14
  emotional uncertainty 176
  Fox's components of 269
  functional responses to 14
  living with 6, 299–306
    pain of 283–4
  management of 7–8
  medical training and 7, 209, 211–16, 219–25, 227–35, 237–48, 249–58
  metacognition and 14
  'not knowing', perceptions of failure in 6
  patients' responses to 274
  pervasive nature of 6
  pseudo certainty 7
  recognition of 13–14
  reduction of 9
  risk and 8

situations making for 280–1
skills and dealing with 8, 16
as training issue, recognition of 214
uncertainty avoidance 196–7
'what do you do when you don't know what to do?' (WDYDWYDKWTD) 6, 8
see also embracing uncertainty; learning about uncertainty; psychology of uncertainty; WDYDWYDKWTD

uncertainty, training to deal with
aims of training for uncertainty *215–16*
ambiguity, discomfort with 212
approaches to uncertainty during training 213
Associates-in-Training (AiTs) 215
attitudes for uncertainty *216*
decision-making, anxieties about 212
difficulties in current training 212–14
educational AIMS of training 215–16
evidence-based practice 215
experience, coping with uncertainty and 213–14
goals 214
'good practice', exploration of 214
knowledge about uncertainty *215*
Less Than Full Time Training (LTFT) roles 214
management of uncertainty, training and 213, 214
medical school, problems in 212
personal inadequacy in face of uncertainty 212
personality traits 212
professionalisation, components of 213
RCGP core curriculum 215
'self-regulated' learners 214
skills for uncertainty *216*
specialisation 213
Specific Problem Solving 215
training for uncertainty, overall aim of 215
treatment philosophies, development of 214
uncertainty as training issue, recognition of 214
WDYDWYDKWTD
dealing with situations of 211–12
expertise and 211
recognition of situations of 211–12

unconscious incompetence 28
uniformity, pressures for 199
unkindness 141–2

variables 5–6

WDYDWYDKWTD 6, 8, 14, *15,* 17, 18–19
application of thinking types to 31–2
dealing with situations of 211–12
experiences in training context 237, 241, *242,* 247
expertise and 211
helping learners in situations of *223*
identification of difficulty with 221
moments in patients 274, 292–3
performance of colleague as cause 249
recognition of situations of 211–12

When Doctors and Patients Talk (Health Foundation, 2012) 270–1, *273,* 282
'why don't you … ?' and 'yes, but …', game of 104, 106, 117–18
'wicked' problems 271
Working with Vulnerable Groups (Gill, P., Wright, N. and Brew, I., eds) 93

www.ingramcontent.com/pod-product-compliance
Lightning Source LLC
LaVergne TN
LVHW071200210926
848482LV00014B/698